MEDIEVAL ISLAMIC MEDICINE AND MEDICAL LUMINARIES

ADEL K. AFIFI, M. D., M. S., AND RONALD A. BERGMAN, PH.D. (PROFESSORS EMERITI, CARVER COLLEGE OF MEDICINE, UNIVERSITY OF IOWA)

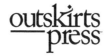

TO

LARRY ANNA

WHOSE

LOVE AND SUPPORT WERE BOUNDLESS

Acknowledgment

This work could not have been possible without the many authors whose works are cited in the references,

And would not have been completed without the patience, support, and love of our families.

Electronic editing of the manuscript could not have been possible without the expertise of Drs. Rema and Walid Afifi, Zuhair Ballas, and Riad Rahhal.

The professional guidance and support of Dana Nelson, Laura Stewart, and Pat Wilson of Outskirts Press during the publication process brought this book to fruition.

To all of them we owe much gratitude.

Table of Contents

Introduction

Of the three great religions, only Christianity and Islam competed for worldwide acceptance, and both almost achieved their goal. The work of Catholic Jesuits and the disciples of Islam was educational, political, social, and, at times, harsh.

The acts of horror committed in the name of God through the ages by the Christian, Jewish, and Muslim radical fringe should not be carried over to other members of a sect or a religion today.

Because of the onslaught of Western media on Islam, the use of such derogatory terms as Islamic terrorism and conflict of civilizations, it is useful to be introduced to, and to consider, the contributions of Muslims and Arabs to science and civilization.

A recent public opinion poll (Lyons, 2009) found that a majority of Americans see "little" or "nothing" to admire in Islam or the Muslim world. An old Arabic saying states, "Medicine was non-existent before Hippocrates (who created it), dead before Galen (who revived it), scattered before Al-Razi (who collected it) and incomplete before Avicenna (who completed it)" (Al-Mahi, 1959).

The thirteenth-century philosopher, Roger Bacon, one of the early

Western proponents of the scientific method, praised the Muslims for their intellectual innovations (Lyons, 2009).

Islamic civilization once extended from China to the Atlantic Ocean; less remembered is its impact on Western science and medicine between the ninth and fifteenth centuries (Majeed, 2005). It was through Arabic translations that the West learned of Hellenic medicine, including the works of Galen and Hippocrates (Islamic Medicine, http://encyclopedia. thefreedictionary.com/Islamic+medicine;Tarabay, 2011).

The wave of the renaissance of Arab science reached America about turn of the twentieth century, when wealthy Americans began to buy manuscripts from the Near East. The Army Medical Library in the USA had, in 1942, over five hundred manuscripts of Arab medicine. Manuscripts of Arabic science and medicine are scattered all over the world in public and private libraries. The Garrett Collection at Princeton University, the Prussian State Library in Berlin, and the British Museum possess the largest collection of manuscripts (Mayer, 1942).

Medicine was a central part of medieval Islamic culture. Until the rise of modern science, no other civilization engaged as many scientists or produced as many scientific books (Dallal, 2010;Tarabay, 2011).

Contrary to some historians' narrative, Islamic science developed in the context of Islamic culture, not despite it (Dallal, 2010). The Quran considers scientific inquiry a virtue and calls on Muslims to reflect on the outside world and the world within where they would find evidence of God's creation and deepen piety (Dallal, 2010). The Hadith (sayings of the Prophet) also encourages science and the state of good health. "The best gift from Allah, after belief, is health" (Freely, 2011). "The ink of the scholar is more holy than the blood of the martyr" (Bushrui, 2002). "The superiority of the learned man over the devout is like that of the moon, on the night when it is full, over the rest of the stars" (Abu el Aish, 2010).

What is known about the status of the medical profession in medieval Islamic civilization suggests that physicians were very highly respected, highly remunerated. In Baghdad in 931 AD, there was a minimum of one physician for at most three hundred inhabitants, a very high ratio in to-day's standards (Rosenthal, 1978). Islamic medicine refers to medicine developed in the medieval Islamic civilization and written in Arabic. It is not purely Arab, since contributions to it were made by Persians (Al-Razi/Razes, Al Majusi/Haly Abbas, Ibn Sina/Avicenna), Greek, Syriac, Turks, and Kurds.

Neither was it purely Islamic, since there were Christians (Hunayn ibn Ishaq) and Jews (Maimonides) who played critical roles in science and medicine. All (Arabs, Persian, Christians, Jews, Muslims) lived within the sphere of Islamic culture, which was welcoming for science and inquiry and which absorbed many different cultures, integrated them, and de-veloped them (Ullmann, 1997; Lyons, 2009). No matter the ethnic origin or religious affiliation, their work was written in Arabic, and frequently under the patronage of an Arab Muslim caliph (Lyons, 2009).

Medical knowledge acquired under Islamic civilization was built on the theoretical and practical knowledge of Greece and Rome. Galen and Hippocrates were major references for it (Siraisi, 1990).

Scholars under Islam did not only translate Greek and other knowledge into Arabic but produced new medical knowledge, which they preserved and transmitted later to Europe by reverse translation, and thus contrib-uted to the European renaissance. Avicenna's "Canon of Medicine" was translated into Latin and was disseminated throughout Europe (http://www.nlm.nih.gov/hmd/arabic/med_islam.html; Lunde, 1982).

The major contribution of Muslims and Arabs to medicine was to put the study of medicine on a scientific footing and eliminate superstition and folk practice (Lund, 1982).

The contributions of Islamic civilization to medicine were not limited to translation and preservation of medical knowledge of the ancients but, in addition, were characterized by the development of a health system that included systems of medical education with different paths to become a physician. This included self-study, shadowing a medical scholar, as well as the traditional path in medical schools. Well-developed hospitals existed with separate facilities for genders and type of illness; libraries; conference rooms for teaching; and pharmacies. To address the psychological needs of patients, hospitals were frequently surrounded by gardens, and what we now call "music therapy" was part of the treatment of patients. To ensure quality of care, physicians had to take qualifying examinations and be licensed before being allowed to practice. They had to abide by a code of medical ethics with well-defined obligations on the physician towards patients, colleagues, assistants, and the community.

ONE

Ancient Pre-Islamic Medicine

EGYPTIAN MEDICINE (Beginning 2900 BC)

The early healing practices in ancient Egypt were entrusted to priests and later to specialists who confined their practice to surgery, gastrointestinal upsets, obstetrics, or eye disorders. General health and hygienic issues were left to uneducated practitioners (Al-Samerra'i, 1989; Laws, 1998).

The father of medicine in Ancient Egypt (Imhotep) lived in the twenty-eighth century BC. The name means "He who comes with peace," and to him is attributed the saying "Eat, drink, and be merry, for tomorrow we shall die" (Al-Samerra'i, 1989; Taylor, 2008).

Knowledge about ancient Egyptian medicine was obtained primarily from study of nine papyri, of which three are best known: the Edwin Smith, Ebers, and Kohn, named after the archeologists who discovered them (Al-Samerra'i, 1989).

The oldest known surgical treatise, The Edwin Smith Surgical Treatise (named after the American Egyptologist who found it in London), dates back to the seventeenth century BC. Some attribute the treatise to Imhotep, the Egyptian God of medicine (Al-Samerra'i, 1989). In it, data is presented in a systematic way (presentation, physical examination, assessment, and verdict). The verdict, in some cases, consisted of "nothing can be done" (Taylor, 2008). The treatise contains information on joint displacement, bone fractures, disorders of the brain and spinal cord, signs of fractures of the vertebral column, and their effects on movement and bladder function (Al-Samerra'i, 1989).

The Ebers treatise is the largest and most complete of the three papyri. It was written around 1550 BC and includes anatomical and physiological information, in addition to information about gastrointestinal diseases; eye, ear, and nose disorders; skin diseases; bone disease; and burns. It has information about heart movements and its relations to pulse and treatment of aneurysms. It also includes information about seven hundred drugs used at that time, including squille and Sinna (Al-Samerra'i, 1989).

The Kohn treatise dates back to 1950 BC and deals mainly with women's diseases. It includes nineteen treatments for women's diseases, care of the pregnant woman, and attempts to find the gender of the infant in utero (Al-Samerra'i, 1989).

From study of papyri, we learn that ancient Egyptians practiced trephination for head injuries, filled teeth with a type of mineral cement, and had extensive pharmacopeia of medicines for various ailments, and through the practice of surgery, autopsy and embalming, they understood human anatomy (Taylor, 2008).

The early Egyptians knew about the hemostatic properties of muscle, and used a dressing impregnated with honey after bleeding had stopped (Laws, 1998).

Among the herbal medicines used were digitalis (for heart disease), Senna and coriander (for gastrointestinal diseases), as well as honey for a variety of disorders (Al-Samerra'i, 1989).

CHINESE MEDICINE (Beginning 2700 BC)

The founder of Chinese medicine is Emperor Shen Nung (2737 BC) who wrote "Pen Tsao," a book describing a number of botanical remedies, one of which is a compound from which ephedrine is derived. In desperate cases, they complemented herbal medicines with certain poisons such as arsenic and nux vomica (Laws, 1998; Taylor, 2008). Herbal medicines used included rhubarb, castor oil, kaolin, aconite, camphor, cannabis, indica, and ephedra vulgaris (Laws, 1998).

Acupuncture, another signature of Chinese medicine, can be traced to the time of the Stone Age. Acupuncture was practiced to maintain the balance (a constant theme in ancient Chinese medicine) among the forces of the "yang" and the "yin," representing "plus," "minus," "light," and "dark" (Laws, 1998; Taylor, 2008).

The Chinese healer examined the body, paying special attention to body temperature as determined by palpation and the character of the pulse (Laws, 1998).

In the second century AD, a textbook about fever became the standard reference for hundreds of years (Laws, 1998).

The interest of the Chinese in the healing art is seen in the attitude of Emperor Wu Ti in the second century BC, who had 850 volumes on medicine in his library (Laws, 1998).

The ancient Chinese are known to have contributions besides acupuncture. They practiced inoculation for smallpox in the eleventh century and used anesthesia for surgical procedures (Laws, 1998).

BABYLONIAN MEDICINE (Beginning of 2250 BC)

Ancient Babylonian medicine was characterized by its regulation by the government. Fees for various types of care were set by law, taking into consideration the quality of care provided and the ability of the patient to pay. If a physician error caused the patient to lose an eye, the physician might also lose an eye (Al-Samerra'i, 1989; Taylor, 2008). Babylonians attributed illness to anger of the gods for a sin that the patient committed. Such sins included theft, lies, lack of respect for places of worship, killing, and spitting in rivers from which people drink (Al-Samerra'i, 1989). On the other hand, Babylonian physicians knew the importance of cleanliness, transmission of disease, and dangers of flies on health (Al-Samerra'i, 1989). It is believed that the Babylonians knew about malaria, bilharzias and ankylostomatitis because these diseases were prevalent in their land (Al-Samerra'i, 1989).

Babylonian physicians used herbal medicines and secretions of some animals for treatment purposes. They used close to 250 herbal drugs, and 180 drugs from animal sources. They used to include several drugs in the same prescription to be used in the order in which they were listed until the patient found the one that benefitted him (Al-Samerra'i, 1989).

From their animal sacrifices, the Babylonians had a good knowledge of anatomy. They gave special attention to the liver, which they considered the source of blood and center for emotion. They considered the heart the center of intelligence, the stomach the center of excellence, the uterus the center of love, and the eyes and ears centers of alertness and awareness (Al-Samerra'i, 1989).

Babylonian practitioners usually confined their practice to one disorder and did not practice their profession on the seventh, fourteenth, nineteenth, twenty-first, and twenty-ninth days of the month (Al-Samerra'i, 1989).

In the early Babylonian times, the sick were exposed in the marketplace for passersby to tell of cures that they had attained for a similar affliction. Priests recorded these testimonials in a book, "the Sacred Book," which became the accepted medical code. Physicians trained in government schools and licensed by examination performed surgery and midwifery in their offices or homes because letting blood in the temple was taboo (Al-Samerra'i, 1989; Laws, 1998).

PERSIAN MEDICINE (Beginning 678 BC)

In ancient Persia, priests attended to the spiritual and physical ills of people. By the late fifth century BC, Persians had access to Greek medicine and social life. The practice of medicine was regulated. The apprentice physician had to gain experience by treating infidels and foreigners for one to two years before he was deemed qualified to attend to Persian citizens (Laws, 1998). By the end of the sixth century, the city of Ghondi-Shapour had become the intellectual and medical center of the East. The Ghondi-Shapour Hospital became a model for subsequent hospitals in Baghdad and Damascus and the center of training of Islamic physicians (Al-Samerra'i, 1989; Laws, 1998). When Muslims conquered Persia in 633 AD, interest in medicine shifted to Baghdad (Laws, 1998).

ASSYRIAN MEDICINE

The Assyrians codified medical care, and were aware of the effects of a blow to the head and the fatal outcome of injury to the upper cervical spine. They produced unconsciousness by compressing the neck to occlude the carotid arteries (Laws, 1998).

GREEK MEDICINE (Beginning 460–377 BC)

Ancient Greek medicine is dominated by the teachings and scientific observations of Hippocrates. Hippocrates envisioned the outer body as a shell, within which humors, in constant flux and in need of constant cleansing, circulated. Bodies were healthy if there was a balance between humors entering the body and those exiting it. Disease was caused by blockages that prevented the circulation of humors, and healing was "getting rid of the viscous and hardening matter" inside the body in order to restore the normal "flux" of secretions and excretions (Miles, 2008). About seventy works composing the Hippocratic Corpus exist, some in the form of aphorisms (Taylor, 2008). Some of the aphorisms are (Al-Samerra'i, 1989):

"The old tolerate hunger, followed by the young, but children, especially the active among them are less tolerant to hunger."

"Laxatives should not be used in acute illnesses."

"Pain is relieved by rest if movement is the cause."

"Life is short, knowledge is wide, opportunities are limited, judgement is difficult, and so the physician should be always ready to do his duty."

"Not only should the physician carry out his duty, but the patient too."

"Better to fill your stomach with water than with food."

"Sudden death is more common in obese people than in the skinny."

"The most important in the healing of epilepsy in children is the age."

"If the patient does not respond to your treatment, do not change the treatment, but find out the correct diagnosis."

"Medicines can be given during the fourth and seventh months of pregnancy. After that, the lesser medicines the better."

Hippocrates was born in the island of Cos in 460 BC. He taught that hygienic methods and proper diet will enhance patient's vitality. He and his disciples practiced critical observations and deductive reasoning to separate mysticism from medicine. He and his colleagues healed, taught, and recorded their observations in the temple of Aesculapius on a hillside outside of Cos (Taylor, 2008). Aesculiades, the physician priest, became so skilled and known for his achievements that it was said that he cured so many people, even raising a man from the dead (Laws, 1998).

All matters of ills were treated by diet, baths, mineral waters, suggestions, manipulation, and some herbal drugs (Laws, 1998).

The Greeks believed the epilepsy was caused by the gods and called it the "sacred disease." Hippocrates disagreed with this concept, arguing that if epilepsy is caused by the gods, then all diseases are caused by gods, and taught that epilepsy is a hereditary disorder (Al-Samerra'i, 1989).

The Hippocratic teachings include a description of malaria and eradication by destroying the breeding waters—post-partum depression, anthrax, melancholy, paralysis contralateral to the brain lesion (Al-Samerra'i, 1989).

Greek physicians negotiated their fees with their patients before providing care. The fee varied depending on the complexity of the disease, expected duration of treatment, the social and financial status of the patient. It was customary for the physician to visit the patient in his home or for the patient to consult the physician in the physician's home (Al-Samerra'i, 1989).

The Greeks did not have medical schools. Candidates for the profession of medicine were mentored by established physicians after they paid their fees.

ROMAN MEDICINE (first century BC–500 AD)

In Roman times, medicine was divided into three areas: one used diet as a cure, another used medicines for treatment, and the third used manipulation (Laws, 1998).

Roman medicine was characterized by its emphasis on public health measures. The Romans valued personal cleanliness and physical exercise.

They worked to ensure pure water by building aqueducts to transport clean water, constructing public baths, building sewers to remove waste, and espousing cremation of the dead (Taylor, 2008).

The luminary of ancient Roman medicine was Claudius Galen (129–200 AD). Early in his career, Galen was a physician to gladiators. It gave him the opportunity to examine the workings of the human body when human dissection was forbidden.

Galen adopted Aristotle's model of the body as a system of solid organs, a view that dominated medical therapy long after the theory had come into question (Miles, 2008). Galenic doctrine emphasized the hygienic, preventive role of medicine rather than remedial medicine. Ordered living and good diet were paramount (Miles, 2008).

He dissected a wide range of animals, including pigs, dogs, and monkeys. He described the value of measuring the pulse during physical examination and described cardiac arrhythmias. He wrote his personal observations along with the available medical knowledge at the time in hundreds of books, of which only two hundred survived (Taylor, 2008).

In the absence of some type of agent to anesthetize and immobilize an animal, he found that cutting the recurrent laryngeal nerve would eliminate the squealing of the pig (Laws, 1998).

Galen gave a precise account of removing the brain and a clear description of the cranial nerves known at the time (Laws, 1998).

Galen also gave a description of operating conduct, including personal preparation, clothing, fingernails, position of the patient and the surgeon, and lighting of the operating field, as well as the position of the operating instruments such as hammers, knives, chisels, drills, trephines, and elevators (Laws, 1998).

Some of Galen's work turned out to be wrong. Among them: his consideration that the heart is made up of only two (instead of four) chambers; that the human liver is five lobed (like dogs') instead of two; and that the brain secreted "vital spirits" carried via hollow nerves to the muscles, permitting movement (Taylor, 2008).

The fall of the Roman Empire in 476 AD marked the beginning of the dark age of medieval times, which lasted from 476 AD to the beginning of the Renaissance in the fourteenth century. During this time, Galen's teachings, with its truth and errors, constituted the medical references for a millennium (Taylor, 2008). During the medieval period, there were "medical healers" using herbs, religion, and mysticism.

During the dark age of Europe, a golden age was appearing in the East, with the critical observations of Al-Razes (850–923), the systemization of medicine by Avicenna (980–1037), and the scholarly approach to disease by Maimonides (1135–1204), all of which contributed to the rise of the Renaissance in Europe (Taylor, 2008).

INDIAN MEDICINE

Long before the Europeans established public health systems, the Hindus had established sanitation and health care for their people (Laws, 1998).

As early as 600 BC, Hindu physicians had knowledge of muscle, nerve, ligament, fascia, nerve plexuses, vascular and fatty tissue, and lymphatic tissue. They had insight into the reproductive system and some knowledge of the digestive system. They had limited knowledge of the head and brain. The head narrative was limited to one sentence: "the head is three fold, skin, bone, and brain" (Laws, 1998).

The Hindus' knowledge of anatomy was not based on dissection. They taught that the skeleton is made up of 360 bones. They estimated that the body has 500 muscles and 300 vessels (Al-Samerra'i, 1989).

The Hindus were familiar with several diseases, among them malaria and diabetes (they called the honey urine). They used the color, density, and precipitates of urine in diagnosis (Al-Samerra'i, 1989).

Illness was attributed to disorder of the humors (air, phlegm, water, and blood) and treated with herbs and charms (Laws, 1998).

Diagnosis of disease was made by inspection and auscultation of the heart. In the compendium of Susruta, written several centuries before Hippocrates, a physical examination is described, pulse variations are described, and urine tests are outlined. Treatment consisted of diet, enemas, fasting, baths, and application of leeches (Laws, 1998). They used Belladonna for sedation and anesthesia, as well as leaves and herbal products in treatment (Al-Samerra'i, 1989).

They are reported to have practiced plastic surgery, caesarian sections, and extraction of bladder stones, and to have had over a hundred surgical instruments. They used pressure and cautery to stop bleeding (Al-Samerra'i, 1989).

TWO

Prophetic Medicine

Prophetic medicine refers to a body of medical knowledge assembled across time and purported to contain recipes and cures taught by Prophet Muhammad (Khalidi, 2009). Some argue that the tradition was in reality Arabian folk medicine interacting with the newly arrived Greek medical tradition (Ullmann, 1997).

Several treaties were written on prophetic medicine, including those by al-Dhahabi (d.1348), al-Sanawbari (d.1412), al-Suyufi (d.1505), al-Hanafi (sixteenth century), al-Qalyubi (d. 1659), al-Simillawi (d. 1698), Al-Naishapuri (d. 1750), and Al-Tafilati (d. 1777) (http://www.nlm.nih.gov/hmd/arabic/propheticmed/html.

According to Ibn al-Qayyim (Khalidi, 2009), prophetic medicine "is unlike that of the physicians, for it is certain, positive, and divine, issuing from inspiration, the niche of prophecy and perfection of mind, whereas ordinary medicine is mostly guessing, intuition, and experience. One cannot deny that many sick people derive no benefit from prophetic medicine, for it can only benefit those who accept it inwardly and believe in its curing potential through unwavering and obedient faith."

The practitioners of prophetic medicine were clerics. They advocated the traditional medical practice of Prophet Muhammad days, and those mentioned in the Quran, in preference to those assimilated from Hellenistic society (http://www.nlm.nih.gov/hmd/arabic/prophetic med. html).

The therapy recommended in those treaties included diet and simple drugs, honey, bloodletting, and cautery.

They provided prayers and pious invocations to be used by devout patients in such conditions as snake bites, poisons, depression, and insomnia, among many others (Ibn al-Qayyim al- Jouzieh, undated).

Superstitions and magical cures were also prescribed, remnants of earlier practices. Such superstitions continued to appear in later scientific treatises to avoid criticism of the scientific work by charlatans of the time (Wakim, 1944).

There was prohibition against the use of wine and soporific drugs as medicament. According to a reliable narrator of Hadith (Moslim), the Prophet responded to a question about the use of wine as a medicament by answering, "It (the wine) is not a cure, it is the disease" (Ibn al -Qayyim Al-Jouzieh, undated).

(http://www.nlm.nih.gov/hmd/arabic/prophetic med.html)

Islam places a premium on personal hygiene, as demonstrated by the ritual washing of hands, feet, and face before each of the five daily prayers (Lyons, 2009).

Prophetic medicine was not considered detrimental for, or competitive with, medical practices based on Hellenistic medicine. It flourished for centuries alongside that of Greek-based humeral medicine (http://www.nlm.nih.gov/hmd/arabic/prophetic med.html).

Imam Bukhari (810–870), a noted authority on the Hadith (sayings of the Prophet), in his book "Kitab al Tibb" (Book of Medicine) attributed the following Hadith about healing to the Prophet, "gulp of honey, cupping, and branding with fire, cauterization," but he forbid his followers from using cauterization unless the other two failed (Deuraseh, 2004).

According to Imam Bukhari, "a man came to the Prophet and said: 'My brother has some abdominal trouble.' The Prophet replied, 'Let him drink honey.' The man came back and the Prophet told him again, 'Let him drink honey.' The man returned for the third time and said, 'I have done that.' The Prophet said, 'Allah has said the truth, but your brother's abdomen has told you a lie. Let him drink honey.' He made him drink honey, and he was cured" (Deuraseh, 2004). Sahih Al-Bukhari also included the following Hadith "Li Kulli Daen Dawa'" (there is no disease that Allah has created, except that He also has created its treatment), suggesting that the Prophet believed and taught that there is a cause and a cure for every disease (http://www.usc.edu/dept/msa/fundamentals/hadithsunna/bukhari/071.sb1). Reportedly, this was a response of the Prophet to a Bedouin man who asked him if he should seek treatment for an ailment.

Other Hadiths attributed to the Prophet include (Ajlouni, 2003):

"Body health supersedes religious health."

"Necessities validate prohibitions."

"Preventing harm is preferable to procuring benefits."

"The basic concept in useful matters is permissiveness."

"The basic concept in harmful matters is prohibition."

"Science is twofold, theology and medicine" (Bayon, 1952), equating the importance of the study and practice of medicine with that of theology and Islamic jurisprudence.

Other hadiths quoted by Ibn al-Qayyem al-Jouzieh in his book "al-Tibb al Nabawi" (Phrophetic Medicine) (Ibn al-Qayyem al-Jouzieh, updated) include:

On another occassion, the Prophet is reported to have said, "God created a medicine for every disease except one, old age" (Ibn al-Qayyem al-Jouzieh, undated).

"To you I recommend two healing agents, honey and the Quran" (Ibn al-Qayyem al-Jouzieh, undated).

The value of honey is also emphasized in many verses in the Quran. Surah al-Nahl, verses **68–69**, refers to honey as "shifa' li al Nas" (cure for people).

"La Tukriho Mardakum 'ala al Ta'am wal Sharab" (Don't force food and fluids on the sick).

"Salo Allah al Yaqeen wal 'Afiya, Fama Outieh Ahadon, ba'dal Yaqeen Khayran minal Afiyah" (Ask God for faith and health, for nothing better after faith than health).

There is no clear rational explanation for the popular use of cupping at the time of the Prophet. It is, however, easy to perform, using a hot jar attached to the skin surface to extract toxins and other harmful substances from the body to the skin surface. With time, people found that the use of leech, as a means of sucking blood, was similar to cupping (Deuraseh, 2004).

Cauterization (al Kay) by hot metal was used as a way to burn a wound in order to stop bleeding and prevent infection (Deuraseh, 2004).

THREE

Preserving and Expanding Ancient Heritage

TRANSLATIONS

Translations were few prior to 800 AD. The Umayyads were busy with conquest and administrative matters and did not concern themselves with translations. However, translation of the first medical books into Arabic occurred during the Umayyad rule. Not until caliph Al-Mamoun established Bayt al-Hikma in Baghdad did serious translations of sciences from other languages began in earnest (Landau, 1959; Al-Samerra'i, 1989; Ullmann, 1997).

Over the course of 150 years, all available Greek books of science and philosophy were translated, and Arabic replaced Greek as the language of science (Landau, 1959; Lyons, 2009).

Probably the centerpiece of translations in Bayt al-Hikma, under the patronage of caliph Al-Mamoun, was that of Ptolemy's book of astronomy, "Megale Syntaxes" (The Great Composition), recognized later by its Arabic name "Almagest." The Almagest constituted a road map for Arab scientists for research and study. Among Arab and Muslim scholars, Almagest was the most important book after the Quran (Lyons, 2009).

The first translator and writer of independent medical works in Arabic was a Christian, Ibn Masaweh, and after him, his student Hunayn Ibn Ishaq. Those Christian pioneers were followed by the first notable Muslim physician in the first half of the ninth century, Al-Tabari (Athar, 1993).

The most important translator in Bayt al Hikma was Hunayn Ibn Ishaq (808-873), who directed Bayt al Hikma, followed by his son Ishaq, his nephew Hubaysh Al-A'sam, and Isa Ibn Yahya (Ullmann, 1997).

Arab scholars added knowledge to translated materials from Babylonian, Greek, Egyptian, Indian, and Persian civilizations. Translators came from different ethnic origins and religions.

Translations in Bayt al Hikma took several routes: from Greek directly to Arabic, indirectly via Syriac or from Indian to Persian to Arabic (Ullmann, 1997).

A major problem that faced translators of Greek medicine and its adoption by Muslims was the fact that Greek medicine was based on mythology and the Greek religion recognized multiple Gods in comparison to scientific medicine and the concept of one God of Islam (Ullmann, 1997).

While Aesculapius played the role of God of Healing in Greek medicine, he was honored by Muslims as the discoverer and originator of medicine (Ullmann, 1997)

The Hippocratic Oath, which reads in Greek, "I swear by Apollo physician and Aesculapius and Hygiea and Panaceia and all the gods and Goddesses..." was transformed in the Muslim oath to read, "I swear by God, lord of life and death, the giver of health... and swear by Aesculapius and the saints of God be they men or women..." (Ullmann, 1997).

Problems were also encountered when it came to practical applications of Greek medicine. While the Greek sprayed umbilical hernias of infants with ashes of pig bones, Muslims practitioners replaced pig ashes (forbidden in Islam) by ashes from calf Achilles tendon (Ullmann, 1997).

Besides bringing pre-Islamic science and philosophy to the Arabs, translations played a very significant role in preserving such knowledge for reverse translations later on to Latin.

Of Galen's chief anatomical work, "Perianatomikon Egkheireseon," only volumes 1–8 and part of volume 9 are available in Greek, while the entire volumes of the book was preserved in its Arabic translation (Ullmann, 1997).

Similarly, of Galen's commentary on the Hippocratic work "About the Atmosphere, De Aere Acquis Locis," only four short passages are preserved in Greek, compared to the whole commentary preserved through Arabic translation (Ullmann, 1997).

The magnitude and vigor of translation is evident in the number of translators and the manuscripts they translated. Chapter 9 of Ibn Abi Usaibiah, book "Tabakat Al Attiba," contains an impressive list of translators from Greek into Arabic, as well as what was translated (Ibn Abi Usiabiah, 1245/1246). It is worth remembering that translation did not begin with the establishment of Bayt Al-Hikma. Earlier translations of Galen's books were done by Abu Yuhanna Al-Batriq and Georges Ibn Jibrail Bukhtishu for Caliph Al-Mansour, and by Theophile Ibn Tuma Al-Rahawi for Caliph Al-Mahdi (Al-Samerra'i, 1989).

It is important to recognize that Muslim scientists did more than simply translate and preserve the works resulting in the future transmission to Europe. The translation activity went hand in hand with scientific research. In many instances, the translated works were reformulated and transformed (Dallal, 2010). A strong emphasis on experimentation and empiricism led to new results and new observations, which were contrasted and combined with those of Galen by writers such as Al-Razi,

Al-Majusi, Al-Zahrawi, Ibn Sina, Ibn Zuhr, and Ibn al-Nafis. The experiments carried out by Al-Razi and Ibn Zuhr contradicted the Galenic theory of humorism, while Ibn al-Nafis's discovery of the pulmonary circulation contradicted the Galenic theory on the heart (http://en.wikipedia.org/wiki/galen).

TRANSLATORS

Bukhtishu, Georges Ibn Jibrail, one of the early translators of Greek books into Syriac and from Greek and Syriac into Arabic, was employed by caliph Al-Mansour (Ibn Abi Usaibiah, 1245/46; Al-Samerra'i, 1989)

Hunayn Ibn Ishaq, fluent in Arabic, Syriac, Greek, and Persian, was known for his accurate and meticulous translations (Ibn Abi Usaibiah, 1245/46; Al-Samerra'i, 1989). Some of the translations attributed to Hunayn Ibn Ishaq were actually translated by his students and edited by Hunayn (Al-Samerra'i, 1989). While translating, Hunayn composed medical treatises of his own, including "Al-Masa'il fil Tibb lil Muta'allimin" (Questions on Medicine for Students) and "Kitab al'Ashr Maqalat fil Ayn' (Ten Treatises on the Eye) (Dallal, 2010).

Ishaq Ibn Hunayn, son of Hunayn Ibn Ishaq, fluent in his father's four languages, and similar to his father, was reputed for clear and accurate translations and tendency towards classifications (Ibn Abi Usaibiah, 1245/46; Al-Samerra'i, 1989).

Al-A'sam, Hubaysh, nephew and student of Hunayn Ibn Ishaq, was similarly noted for accuracy in his translations (Ibn Abi Usaibiah, 1245/46; Al-Samerra'i, 1989). Most of his translations were into Arabic (Al-Samerra'i, 1989).

Isa Ibn Yahya Ibn Ibrahim was one of the student of Hunayn Ibn Ishaq. He was one of the prolific translators. All his translations were into Arabic, including some of Galen's books (Ibn Abi Usaibiah, 1245/46; Al-Samerra'i, 1989).

Qusta Ibn Luqa al Baalbaki was fluent in several languages. He translated books in different disciplines, including medicine (Ibn Abi Usaibiah, 1245/46; Al-Samerra'i, 1989).

AL-Abrash, Ayyoub (Abu Ibrahim) provided a small number of translations into Syriac. His translations were as good in quality as those of Hunayn Ibn Ishaq. Some mix-up between the names Ayyoub Al-Abrash and Ayyoub Al-Rahawi suggest that the two are the same person. Ibn Abi Usaibiah, however, reported them as two different people. Al-Abrash translated over thirty-five books from Greek into Syriac (Ibn Abi Usaibiah, 1245/46; Al-Samerra'i, 1989).

Mesergese(Masergueh) was a Syriac physician who lived during the rule of Haroun Al-Rashid. He translated from Syriac into Arabic. Among his books was one about food benefits and harm and a book on the benefits and harm of drugs (Ibn Abi Usaibiah, 1245/46; Al-Samerra'i, 1989).

Ibn Masergese (Masergueh) was a practicing physician and translator. His translations were as good as his father's. Following in his father's steps, he wrote a book titled "Colors and Smells" (Ibn Abi Usaibiah, 1245/46; Al-Samerra'i, 1989).

Al-Kharkhi, Shahdi, a Syriac from Karkh in Iraq, provided a modest amount of translations from Syriac into Arabic (Ibn Abi Usaibiah, 1245/46; Al-Samerra'i, 1989).

Al-Kharkhi, Ibn Shahdi, a Syriac from Karkh, translated from Syriac into Arabic. He translated Hippocrates's book "On Embryos" and Galen's books "Kitab Al-Nabd" (On Pulse) and "Kitab Al-Sina'a Al-Tibbiya" (Medical Profession) (Ibn Abi Usaibiah, 1245/46; Al-Samerra'i, 1989).

Al-Hajjaj Ibn Yusef Ibn Matar worked for Caliph Al-Mamoun. He translated Ptolemy's "Almagest" and two translations of Euclides book, one under the title "Al-Harouni," after Caliph Haroun Al-Rashid, and the other "Mamouni," after Caliph Al-Mamoun. The Euclid book translations were later corrected by Thabet Ibn Qurra (Ibn Abi Usaibiah, 1245/46; Al-Samerra'i, 1989).

Ibn Na'meh Al-Homsi, Abdel Masih Ibn Abdallah had few but quality translations. He was originally from Homs in Syria but lived in Baghdad during the rule of Caliph Al-Mu'tasim (Ibn Abi Usaibiah, 1245/46; Al-Samerra'i, 1989).

Al-Na'meh Al-Homsi, Zorba Ibn Manho made translations that were not highly valued (Ibn Abi Usaibiah, 1245/46).

Al-Homsi, Hilal Ibn Abi Hilal was a Nestorian from Homs in Syria. He provided accurate translations, but they were average quality of Arabic presentation (Ibn Abi Usaibiah, 1245/46).

Al-Turjuman, Fathiun had poor mastery of the Arabic language even though "al-Turjuman" is the Arabic word for "translator." His translations were described as melodic. He translated from Greek and Syriac into Arabic (Ibn Abi Usaibiah, 1245/46; Al-Samerra'i, 1989).

Abu Nasr Ibn Nari Ibn Ayyoub provided few translations of relatively poor quality (Ibn Abi Usaibiah, 1245/46).

Al- Mutran, Baseel (Basilos) translated several books of high quality (Ibn Abi Usaibiah, 1245/46).

Ibn Baseel, Istifan was the son of Basilos Al-Mutran. His translations were as good as those of Hunayn ibn Ishaq but not as eloquent. He translated from Greek to Arabic (Ibn Abi Usaibiah, 1245/46; Al-Samerra'i, 1989).

Al-Turjuman, Musa Ibn Khalid translated many (estimated at sixteen) of Galen's books from Syriac into Arabic. His translations do not match in quality those of Hunayn Ibn Ishaq (Ibn Abi Usaibiah, 1245/46; Al-Samerra'i, 1989).

Istath (Istalion) was the Patriarch of Alexandria. He is listed among the average translators. He translated for Yahya Al-Barmaki, one of the Baghdad supporters of translations (Ibn Abi Usaibiah, 1245/46; Al-Samerra'i, 1989).

Ibn Rabita, Hairoun had an average reputation as translator (Ibn Abi Usaibiah, 1245/46).

Al Sanqal, Tadros translated books on philosophy of above-average quality (Ibn Abi Usaibiah, 1245/46).

Al-Rasi, Surjius (Al-Rasi'in) translated several books into Syriac. Those later corrected by Hunayn Ibn Ishaq are of good quality but the rest are of average quality (Ibn Abi Usaibiah, 1245/46; Al-Samerra'i, 1989)..

Al Rahawi, Ayyoub was multilingual, had better mastery of Syriac than Arabic. He translated from Greek into Syriac. Some of his translations into Syriac were redone by Hunayn Ibn Ishaq (Ibn Abi Usaibiah, 1245/46; Al-Samerra'i, 1989).

Al-Naqel, Yusuf (Abu Yacoub) Ibn Isa al-Mutatabib, nicknamed "The Sleepy," was a quality translator (Ibn Abi Usaibiah, 1245/46; Al-Sammera'i, 1989).

Ibn Al- Salt, Ibrahim was proficient in Greek, Syriac, and Arabic. He was an average translator (Ibn Abi Usaibiah, 1245/46; Al-Samerra'i, 1989).

Al-Naqel, Thabe was an average translator but better than Ibrahim Ibn Al-Salt; he translated few books, including one of Galen's (Ibn Abi Usaibiah, 1245/46; Al-Samerra'i, 1989).

Al-Kateb, Abu Yusuf was an average translator and translated several books by Hippocrates into Arabic (Ibn Abi Usaibiah, 1245/46; Al-Samerra'i, 1989).

Ibn Bukhtishu, Yuhanna was the physician of the Abbasid Caliph

Al-Mu'tadid. He translated several books from Greek into Arabic (Ibn Abi Usaibiah, 1245/46; Al-Samerra'i, 1989).

Al Batriq, Abu Yuhanna served Caliph Al Mansour, who asked him to translate several old books, including medical treatises by Galen and Hippocrates (Ibn Abi Usaibiah, 1245/46; Al-Samerra'i, 1989).

Al-Batriq, Yuhanna (Abu Zacharia) mastered Latin, Greek, and Syriac but not Arabic languages. He was a philosopher but not a physician. He had enough knowledge of medicine to be able to translate books by Aristotle and Hippocrates (Ibn Abi Usaibiah, 1245/46; Al-Samerra'i, 1989).

Al-Rahawi, Qabda was trusted by Hunayn Ibn Ishaq to help him translate some books, which Hunayn later edited (Ibn Abi Usaibiah, 1245/46; Al-Samerra'i, 1989).

Ibn Banas, Mansour was another translator trusted by Hunayn Ibn Ishaq. He had better mastery of Syriac than Arabic . He translated from Syriac into Arabic and from Arabic into Syriac (Ibn Abi Usaubiah, 1245/46; Al-Samerra'i, 1989).

Ibn Hirmiz, Abd Yasho' was Archbishop of Mosul in Iraq and a friend of Gabriel Ibn Bukhtishu, who trusted him to help him in translation (Ibn Abi Usaibiah, 1245/46; Al-Samerra'i, 1989).

Al-Dimashki, Saeed Ibn Yacoub ((Abu Uthman) was considered among the best translators. He wrote most of his works for Ali Ibn Isa Al-Jarrah, the Vezier of Caliph Al-Muqtadir. He was appointed head of hospitals in Baghdad, Mecca, and Medina (Ibn Abi Usaibiah, 1245/46; Al-Samerra'i, 1989).

Ibn Biks, Ibrahim (Abu Ishaq) was one of the well-known Baghdad physicians. He had very good command of the Arabic language and translated many books into Arabic. His translations were of good quality and popular. He worked in the Udadi hospital in Baghdad. He became blind late in his life (Ibn Abi Usaibiah, 1245/46; Al-Samerra'i, 1989).

Ibn Biks, Ali Ibn Ibrahim (Abu Al-Hasan) was like his father, a practicing physician and good translator. He worked at the Udadi hospital in Baghdad (Ibn Abi Usaibiah, 1245/1246; Al-Samerra'i, 1989).

Al-Rahawi, Theophile Ibn Touma was among the translators of Greek books for Caliph Al-Mahdi (Al-Samerra'i, 1989).

Al-Rumi, Sirjius Ibn Elia translated books by Hippocrates and Galen (Al-Samerra'i, 1989).

Ibn Saharbakht, Isa translated books by Hippocrates and Galen, as well as writing a book on simple drugs (Al-Samerra'i, 1989).

Ibn Ali, Abdullah was well versed in Persian language and translated a book from Indian into Arabic (Al-Samerra'i, 1989).

Al-Natili Al-Tabari, Al-Hussein Ibn Ibrahim Ibn Al-Hasan Ibn Khorshid was translating in 990 AD. Among his translations is a book on plants (Al-Samerra'i, 1989).

Isa Ibn Yahya Ibn Ibrahim was a student of Hunayn Ibn Ishaq. He assisted Ibn Ishaq in translating a number of books by Hippocrates and Galen (Al-Samerra'i, 1989).

Ibn Sayyar, Yahya translated Galen's book on "Sleep and Wakefulness" (Al-Samerra'i, 1989).

Ibn Zar'a, Isa Ibn Ishaq (Abu Ali) was a philosopher, physician, and translator. He died in 1008 AD. He translated books by Galen (Al-Samerra'i, 1989).

Nazif Al-Qiss was originally a Greek. Al-Qiss in Arabic was a clergyman. He combined medicine, theology, and translation. He practiced medicine in Al-Udadi Hospital in Baghdad (Al-Samerra'i, 1989).

Al-Jawhari, Al-Abbas Ibn Said translated a book on poisons from Persian into Arabic for Caliph Al-Mamoun. The book was originally written in Hindu and translated into Persian by Abu Hatem Al-Balkhi (Al-Samerra'i, 1989).

Ibn Aseed, Isa was a Syriac from Baghdad. He was a student of Thabet Ibn Qurra and translated for him (Al-Samerra'i, 1989).

Al-Takriti, Abu Zacharia Ibn Adi was a student of Farabi. He translated philosophical treatise from Greek into Arabic (Al-Samerra'i, 1989).

Ibn Yunis, Matta (Abu Bishr) was among the best philosophers in his time. He translated books by Aristotle from Greek to Syriac. The book was then translated into Arabic by Hunayn Ibn Ishaq (Al-Samerra'i, 1989).

Al-Hadithi, Musa translated a book by Serapiun into Arabic (Al-Samerra'i, 1989).

Ibn Al-Bahloul, Abu Al-Hasan translated a book by Ibn Serapiun into Arabic (Al-Samerra'i, 1989).

SPONSERS OF TRANSLATORS

Besides the above translators, most of whom translated for caliphs, there were freelance translators hired by members of well-known families who had attained power and wealth, such as:

The Al-Barmakids, who paid thousands of Dirhams to translators of books (Afnan, 1958).

The Nowbakht family, who were distinguished authors themselves and supported translators from the Greek language (Afnan, 1958).

The Munajjem family (family of the astronomers) were interested in astronomy and were among the authors and famous patrons of translation. Mohammad Ibn Musa Al-Munajjem, one of the famous Bani Musa tribe members who were close to the caliphs, was most interested in translation of Hunayn Ibn Ishaq, who had translated for him a number of medical books. Another member of this family, Ali Ibn Yahya, known as Ibn Al Munajjem, one of the recorders and confidant of Caliph Al Mamoun, was interested in medical books (Afnan, 1958).

In addition, bookkeepers and intermediaries recruited and supported translators, such as (Ibn Abi Usaibiah, 1245/1246):

Shirsho' Ibn Qatrab, from Ghondi-Shapour (Iran), who pampered translators and bought their translated books, preferring books in Syriac than Arabic.

Thadrus Al-Usquf, pastor of Al Karkh quarter in Baghdad, interested in book collection, and asked a number of Christian translators to translate some valuable books.

Muhammad Ibn Musa Ibn Abdel Malek engaged translation of medical books and was conversant in medical subjects.

Isa Ibn Yunis Al-Kateb Al-Hasib, among the dignitaries in Iraq, was interested in obtaining ancient books, in particular those related to Greek sciences.

Ali, known by "Al Fayyoum", engaged several translators.

Ahmad Ibn Muhammad, known as "Ibn Al-Mudir Al-Kateb", overwhelmed translators with gifts and money.

Ibrahim Ibn Muhammad Ibn Musa Al-Kateb sought the friendship of scholars and translators and was interested, in particular, in translations of Greek books into Arabic.

Abdullah Ibn Ishaq was enthusiastic about translation and in the acqusition of books.

Mohammad Ibn Abdel Malek Al Zayyat spent close to 2,000 dinars monthly on translated books, especially those of Greek origin. He engaged several luminaries in translations, such as Yuhanna Ibn Masaweh, Gabriel Ibn Bukhtishu, and many others.

In general, the professional translators, most of who were Christians, fell into three groups (Afnan, 1958): the pre-Hunayn school; the school of Hunayn; and the post-Hunayn school. Their activities included translations from Greek to Syriac, Greek to Arabic, Syriac to Arabic, and Arabic to Syriac (Afnan, 1958). The same work was frequently translated by different people, different works translated by the same person, revisions of translations by the same author or other authors, and translation of one or different works by one person into both Syriac and Arabic (Afnan, 1958).

FOUR

Bayt Al-Hikma (House of Wisdom)

Established in Baghdad in 832 AD by the Abbasid Caliph Al-Mamoun (813–833 AD), son of Caliph Haroun Al-Rashid of *Thousand and One Nights* fame, Bayt Al-Hikma was a center for translation, writing, and study (Al-Mahi, 1959; Landau, 1959; Ullmann, 1997). It was originally established by Caliph Al-Mansur as a repository for Pahlavi (scholarly language of pre-Islamic Persia) manuscripts and the translation from Persian to Arabic of Sasanian history and culture. It developed under Caliph Al-Mamoun into an unrivaled center for the study of humanities and for sciences, including mathematics, astronomy, medicine, chemistry, and geography. Drawing on Persian, Indian, and Greek texts, including those of Aristotle, Euclid, and Pythagoras, among others, scholars in Bayt Al-Hikma accumulated the greatest collection of knowledge and added to it their own observations and commentaries (Al-Samerra'i, 1989; Eknoyan, 1994; Whitaker, 2004; Al-Khalili, 2011; Freely, 2011). As part of a treaty with the king of Cyprus, Caliph Al-Mamoun demanded the transfer of Greek scholarly books in the Cyprus repository to Baghdad's Bayt Al-Hikma (Al-Samerra'i, 1989).

Caliph Al-Mamoun's passion for Bayt Al-Hikma was ascribed by Ibn Al-Nadim, a chronicler of medieval Arab history, to a mystical dream in which Aristotle appeared to Al-Mamoun. After his initial shock, Al-Mamoun asked Aristotle to define "that which is good," to which Aristotle answered, "Whatever is good according to the intellect, religious law, and the good of the masses." The dream was interpreted by the Caliph to mean that promoting scientific scholarship is a religious duty (Al-Samerra'i, 1989; Lyons, 2009; Freely, 2011).

The first director of Bayt Al-Hikma was Ibn Masaweh, followed by Hunayn Ibn Ishaq and Ishaq Ibn Hunayn (Myers, 1964; Al-Samerra'i, 1989).

For two centuries, works of mathematics, astronomy, physics, and medicine were translated from Greek, Persian, and Hindu, and further developed by Islamic scholars under the caliph's patronage (Brown, 2010).

Bayt Al-Hikma emerged as the battleground for the conflict between the dictates of science and the then prevalent medieval conception of God. Among the early translation work of Bayt Al-Hikma was Aristotle's work on the use of dialectics, which was used by Abbasid theologians against Muslim heretics (Lyons, 2009).

Important figures under Caliph Al-Mamoun, who facilitated translations, were three brothers from the Banu Musa tribe (Mahmoud, Ahmad, and Al-Hasan), sons of an ex-highway robber who became an astrologer and who befriended Caliph Al-Mamoun, before the latter assumed the caliphate. When the father died, his sons were taken under the patronage of Caliph Al-Mamoun. They became rich and powerful and developed a passion for collecting ancient manuscripts. They also supported a group of translators that included Hunayn Ibn Ishaq and Thabet Ibn Qurra, who were paid generously for their work (Al-Samerra'i, 1989; Al-Khalili, 2011; Freely, 2011).

It is said that Caliph Al-Mamoun used to pay translators the weight of a translated manuscript in gold. Reportedly, Hunayn Ibn Ishaq used large letters and triple or quadruple spacing on heavyweight paper to increase the weight of the manuscript (Al-Mahi, 1959).

Scholars in Bayt Al-Hikma were sent by the caliph everywhere in search of manuscripts to translate. Hunayn Ibn Ishaq, the chief translator at Bayt Al-Hikma from 847 to 861, looked for a medical text by Galen (second century AD) in Mesopotamia (now Iraq), all of Syria, Palestine, and Egypt. He found a partial copy in Damascus. Additional chapters were located elsewhere, and translated into Arabic (Al-Samerra'i, 1989; Brown, 2010).

Thabit Ibn Qurra translated nearly two hundred books on medicine, mathematics, and astronomy (Brown, 2010).

In Bayt Al-Hikma, great books were not only translated but reworked, corrected, refined, and improved, leading to the emergence of new scientific terminology (Eknoyan, 1994; Lyons, 2009). Many of the books were translated multiple times by different translators, either to improve the quality of previous translations or to add new material (Al-Samerra'i, 1989).

Thus, Bayt Al-Hikma became a repository for the translated important works of such as Euclid, Archimedes, Aristotle, Ptolemy, among classical thinkers (Brown, 2010).

Another luminary of Bayt Al-Hikma was Musa Al-Khawarizmi, the most famous mathematician of Bayt Al-Hikma, known as the "Father of Algebra." The word "algebra" is derived from his book "Kitab Al-Jabr." "Jabr" in Arabic is "algebra" in English (Whitaker, 2004). Khawarizmi wrote the first book on Arabic numerals, titled "On Indian Calculations." Another book by Al-Khawarizmi "Kitab al-Mukhtasar fi Hisab al-Jabr Wal Muqabalah" (Compendium Book on Calculations by Completing and Balancing) is believed to be the origin of modern-day algebra. Khawarizmi also is reported to have calculated the circumference of the Earth at 23,220 miles (actual is 24,900 miles) (Brown, 2010).

Close by Bayt Al-Hikma was an observatory to watch the stars, a central interest of Caliph Al-Mamoun (Brown, 2010; Al-Khalili, 2010).

The program of translation in Bayt Al-Hikma and dissemination of its products were facilitated by the presence of paper mills in Baghdad (Eknoyan, 1994; Freely, 2011).

Translators and scholars in Bayt Al-Hikma were provided with working space as well as administrative and salary support (Al-Samerra'i, 1989).

With time, Bayt Al-Hikma developed into a translation center, library, manuscript repository, and scholarly academy. It earned the title of "Treasury of the Books of Wisdom," and "The Treasury of Wisdom" (Lunde, 1982; Lyons, 2009). By the middle of the ninth century, Bayt Al-Hikma became the largest repository of books in the world (Al-Khalili, 2011).

Activities in Bayt Al-Hikma almost came to a standstill during the rules of Caliphs Al-Mu'taz and Al-Musta'in due to their rivalries and disinterest in scholarship. Activities in Bayt Al-Hikma were resumed during the rule of Caliph Al-Mu'tamid (Al-Samerra'i, 1989).

In addition to Bayt Al-Hikma, several private libraries were scattered all over Baghdad so that Baghdad was, so to speak, "Medinat Al-Hikma" (The City of Wisdom) (Al-Khalili, 2011).

Bayt Al-Hikma was destroyed along with all of Baghdad during the Mongol invasion in 1258 (Al-Samerra'i, 1989).

FIVE

Medical Luminaries, Their Lives and Works

PRE-ISLAMIC/EARLY ISLAMIC PERIOD (500–660AD)

IBN HEZEEM

Ibn Hezeem was well-known for his general practice of medicine, but in particular his expertise in cautery. He lived before Ibn Kilda Al-Thaqafi (Al-Samerra'i, 1989).

AL-ASLAMIYYAH (ASLAMIA), RAFEEDA (RAFAIDA), BINT SAAD (born in approximately 620 AD)

Al-Aslamiyyah was the first health nurse and social worker in Islam. She came from the Bani Aslam tribe of the Khazraj tribal confederation in Medina. She was born in Yathrib (Medina) before the migration of the Prophet to it. She was among the first in Medina to accept Islam and used to accompany the Prophet on his missions to attend to the wounded. She participated in the battles of Badr, Uhud, Khandaq, among others. A tent was made for her in the proximity of the Prophet's mosque in Yathrib (today's Medina in Saudi Arabia) to attend to patients. The tent is considered the first hospital in Islam. Al-Aslamiyyah's father, Saad Al

Aslamy, was a physician from whom she learned medical care. Her contributions were not limited to nursing care. She was involved in social work in the community. She came to the assistance of every Muslim in need, the poor, the orphaned, or the handicapped. She was an empathic, kind person and a good organizer. With her clinical skills, she trained other women to be nurses and to work in the area of health care. She used her clinical skills and medical experience to develop the first ever documented mobile care units that were able to meet the medical needs of the community. An award is given in her name every year to a graduate of the School of Nursing of the University of Bahrain who consistently excels in delivering superb nursing care to patients (Al-Samerra'i, 1989; http://en.wikipedia.org/wiki/Rufaida_Al-Aslamia).

AL-SHIFA' BINT ABDULLAH AL-QURAYSHIAH AL- ADAWIYAH (d. 640 AD)

Al-Shifa' was especially competent in dermatologic disorders. She was called "al-Shifa" (healing) because of her professional expertise in medicine. Her original name was Layla, and her kunya (title) was Umm Suleiman. She was an early Muslim convert, having converted to Islam before the Hijra to Medina, when it was a dangerous thing to do. It is reported that the Prophet asked her to teach his wife Hafsa reading and writing, some say teaching her healing by "ruqyah." She was highly regarded by Caliph Omar, who used to ask for her opinion and entrusted her to monitor the salesmen in the marketplace, thus becoming the first Muslim woman to hold an official position in public administration. Her duties were to ensure that business practices would always be consistent with Islamic values. She also had an impact on Islamic history, having narrated many hadiths (sayings) of the Prophet (Al-Samerra'i, 1989; http://www.daralhadith.org.uk/?p=164; http://theislampath.com/smf/index.php?topic=6955.0).

UM ATTIYAH AL-ANSARIYYAH

Um Attiyah was another female early convert to Islam. She practiced circumcision and is reported to have accompanied the Prophet in battle and took care of the injured (Al-Samerra'i, 1989).

IBN THA'LABA AL-AZDI, DAMMAD

Ibn Tha'laba was a personal friend of the Prophet before the onset of Islam. It is reported that he interviewed the Prophet to ensure his sanity, and on that basis, he committed himself to Islam and started to treat the converts to Islam (Al-Samerra'i, 1989).

IBN KA'AB, AL-HARITH

Ibn Ka'ab lived in the days of the Prophet and is reported to have attended to the second Caliph Omar Ibn Al-Khattab for his fatal stab (Al-Samerra'i 1989).

IBN KILDA AL-THAQAFI, AI HARITH IBN UMAR IBN ILAJ (ABU WA'EL) (d. 634/635)

The name Al-Thaqafi relates to his origin from Thaqif, in the Taif region in Saudi Arabia. Ibn Kilda is the best known of the luminaries in the pre-Islamic and early Islamic period and earned the title of "the physician of the Arabs" (Al-Samerra'i, 1989). The first recorded contact of the Arabs with medicine begins with Al Harith ibn Kilda, the Prophet's cousin, and his personal physician. He travelled all the way from Mecca to Ghondi-Shapour in Persia (1,400 kilometers) to study medicine just before the rise of Islam. Remembering that in that time this distance had to be crossed on camel reflects the difficulties Ibn Kilda had to go through in search of medical knowledge (Haddad, 1993).

He is the author of a book "Al-Muhawir" (The Dialogue), describing medical discussions with Kisra Al- Shirwan. Among his recommendation for longevity were early meals, light clothing, and moderate sex (Ibn Abi Usaibiah, 1245/46; Al-Mahi, 1959; Haddad, 1975; Al-Samerra'i. 1989).

Before studying medicine, Ibn Kilda played the Oud, a string instrument popular in Arab culture, which he learned in Persia, some say in Yemen (Ibn Abi Usaibiah, 1245/46; Samerra'i, 1989). He converted to Islam and stayed in Arabia throughout the rule of the four caliphs: Abu Bakr, Omar, Uthman, and Ali (Ibn Abi Usaibiah, 1245/46; Haddad, 2003).

Famous quotes from Harith Ibn Kilda include (Ibn Abi Usaibiah, 1245/46; Al-Samerra'i, 1989; Haddad, 1993):

"The body is like the earth. If you take care of it, it will last, and if you neglect it, it will be ruined."

"Staying on diet is controlling your lips and being moderate with use of your hands."

"Do not enter a bath on a full stomach."

"Do not eat when angry."

"The most harmful thing for an elderly man is to have a good cook and a pretty and sexy consort."

IBN AL-HARITH IBN KILDA AL-THAQAFI, AL-NADER IBN MANAF IBN ABDEL DAR (d. 670 AD)

Al Nader Ibn Al-Harith Ibn Kilda was the cousin of the Prophet and the son of Al-Harith Ibn Kilda. He lived in Mecca and traveled wide and far. He met and learned from rabbis and priests philosophy and wisdom. From his father he learned medicine (Ibn Abi Usaibiah, 1245/46).

In spite of his relations to the Prophet, Ibn Al-Harith was jealous of the Prophet and worked with the Prophet's adversaries in Mecca to challenge his prophecy (Ibn Abi Usaibiah, 1245/46; Al-Samerra'i, 1989).

AL-SUKUTI, ATHIR IBN AMR

Not much is known about Al-Sukuti other than he participated in the treatment of Caliph Ali Ibn Abu Talib from the stab wound that killed him (Al-Samerra'i, 1989).

UMAYYAD PERIOD (661–750 AD)

The Umayyads showed little or no interest in science. They had a passion for architectural projects and were occupied in protecting and expanding their empire and subduing internal revolts. Among the Umayyads' architectural projects are the Al-Aqsa and Dome of the Rock mosques in Jerusalem; the Umayyad mosque in Damascus; the three religious monuments of Islam (Bayon, 1952; Williams, 2006; Al-Khalili, 2011; Tarabay, 2011).

IBN UTHAL

Ibn Uthal, of the Christian faith, studied medicine in in the medical school of Ghondi-Shapour and was one of the prominent physicians in Damascus and personal physician to the first Umayyad caliph, Mu'awiya Ibn Abi Sufian (661–680), who kept him close to him and had great trust in him (Ibn Abi Usaibiah, 1245/46; Al-Samerra'i, 1989).

Ibn Uthal was well versed in simple and compound drugs as well as poisons. His expertise in poisons was used by the caliph to poison and kill a competitor to the throne, Abdul Rahman Ibn Khalid Ibn Al-Walid, by feeding him honey mixed with poison prepared by Ibn Uthal. Upon hearing of his death, Abdul Rahman's nephew, who lived in Mecca, Saudi Arabia, traveled to Damascus, where he revenged his uncle's death by assassinating Ibn Uthal (Ibn Abi Usaibiah, 1245/46)

IBN ABJAR AL-KANANI, ABDUL MALEK

Ibn Abjar was a Christian, learned physician who studied and taught in the medical school in Alexandria. He was also a philosopher and chemist. He converted to Islam when the Arabs occupied Egypt. He was consulted by Prince Omar Ibn Abdul Aziz, before the latter became the Umayyad

Caliph in 717 AD. It is said that Omar Ibn Abdul Aziz was instrumental in his conversion to Islam and in transferring him to Damascus when he became Caliph. He is quoted to have said, "Avoid using a drug as long as your body is fighting the disease on its own," which is a reflection of prophetic medicine (Ibn Abi Usaibiah, 1245/46; Al-Samerra'i, 1989).

IBN ABI RAMTHA AL-TAMIMI

Ibn Abi Ramtha practiced medicine and surgery during the time of the Prophet. It is reported that he entered the house of the Prophet and offered to treat him from an ailment he had. The Prophet told him that the physician is a helper to God the healer (Ibn Abi Usaibiah, 1245/46; Al-Samerra'i, 1989).

TIAZOUQ

Tiazouq was a well-known physician during the early Umayyad rule in Damascus. His medical practice emphasized general hygiene and avoidance of drugs until necessary. He served the ruler Al-Hajjaj Ibn Yousuf Al-Thaqafi, who trusted his advice, including his advice to soak his feet in hot water as a treatment for headache. His other suggestions to Al-Hajjaj for maintaining good health included the following (Ibn Abi Usaibiah, 1245/46); Al-Samerra'i, 1989):

1. Avoid eating when your stomach is full.

2. What your teeth cannot chew easily, your stomach cannot digest easily.

3. Wait two hours after a meal to drink water.

4. Avoid excessive intercourse.

5. Avoid intercourse on a full stomach.

6. Intercourse with old women shortens life.

Al-Hajjaj is reported to have asked his secretary to write these recommendations in gold and save them in a gold box (Ibn Abi Usaibiah, 1245/46).

SCHOLARSHIP

Tazoq wrote an exhaustive book to his son, referred to in Al-Hawi fil Tibb, in which he addressed topics on stomach ailment, lung disorders, colitis, disorders of the liver and spleen, and the approach to placental disorders (Samerra'I, 1989). He also wrote a book on mixing of drugs, another defining the name of drugs, as well as "Al-Fusul fil Tibb," and a poem on how to preserve health (Ibn Abi Usaibiah, 1245/46; Al-Samerra'i, 1989).

Tiazoq died at an old age in the year 90 AH (708 AD) (Ibn Abi Usaibiah, 1245/46).

At his death bed, he is quoted to have said (Al-Samerra'i, 1989):

"Do not buy a medicine unless you need it."

"Do not eat food if your stomach is full of food."

"After you eat, walk about forty steps."

FURAT IBN SHUHNATA

Ibn Shuhnata was a Jewish physician and one of the best students of Tiazoq, and the closest of his students to him. He served Al-Hajjaj after his teacher Diazoq passed away. He also served Caliph Abu Jaafar Al-Mansour, and his son Isa Ibn Musa (Al-Samerra'i, 1989).

AL-MUHANDIS, MUHAMMAD

Al-Muhandis ("engineer" in Arabic) was so named because of his knowledge of geometry and reputation as an engineer and carpenter prior to his study of medicine. Most of the doors of Al-Nuri Hospital in Damascus were made by him. He studied medicine under Ibn Abi Al Hakam, chief physician at Al-Nuri Hospital where he also practiced medicine (Jadon, 1970).

ABUL-HAKAM AL-DIMASHKI, MOHAMMAD

Abul-Hakam Al-Dimashki was the first of three physicians in the family; the others include his son, Hakam, and his grandson, Ibn Al-Hakam.

Abul-Hakam was of the Christian faith, well versed in drugs and their use (Ibn Abi Usaibiah, 1245/46). He served Caliphs Muawiya Ibn Abi Sufian (661–680), Yazid Ibn Muawiya, Abdul Malik Ibn Marwan, and his son Al-Walid Ibn Abdel-Malik (d. 715) (Al-Samerra'i, 1989).

Abul-Hakam served as chief physician of Al-Nuri Hospital in Damascus. In addition to his duties at Al-Nuri Hospital, he was assigned to visit the Citadel of Damascus to attend to the sick dignitaries of the Umayyad State and to lecture at the great lecture hall of Al-Nuri Hospital, where his teaching sessions lasted three hours. He learned the profession of medicine from his father, who was a famous physician and had a dispensary in Damascus. Al-Hakam is known to have successfully treated a case of severe hemorrhage caused by an unskillful surgeon barber (Jadon, 1970).

Abul-Hakam is reported to have lived beyond the age of a hundred (Ibn Abi Usaibiah. 1245/46; Al-Samerra'i, 1989).

No publications are known for Abul-Hakam (Al-Samerra'i, 1989).

MASARJAWAIH AL-BASRI

Masarjawaih was one of the earliest Jewish physicians in the Arab and Muslim worlds, and the earliest translator from Syriac. He studied medicine in the school of medicine in Ghondi-Shapour (Persia) but lived and practiced in Basra, Iraq, around 683 AD (64 AH) during the Umayyad dynasty. His son, Issa, also a translator and author of two treatises (on color and on food) must have converted to Christianity, judging from his name (Ibn Abi Usaibiah, 1245/46; Al-Samerra'i, 1989; http://en.wikipedia.org/wiki/Masarjawaih).

SCHOLARSHIP

Masarjawaih translated the thirty-chapter medical pandects of the arch- deacon or prespyter Aaron Bin A'youn (610–641 AD) from Syriac into Arabic and added two chapters of his own. It is believed that this was the first scientific book to be translated into Arabic. The book was translated during the rule of the Umayyad Marwan Ibn Al-Hakam but kept in the government archives until the rule of Caliph Omar Ibn Abdel Aziz (710 AD) who ordered its distribution for the benefit of the public, having found in it nothing contrary to Islamic Shari'a (Ibn Abi Usaibiah, 1245/46; Al-Samerra'i 1989; http:/en.wikipedia.org/wiki/Masarjawaih).

Among his books are:

The Virtues of Food, Their Advantages and Their Disadvantages

This book was written in Arabic (Ibn Abi Usaibiah, 1245/46; http://en.wikipedia.org/wiki/masarjawaih).

The Virtues of Medicinal Plants, Their Advantages and Disadvantages

This book was also written in Arabic (Ibn Abi Usaibiah, 1245/46; http://en.wikipedia.org/wiki/Masarjawaih).

The above books are known to a certain extent by quotations, since none has been preserved or were preserved in fragments (http://en.wikipedia.org/wiki/Masarjawaih).

HAKAM AL-DIMASHKI

Hakam Al-Dimashki, son of Abul-Hakam Al-Dimashki, lived in Damascus, and kept the reputation of his father as a good physician. Like his father, he lived a long life. He died in the year 210 AH (825 AD) at the age of

105 and according to his son, Ibn Al-Hakam, in full control of his mental health. The last part of his life, he served under the Abbasid dynasty. Like his father, he did not leave any scholarly contributions (Ibn Abi Usaibiah, 1245/46; Al-Samerra'i, 1989).

IBN HAKAM AL-DIMASHKI, ISSA (d. 839 AD)

He was the son of Hakam Al-Dimashki and grandson of Abul-Hakam Al-Dimashki. He was called Abi Al-Hasan. He was known to be pious, hence his name Jesus (Issa in Arabic). He lived most of his life in the Abbasid period, and served Caliph Haroun Al-Rashid, including treating Al-Rashid's favorite jariya (concubine) Ghadid Musfa (Ibn Abi Usaibiah, 1245/46; Al-Samerra'i, 1989). He died around 839 AD during the rule of Caliph Al-Mu'tasim Bi Allah' (Al-Samerra'i, 1989).

SCHOLARSHIP

Kitab Manafi' aL-Hayawan (Book of Animal Benefits) (Ibn Abi Usaibiah, 1245/46; Al-Samerra'i, 1989)

Al-Risala al-Kafiyah al-Haroniyyah

The manuscript is kept in the Libraries of Paris, Cambridge, and the Vatican (Al-Samerra'i, 1989)

Kitab fil A'shab wal-'Aqaqeer (book on plants and medicines (Al-Samerra'i, 1989).

Kunnash al-Yaqouta (Book of Rubis)

This book was referred to by Al-Razi in his "Al-Hawi fil Tibb" in connection with treatment of asthma, pulse irregularity, liver jaundice, gall bladder pain, methods of preventing pregnancy, treatment of bladder ulcer, treatment of renal stones, hemorrhoids, among many others (Al-Samerra'i, 1989).

ZEINAB TABIBAT BANI AWD

Zeinab was a woman physician from the Bani Awd (Aoud) tribe. She was known for her expertise in ophthalmology and treatment of wounds (Ibn Abi Usaibiah, 1245/1246; Cumston, 1921). It is reported that an Arab man went to her to treat his trachoma. After she treated him, he recited a poem written by an Arab poet about a woman physician. When he finished reciting the poem, Zeinab asked him if he knew the author of the poem and the name of the physician about whom the poem was written. It turned out that it was written about her by the patient's uncle, Abu Samak Al-Asadi (Ibn Abi Usaibiah, 1245/46). The precise epoch in which she lived is not clear. Cumston (Cumston, 1921) suggests that it was before the time of the prophet.

THE ABBASID PERIOD (750–1258 AD)

In 750 AD, descendants of the Prophet's uncle, Abul-Abbas Ibn Abdel Muttalib, led a revolution against the Umayyads and established a multiethnic, learned dynasty, the Abbasid dynasty. The Abbasids moved their capital from Damascus to Baghdad (City of Peace) and initiated the most ambitious process in history by translating Greek, Persian, and Indian literature into Arabic in order to gather and assimilate the world's learning. Thus, the Abbasids became known as "The Patrons of Learning" (Bayon, 1952; Williams, 2006; Lyons, 2009; Feiler, 2011; Freely, 2011; Al-Khalili, 2011; Tarabay, 2011). According to Arabic legends, Caliph Al-Mansour journeyed several times to the banks of the Tigris and Euphrates Rivers in search of a capital for his empire. He finally selected a village on the Tigris where a Christian monastery stood and named it Baghdad, meaning the "City of God" (Cortas, 2009).

Several factors helped the Abbasids realize their ambitions (Afnan, 1958). Their newly established capital in Baghdad attracted scholars from different countries. The liberal and tolerant environment in Baghdad allowed the mixing of Persian culture, Christian Syriac linguistic versatility, and Hellinistic heritage in the search for knowledge and the creation of a new civilization to which all made important contributions. The Abbasid caliphs enhanced the process by their love of learning, the establishing of their own libraries, and their search for and acquisition of ancient books, culminating in the establishment, in Baghdad, in 830 AD, of Bayt Al-Hikma (The House of Wisdom), a beehive of translation, and the repository of Greek, Syriac and Byzantine books of philosophy and medicine (Al-Kurdi, 2004; Al-Khalili, 2011).

From the ninth to the twelfth centuries, Baghdad was a city with no peer in the world, a center for scholars and mystics, abundant with entice-ment of wealth and spiritualism, of poets, the likes of the Sufi Al-Ghazali and the poet Abu Ala' al-Maari (cortas, 2009). Thus, the Abbasid period is known as "the Golden Age of Islamic Medicine."

EARLY ABBASID PERIOD (750–900 AD)

THE BEKHTIYASHU (BUKHTISHU) FAMILY

Members of the Bekhtiyashu family were the first physicians to come to Baghdad from the School of Ghondi-Shapour and to practice medicine in a scientific way. Unlike other physicians of the time who mixed interests in medicine and other disciplines such as philosophy, mathematics, and astrology, they devoted their energies solely to the study and translations of medical books. They were also known for their skill to please rulers (Al-Samerra'i, 1989).

Not much is known about the origins of the family. They were Nestorian Christians. The first part of their name, "Bekht," is a Persian word that means "saved" or "servant"; the other part of the name, "Yashu," means "Jesus" in Persian, thus, "saved by or servant of Jesus" (Al-Samerra'i, 1989; http://en.wikipedia.org/wiki/Bukhtishu). The family name is spelled "Bukhtishu" and "Bukht-Yishu." The family was originally from Ahwaz near Ghondi-Shapour. They eventually moved into Baghdad and later to Nisbin in northern Syria (http://en.wikipedia.org/wiki/Bukhtishu).

Several members of this family served caliphs for over three centuries (seventh, eighth, and ninth), spanning six generations and 250 years (http://en.wikipedia.org/wiki/Bukhtishu). Among them are the following:

JURJIS IBN JIBRAIL, BUKHTISHU the 1st; JURJIS the 1st (d. 769 AD)

He was the most known physician in the Persian medical school of Ghondi- Shapour. He was called upon in 765 AD to treat Caliph Al-Mansour in Baghdad from a stomach ailment that his court physicians could not cure. Being advanced in age, Ibn Jibrail apologized, so he was taken by force to Baghdad. When he successfully cured the caliph, he was asked by the caliph to be his court physician and provided him all he needed, including ordering his servants to provide him with alcoholic drinks. The caliph offered to provide him wiht three of his best concubines, but Jurjis returned them to the caliph, saying, "As a Christian, I can maintain one woman until she dies." He stayed in Baghdad to an advanced age, when he asked the caliph to release him. He returned to Ghondi -Shapour where he died in 769 AD (Al-Samerra'i, 1989). Before permitting him to return to Ghondi -Shapour, the caliph asked him to convert to Islam, but he declined, saying that he wanted to be with his father when he died. Amused by Jurjis's obstinacy, the caliph sent an attendant with him to ensure his safe return to Ghondi-Shapour (Ibn Abi Usaibiah, 1245/1246; http://en.wikipedia. org/wiki/Bukhtishu).

SCHOLARSHIP

Al-Kinash

This was the first of the books to be translated in Baghdad into Arabic by Hunayn Ibn Ishaq. The book includes information about stomach and intestinal disorders, acute diseases, urinary disorders, management of difficult labor, disorders of the uterus, liver disorders, chicken pox, joint disorders, sciatica, and diabetes. The book was a major source for Al-Razi's book "Al-Hawi fil Tibb" (Al-Samerra'i, 1989)..

Kitab al-Akhlat

This book was another source for Al-Razi's book "Al-Hawi fil Tibb" (Al-Samerra'i, 1989).

BUKHTISHU IBN JURJIS, BUKHTISHU the 2nd (d. 801 AD)

Bukhtishu Ibn Jurjis matriculated in medicine under his father while the latter was in the School of Ghondi-Shapour. Like his father, he was well versed in medicine and acted for his father in the Ghondi- Shapour Hospital when his father went to Baghdad to treat Caliph Al-Mansour. When his father passed away, Bukhtishu replaced his father as the chief physician in the Hospital in Ghondi-Shapour (Al-Samerra'i, 1989).

Like his father, Bukhtishu was called into Baghdad to treat the gravely ill Caliph Musa Al-Hadi and was retained by the caliph as his court physician. This angered the caliph's mother, Al-Khaizaran, whose personal physician was not consulted by the caliph. She worked to get rid of Bukhtishu and succeeded to have him leave the court and return to Ghondi-Shapour. However, he was called back to Baghdad one year later to treat the severe headaches of Caliph Haroun Al-Rashid. He successfully treated the caliph and, in gratitude, the caliph appointed him physician in chief, a post he held until his death in 801 (Ibn Abi Usaibiah, 1245/1246; Al-Samerra'i, 1989; http://en.wikipedia.org/wiki/Bukhtishu).

SCHOLARSHIP

Al-Tazkara fil Tibb (Notes on Medicine)

The book contained information about arrhythmias, edema, stomach ulcers, urinary stones, and back pain, referred to in Al-Razi's book "Al-Hawi fil Tibb" (Al-Samerra'i, 1989).

JIBRAIL (GIBRAIL) IBN BUKHTISHU (d. 827/829 AD)

Alternate spellings include Jibril Ibn Bekhtishu, Jibril bin Bukhtishu, Jibril ibn Bakhtishu, Jibra'il ibn Bukhtyishu, and Djabra'il b. Bakhtishu (http://en.wikipedia.org/wiki/Bukhtishu).

Jibrail started working at the Ghondi-Shapour's hospital before he moved to Baghdad to be the personal physician of Ja'far Ibn Yahya Al-Barmakid, Vezier of the Caliph Haroun Al-Rashid. Shortly after that, in 805 AD, the favorite concubine of the Caliph Haroun Al-Rashid woke up one day complaining of her inability to move her arm. All the court physicians failed to cure her. Finally, the Caliph sent for Jibrail. After examining her, he brought her to the Palace Hall where the caliph was holding court, and in front of everyone, he suddenly lifted her dress in an attempt to expose her beautiful bare thighs. She immediately put her hand down to prevent public exposure and was thus cured, an astute method of curing hysterical paralysis (Haddad, 1993). Following that feat, he joined the court of Caliph Haroun Al-Rashid and became the confidant of the caliph. It is reported that Caliph Al-Rashid told his friends to consult Jibrail with any problems they had because he (the caliph) did everything Jibrail recommended (Ibn Abi Usaibiah, 1245/46; Al-Samerra'i, 1989; http://en.wikipedia.org/wiki/Bukhtishu).

While in the service of Caliph Al-Rashid, he advised the caliph in the building of the first hospital in Baghdad. The hospital and adjacent observatory were built after those in Ghondi-Shapour. When the hospital was completed, he served as its first director. The hospital was named after Caliph Haroun Al-Rashid (http://en.wikipedia.org/wiki/Bukhtishu).

Jibrail's luck with Caliph Haroun Al-Rashid did not last when he failed to cure the caliph from his final illness, an ailment that Jibrail frankly attributed to excessive sexual intercourse and bad weather in Tus, where the caliph wanted to stay against Jibrail's advice. The caliph condemned Jibrail to death, and the intervention of Al-Fadl Ibn al-Rabi' saved Jibrail's life (Al-Samerra'i, 1989; http://en.wikipedia.org/wiki/Bukhtishu).

SCHOLARSHIP

Jibrail was fond of Greek medicine and sought to learn from Greek medical books. He was the first to discover the contributions of Hunayn Ibn

Ishaq and the translation of Greek books into Syriac and Arabic and asked him to translate for him some of Galen's books into Syriac (Al-Samerra'i, 1989).

Jibrail Ibn Bukhtishu is credited with the following statement:

"Four behaviors are detrimental to health: eating on a full stomach, drinking on an empty stomach, intercourse with an old woman, and while taking a bath" (Ibn Abi Usaibiah, 1245/46).

Kitab al-Bah (Book on the Penis)

This book was written for Caliph Al-Rashid about excess in sexual intercourse, which Jibrail advised him to avoid. A copy of the book is in the private Al-Hakim Library in Aleppo, Syria (Al-Samerra'i, 1989).

Kinash fil Tibb (Book on Medicine)

This book is likely the one that Al-Razi referred to in his book "Al-Hawi fil Tibb" in connection with intestinal, liver, spleen, and kidney diseases (Al-Samerra'i, 1989).

Waram al-Khisa (Swelling of Testicles)

This book was referred to by Al-Razi in his book "Al-Hawi fil Tibb (Al-Samerra'i, 1989).

Risala fil Ta'am wal- Sharab (Notes on Foods and Drinks)

This book was dedicated to Caliph Haroun Al-Rashid, who was obsessed with eating and drinking wine. It describes the benefits and disadvantages of each. A copy of the book is in the Al-Hakim private library in Aleppo, Syria (Al-Samerra'i, 1989).

Risala Mukhtasarah fil Tibb (Brief Summary of Medicine) (Al-Samerra'i, 1989)

BUKHTISHU IBN JIBRAIL, BUKHTISHU the 3rd (d. 869 AD)

Ibn Jibrail was a religious person and at the same time fond of hearing and saying jokes (Al-Samerra'i, 1989).

He was known to practice medicine using consensus rather than counting on his personal experience and to emphasize prevention, as in the following quotes (Al-Samerra'i, 1989):

"Drinking when hungry is bad, and eating when full is even worse."

"Eating a bit of what is harmful is better than eating much of what is beneficial."

Ibn Jibrail served several caliphs, including Caliphs Al-Mutawakkil, Al-Wathiq, Al-Musta'een Bi Allah, and Al-Muhtadi Bi Allah. His relationship with the caliphs fluctuated from being their favorite to being unfavorable.

SCHOLARSHIP

Kitab fil Hijama (Book on Cupping)

This book is written in the form of questions and answers (Al-Samerra'i, 1989).

Nubtha fil Tibb (Synopsis of Medicine) (Al-Samerra'i, 1989)

Nasa'eh al-Ruhban fil Adwiyah al-Murakkabah (Advice of Monks on Complex drugs) (Al-Samerra'i, 1989)

UBAIDULLAH IBN BUKHTISHU, UBAIDULLAH the 1st

Little is known about Ubaidullah. He was the less known of the Bukhtishu family in the medical profession. He served in the court of Caliph Al-Muqtadir Billah (908-932 AD). He, however, fell into disfavor with the caliph and was dismissed, and his property was confiscated after he died (Al-Samerra'i, 1989).

JIBRAIL IBN UBAIDULLAH, JIBRAIL the 3rd (ABU ISA) (d. 1005 AD)

Jibrail matriculated in medicine with Ali Yusuf Al-Wasiti and practiced medicine in Baghdad. He was one of the prominent physicians in the Abbasid court. He spent some time in Shiraz at the invitation of Adud Al-Dawla Al-Buwayhid but returned to Baghdad with him to serve at the Udadi Hospital. He lived a luxurious life while in the court of Adud Al-Dawla and left Baghdad only on short consultations. He even declined an offer from the Fatimid Al-Aziz, who wanted to establish him in Cairo. After the death of Adud Al-Dawla, he finally left Baghdad to spend the rest of his life in Miafarqin (Persia) reading and writing and died there in 1005 AD (Al-Samerra'i, 1989; http://en.wikipedia.org/wiki/Bukhtishu).

SCHOLARSHIP

Kitab al-Kafi (The Complete Book)

This book, in five volumes, was dedicated to al-Sahib Ibn Ibad (Al-Samerra'i, 1989).

Kitab fi A'sab al-Ayn (Book on the Nerve of the Eye)

A copy of this book is in the Al-Jarrah private library in Aleppo, Syria (Al-Samerra'i, 1989).

Kitab fil Tarikh (Book on History)

This book includes a number of references from the Byzantine historian Andonicos (Al-Samerra'i, 1989).

Maqala fi Alam al-Dimagh (Article on Brain Pain)

A copy of this book is in the private Al-Jarrah library in Aleppo, Syria (Al-Samerra'i, 1989).

UBAIDULLAH IBN JIBRAIL, UBAIDULLAH the 1st (ABU SAID) (d. 1058 AD)

Ubaidullah did not stay long in Baghdad. He moved to Miafarqin (Persia) to practice medicine, and while there, he developed cordial relations with Ibn Botlan, who also practiced there. Like Ibn Botlan Al-Baghdadi, he promoted study of medicine by practice not with purely reading books. In this respect, he and Ibn Botlan rebuked Ibn Radwan, who promoted medical education through reading books of the ancients (Al-Samerra'i, 1989).

Ubaidullah was also against those who viewed medicine as a branch of philosophy and taught that medicine was a purely applied science independent of philosophy (Al-Samerra'i, 1989).

His stay in Miafarqin away from busy Baghdad gave him time and space to devote to reading and writing (Al-Samerra'i, 1989).

SCHOLARSHIP

Kitab Manaqib al-Atibba' (Book on Virtues of Physicians)

Kitab Tazkarat al -Hadir Wa Zad al-Musafir (Ticket for the Resident and Provisions for the Traveler) (Al-Samerra'i, 1989).

Kitab al-Rawdah al-Tibbiyah (Garden of Medicine)

This book is a summary of fifty terms in philosophy and medicine. It was published in Cairo in 1927 by Paul Sbat. Copies of the original manuscript are in libraries in Rabat (Morocco) and the British Museum (Al-Samerra'i, 1989).

Kitab al-Tawasul fi Hifz al-Tanasul (Book of Intercourse in Preserving Procreation) (Al-Samerra'i, 1989)

Kitab Nawadir al-Masa'il (Book of Rare Problems)

This book is a brief account of the book "Ilm al- Awael fil Tibb" (Medical Knowledge of the Ancients) (Al-Samerra'i, 1989)

Kitab fi Ilm al-Hayawan, Khawasihi Wa Manaf'i A'daihi (Book on Science of Animals, Qualities, and Benefits of Organs)

A copy of this book is in Morgan Library in New York City (Al-Samerra'i, 1989).

Maqala fi Harakat al-Nafas (Article on Changes in Respiration) (Al-Samerra'i, 1989)

Risala fil Tibb wal-Ahdath al-Nafsaniyyah (Letter on Medicine and Mental Events)

In this book, the author presented his views about mental illness and considered such illnesses the domain of physicians not philosophers as was believed in those days. The book was published in Beirut, Lebanon, in 1979 from an original manuscript in the Library of Leydin (Al-Samerra'i, 1989).

YUHANNA IBN BUKHTISHU

Yuhanna Ibn Bukhtishu served Al-Muwaffak Bi Allah Ibn Ja'far Al-Mutawakkil, and became his preferred physician and confidant (Ibn Abi Usiabiah, 1245/46; al-Samerra'i, 1989).

SCHOLARSHIP

Yuhanna was proficient in Greek language and wrote the following works:

Ma Yahtaju Ilayhi al-Tabib Min Ilm al-Nujum (What the Physician Needs to know from Astronomy)

A copy of the book is in the private Nahhas Library in Aleppo, Syria (Ibn Abi Usaibiah, 1245/46).

Kitab Taqween al-Adwiyah fi ma Stakhara Minha al- A'shab wal-Aghthiya (Book on Evaluation of Drugs from Herbs)

A copy of the book is in the library of Rabat, Morocco (Al-Samerra'i, 1989).

BUKHTISHU IBN YUHANNA (d. 940 AD)

He is the son of Yuhanna. He matriculated in medicine with his father and joined the courts of Caliphs Al-Muqtadir and Al-Radi. He left no scholarly work (Al-Samerra'i, 1989).

IBN AL-BATRIQ, YAHYA (d. 815 AD)

He was an early Abbasid physician credited with translation, from Greek into Arabic, of "The Book of Pustules" (Kitab al-Buthur), a treatise concerned with the prognosis and signs of death based on skin disorders. The book lists twenty-five skin conditions suggestive of impending death.

The original Greek compilation is said to have been found in the tomb of Hippocrates, and thus attributed to him.

The book was circulated under several titles

Risala fil Qadaya

Risala fi 'Alamat al-Mawt

Risala al-Qabriyya

Qadaya al-Ibuqratiyah al-Dallah 'Alal-Mawt

Kitab al-Sirr (http://www.nlm.nih.gov/hmd/arabic/hippocratic.html)

IBN MASAWEH, YUHANNA ABI ZAKARIA
(MASAWAYH, MESUE SENIOR, MESUESR,
JANUS DAMASCENUS) (777–857 AD)

IBN MASAWEH, THE PERSON:

Yuhanna Ibn Masaweh came from a Syriac Christian family of physicians among whom he was the best known (Al-Samerra'i, 1989).

He was born in Ghondi-Shapour (today's Iran). His mother was from Cisily. He mastered the Syriac and Arabic languages and found no difficulty studying books of medicine written in both languages. He matriculated in the Ghondi-Shapour Hospital and moved to Baghdad in search of fame and wealth. The presence of his father among court physicians (pharmacist) in Baghdad helped Yuhanna meet dignitaries and succeed. He was one of the most known physicians in Baghdad during the first half of the second century and served caliphs Haroun Al-Rashid, Al-Amin, Al-Mamoun, Al-Mu'tasim, Al-Wathiq, and Al-Mutawakkil (Ibn Abi Usaibiah 1245,46; Al-Samerra'i, 1989; Campbell, 2011). His devotion in the service of the church helped his promotion in the church hierarchy. Unlike church leaders in general, he was known to have multiple concubines (Al-Samerra'i, 1989).

Ibn Masaweh was fond of reading medical manuscripts in general and those dealing with anatomy in particular. He was known to have been the first to dissect an ape and to have first-hand experience about anatomical structures to argue against the concepts of Galen. The monkey he dissected was given to him by Al-Mu'tasim (Tarabay, 2011).

He was known to have bad temper and a sharp tongue. To a courtier who annoyed him, he is reported to have said, "If the ignorance where with thou art afflicted were converted into understanding, and then divided amongst a hundred beetles, each one of them would be more sagacious than Aristotle" (Browne, 1962).

Ibn Masaweh mentored Hunayn Ibn Ishaq. The latter was inquisitive and asked many questions of his mentor. At one time, Ibn Masaweh burst out in rage and told his student that he was not worthy of the medical profession and advised him instead to follow in the steps of his father, who was a money exchanger. Hunayn, in response, vowed not to return to Baghdad before he became a renowned physician (Al-Samerra'i, 1989).

To a priest who failed to respond to his prescriptions, he got upset and told him to convert to Islam as a cure (Ibn Abi Usaibiah 1245/46).

Ibn Masaweh is reported to have threatened to dissect his feeble- minded son to find out the cause of his retardation and "to relieve the people of him" and probably would have, were it not for the caliph who stopped him (Khairallah, 1942; Ibn Abi Usaibiah, 1245/46).

IBN MASAWEH THE SCHOLAR:

He was the personal physician of Caliphs Haroun al-Rashid, Al-Amin, Al-Mamoun, Al-Mu'tasim, Al-Wathiq, and Al-Mutawakkil (Ibn Abi Usaibiah, 1245/46; Haddad, 1993). He is reported to have been asked by the caliphs to stand by the dinner table when they ate. He was known to provide the caliphs with digestive preparations (Ibn Abi Usaibiah, 1245/46; Al-Mahi, 1959; Haddad, 1975; Al-Kurdi, 2004).

He directed the first hospital built in Baghdad by Caliph Haroun Al-Rashid (Haddad, 2003), was dean of the medical school in Baghdad (Campbell, 2011), and served as Rector of Bayt Al-Hikma (House of Wisdom) in Baghdad (Al-Mahi, 1959; Al-Kurdi, 2004). His role in the House of Wisdom was believed to have been more administrative and less professional (Al-Samerra'i, 1989).

He pioneered the translation of Greek books into Arabic (Haddad, 1975). He translated thirty books from Greek to Arabic, including one on headaches. He wrote the first book on epilepsy (Al-Mahi, 1959; Al-Kurdi, 2004) and a large tome on general pathology, "Kitab Al-Kamel" (The Complete Book) (Ullmann, 1997).

Among his other publications are:

Kitab al-Burhan (The Proof)

A thirty-chapter book

Kitab Tarkib al-Ayn, 'Ilaliha Wa Adwiyatiha (Book on Structure of the Eye, Its Illnesses, and Treatments)

Kitab al-Himmiyat (Book on Fever)

This book includes information on ear disorders, types of headaches and their treatment, jaundice, among others (Al-Samerra'i, 1989).

Kitab al-Aghthiyah (Book on Nutrition),

The book includes information about benefits of some foods, as well as treatment of bloating, constipation, among others. The original manuscript of the book is kept at the Basil Library in Aleppo, Syria (Al-Samerra'i, 1989).

Kitab al-Ashribah (Book on Drinks) (Al-Samerra'i, 1989)

Kitab al-Fasd wal-Hijamah (Book on Venisection and Cupping) (Al-Samerra'i, 1989),

Kitab Islah al-Adwiyah (Book on Medical Treatments)

The book includes information about drugs that are used to treat vomiting, jaundice, sciatica, arthritis, gum diseases, diarrhea, and cough, among many others (Al-Samerra'i, 1989).

Kitab Dukhoul al-Hammam, Manafi'hou Wa Dararuhu (Book on Benefits and Harm of Taking a Bath)

Kitab al-Sumum Wa 'Ilajiha (Book on Poisons and Treatment)

The book is mainly about snake poison and its treatment (Al-Samerra'i, 1989).

Kitab Mihnat al-Tabib (Book on the Profession of Medicine) (Ibn Abi Usaibiah, 1245/46; Al-Samerra'i, 1989)

Kitab al-Tashrih (Book of Dissection)

Ibn Masaweh was the first to write a book on anatomical dissection. His book on the anatomy of the monkey, dedicated to Caliph Al-Mu'tasim, has been lost (Haddad, 1993; Haddad 2003). The monkey he dissected was a gift to the caliph from his representative in Nubia in Africa (Khairallah, 1942; Al-Samerra'i, 1989).

Nawadir al-Tibb (Al-Fusul al-Hikmiyyah wal-Nawadir al-Tibbiyyah) (Rare and Wisdom Cases in Medicine)

This book was written at the request of his student Hunayn Ibn Ishaq. It contains 132 sections (cases of wisdom) along the pattern used by Hippocrates but much more concise. Each hikma does not exceed few lines. It includes a wide variety of topics like pathology, therapeutics, dietetics, and diagnosis (Tarabay, 2011).

Originals are kept in the libraries of Al-Azhar University in Cairo, the Madrid Library, and the Library of Leyden (Al-Samerra'i, 1989).

The book was translated into Latin and used as a reference until the seventeenth century (Tarabay, 2011).

Kitab fil Jizam (Book on Leprosy) (Al-Samerra'i, 1989)

Kitab al-Malinkholia, Asbabiha, Alamatiha, Wa 'Ilajiha (Book on Schizophrenia , Causes, Signs, and Treatment) (Al-Samerra'i, 1989)

Kitab fil Suda' wa Adwiyatihi (Book on Heachache, and its Treatment) (Al-Samerra'i, 1989)

Kitab Daf'a Maddar al-Adwiyah (Book on how to Avoid non-Desirable Side Effects of Drugs)

The original manuscript of this book is kept in the Library of Berlin (Al-Samerra'i, 1989).

Al-Jami' or Jami' al-Tibb (Comprehensive Book of Medicine)

In this book, the author includes consensus opinions of Persian and Roman physicians. It includes their consensus opinions on vomiting, diarrhea, obesity, loss of weight, hard breasts, jaundice, colitis, among many other topics (Al-Samerra'i, 1989).

Kitab al-Kamal Wal Tamam (The Complete Book)

This book includes information on disorders of the mouth and their treatment, drugs used to treat eye disease, disorders of the stomach and intestines and their treatment, diseases of the uterus and pelvic organs and their treatments, disorders of the kidney, sexual intercourse, intestinal parasites and their treatments, sciatica, burn treatment, and arthritis treatment (Al-Samerra'i, 1989).

Kitab al-Ishal (Book on Diarrhea)

This book addresses causes and treatment of diarrhea (Al-Samerra'i, 1989).

Kitab al-Safar Wal Dawar (Book on Travel and Sea Sickness)

This book was used by Al-Razi as a reference for his discussion of the topic (Al-Samerra'i, 1989).

Kitab fi Waja' al-Mafasil (Book on Joint Disorders)

This book includes drugs used in treating joint diseases (Al-Samerra'i, 1989).

Kitab al-Ibdal (Ibdal al-Adwiyah) (Book on Exchange of Drugs)

He wrote this book at the request of Hunayn Ibn Ishaq (Al-Samerra'i, 1989).

Al-Masa'el (The Questions)

This book contains a section on treatment of thirst, effect of humidity on health, and timing of diseases (Al-Samerra'i, 1989)

Kitab al-Tabikh (Book on Cooking)

This is believed to be the first book on the subject written in Arabic (Al-Samerra'i, 1989).

Kitab al-Maedah (Book of the Stomach) (Al-Samerra'i, 1989).

Kitab al-Qoulange (Book on colitis) (Al-Samerra'i, 1989)

Kitab al-Sawt wal-Bahha (Book on Sound and Hoarsness) (Al-Samerra'i, 1989)

Kitab Tadbir al Sihha (Book on Maintaining Health)

This is a book on preventive medicine (Al-Samerra'i, 1989)

Kitab al-Janeen (Book on the Embryo) (Al-Samerra'i, 1989)

Kitab Khalq ai-Insan Wa Ajzaihi (Book on Creation of Man and its Parts)

This book was written for Caliph Al-Mamoun. It lists body parts, the joints, the bones, and the vessels (Al-Samerra'i, 1989).

Aphorisms of which there is a Latin translation. Ibn Masaweh's Aphorisms were published together with those of Maimonides at Bologna in 1489 and at Basle in 1579 (Campbell, 2011).

Ibn Masaweh is also credited for writing the earliest work on agriculture "Kitab Al-Azminah" (Book of the Times), and "The Geoponica," a multivolume collection of agricultural lore compiled for the Byzantine Emperor Constantine VII (Freely, 2011).

In addition to being the first to do anatomic dissection and record it in a book, Ibn Masaweh is credited with being the first to introduce into medicine the use of alum, aloes and antimony. He was also the first to write comprehensively about leprosy and its contagion. He was of the first to describe pruritus due to food allergies (Haddad, 1993).

There are nine Latin editions of Ibn Masaweh's in the British Museum, dated 1462, 1479, 1485, 1495, 1531, 1597, 1603, and 1623 (Campbell, 2011).

IBN MASAWEH, MIKHAIL

Mikhail Ibn Masaweh was the brother of Yuhanna Ibn Masaweh. He was favored by Caliph Al-Mamoun, who called him by his first name and did not use any medicine not approved and prepared by Ibn Masaweh. In his management of disease, he was reluctant to use untried medicines. He insisted on using what his predecessors had tried and proved useful. When asked about the benefits of banana, he responded that he did not see it mentioned by his predecessors. It was said that he never used a treatment method that had not been tried for over two hundred years. He was held in the highest regard by physicians of his time. He did not leave any record of his experience, nor any book (Ibn Abi Usaibiah, 1245/46: Al-Samerra'i, 1989).

QUSTA IBN LUQA Al-BAALBEKI (820–912 AD)

Qusta Ibn Luqa was born near Heliopolis in Syria (now Baalbek in Lebanon) in 820 AD. He was a Melkite Greek Christian who spoke both Syriac and Arabic (Freely, 2011; http://www.levity.com/alchemy/islam13html). From his birthplace, he moved to Baghdad and flourished during the caliphate of Al-Mu'tadid (Al-Khalili, 2011; Freely, 2011).

He was a polymath renowned as a physician and an expert in philosophy, logic, astronomy, geometry, arithmetic, music (Al-Khalili, 2011; Freely, 2011; Ead, H. A. http://www.levity.com/alchemy/islam13html), and one of the prominent translators from Greek to Arabic at Bayt Al-Hikma (Ibn Abi Usaibiah, 1245/46; Myers; 1964; Al-Samerra'i, 1989).

His translations included works of Aristarchus, Aristotle, the mathematicians Diophantus, Galen, and Theodosius, as well as revisions of some of Ishaq Ibn Hunayn's work (Myers, 1964; Al-Khalili, 2011; Freely, 2011).

He was urged to convert to Islam but did not do so (Al-Khalili, 2011).

SCHOLARSHIP

His scholarly output included, in addition to translations of Greek books, fifty-five works in natural sciences, astrology, geometry, mathematics, engineering, social studies, and history. His medical works are brief and most are in the form of letters and do not reflect his wide knowledge of the subject. Among his works are (Myers, 1964; Ullmann, 1997; Al-Khalili, 2011; Freely, 2011):

Risala fil Taharruz Min Al Zukam wal-Nazalat (Letter on Protection from Colds)

Risala fil Adwiyah al-Mushila wal-Ilaj bil-Ishal (Letter on Laxative Drugs and Treatment by Diarrhea)

Kitab fil Bah (Book on the Penis)

This book, in the form of questions and answers, was dedicated to Ibn Mukhlid Abi Al-Hasan Ahmad.

Kitab fi Awja' al-Nuqrus (Book on Gout Pains)

Kitab fil Akhlat al Arba'a wa ma Tashtarik Fihi (Book on the Four Humors and What is Common between Them)

Kitab fi Illat al Mawt al Mufaji' (Book on Sudden Death)

Kitab al-Nabith and Shurbihi fil Wala'em (Book on Wine and Its Use in Parties)

Kitab al-Hammam (Book on Baths)

Kitab fi Du'f al-Asab (Book on Weak Nerves)

Kitab fi Daf' Darar al Sumum (Book on Preventing the Harm of Poisons)

Kitab fil Suda' (Book on Headache)

Al-Madkhal fi Ilm al-Tibb (Book on Introduction to Medicine)

Kitab fi Illat Toul al 'Umr wa qisarihi (Book on Longevity and Short Life)

Treatise on sexual hygiene

Kitab Zad al-Musafir (Book on Medicine for Travelers)

The book consists of fourteen chapters.

Kitab fil-Nawm wal-Ru'ya (Book on Sleep and Dreams)

Kitab fil Himmiyat (Book on Fever)

Risala fi Ikhtilaf al-Nas fi Siyarihim wa Akhlaqihim (On the Diversities of the Character of Man)

The book deals with the relation that exists between constitution and character, conduct of life, the emotion, and aesthetic perception.

Al Farq Bynal Nafs wal-Rouh (On the Difference Between the Spirit and the Soul)

The book was translated into Latin by John of Seville.

Ibn Luqa also wrote a work on magic. He is reported to have come in contact with a noble who attributed his impotence to the work of a witch. Ibn Luqa advised the nobility to rub himself with a concocted aphrodisiac made of a gall of a crow mixed with sesame. This gave the nobility such confidence that he regained his sexual ability (Freely, 2011).

Ibn Luqa spent his last years as a client of King Sancharib of Armenia, where he died (Al-Samerra'i, 1989; Freely, 2011; Ead, H. A. http://www.levity.com/alchemy/islam13html).

IBN ISHAQ AL-IBADI, HUNAYN, ABI ZEID (JOANITUS, JO-HANNITTTUS ONAN, HUMAINUS) (792–873, 809–873 AD)

Hunayn Ibn Ishaq was born in the ancient Christian city of Hirah, just south of Kufa in southern Iraq in 792/809 AD, the year of Caliph Haroun Al-Rashid's death. He was the son of a Nestorian Christian pharmacist. The Al-Ibadi in the name referred to his origin from a Hira tribe, the Ibad tribe (Ibn Abi Usaibiah, 1245/46). He lived for some time in Basra before moving to Baghdad, both cities in Iraq (Ibn Abi Usaibiah, 1245/46; Al-Khalili. 2011; Campbell, 2011).

IBN ISHAQ, THE STUDENT:

He started his medical studies in Baghdad under the direction of Yuhanna Ibn Masaweh in the earliest private medical school in Islam (Tschanz, 2003). As a student, he was known to be inquisitive and to ask too many questions of his teachers. Yuhanna Ibn Masaweh, irritated by his countless questions, dismissed him from class and suggested, instead of studying medicine, he should stick with his town's (Al-Hirah) trade of peddling counterfeit coins, which, he suggested, would earn Hunayn more money than would the profession of medicine (Al-Samerra'i, 1989).

Challenged by his teacher's attitude, Hunayn left Baghdad determined to return to it only after he became a physician. He traveled to Byzantium, where he became fluent in the Greek language. He then returned to

Basra, in Iraq, where he mastered the Arabic language, thus becoming fluent in the four languages of the time, Assyrian, Persian, Greek, and Arabic (Ibn Abi Usaibiah, 1245/46; Brown, 1962; Al-Samerra'i, 1989; Freely, 2011; http://en.wikipedia.org/wiki/hunayn_bin_Ishaq). From Basra, he traveled to Persia and completed his medical studies in the Ghondi-Shapour Medical School around 826 AD during the rule of Caliph Al-Mamoun (Al-Samerra'i, 1989). He was considered the most famous pupil of Masaweh (Haddad, 1993).

IBN ISHAQ, THE PERSON:

His daily routine included taking a Turkish bath after a ride. He would come out of the bath wrapped in a dressing gown. After taking a cup of wine with a biscuit, he would lie down until he had stopped perspiring and would go to sleep. Upon rising from sleep, he would burn perfumes to fumigate his body. Dinner would then be brought to him. Dinner would ordinarily consist of a large feathered pullet stewed in gravy with a half-kilo loaf of bread. After dinner, he would fall asleep. On waking up, he drank four pints of old wine followed by eating some fruits (Freely, 2011). He was a substantial drinker of wine. His preferred fruit is reported to have been apples, pomegranates, and quince (Ibn Abi Usaibiah, 1245/46).

Hunayn Ibn Ishaq had two physician sons, Daud (David) and Ishaq. Daud did not excel in the profession, while Ishaq (see below) translated many Greek texts into Arabic, especially books on philosophy, such as those of Aristotle, among others (Ibn Abi Usaibiah, 1245/46).

IBN ISHAQ, THE PHYSICIAN:

Hunayn was cited by his contemporaries and succeeding generations as the quintessential ethical physician. Hunayn served as physician for Caliphs Haroun Al-Rashid, Al-Amin and Al-Mamoun (Haddad, 2003). He was jailed for one year by Caliph Al-Mutawakkil for refusing to prepare a poison to kill an adversary of the caliph. When he was brought again before the caliph and threatened with death for disobedience, he told the caliph, "I have skill only in what is beneficial and have studied naught else."

He then added "that he awaited the supreme judgement of the Lord." The caliph pardoned him. When he was asked about the reason for disobeying the caliph even under the threat of death, he replied, "Two things, my religion and my profession. My religion commands us to do good even to our enemies, and my profession forbids us to do harm" (Ibn Abi Usaibiah, 1245/46; Al-Mahi, 1959; Meyerhoef, 1989; Tschanz, 2003).

IBN ISHAQ, THE TRANSLATOR:

Proficient in four languages, Syriac, Greek, Arabic, and Persian, Hunayn Ibn Ishaq established himself as a careful, reliable, and scholarly translator and became known as "Sheikh of translators." Within fifty years, he and his students completed the monumental task of rendering in Arabic and Syriac all of the most important Greek medical texts written over a millennium, including all of Hippocrates, Aristotle, Galen, Plato, Paulus, Dioscorides, and all the medical books that he could find (Haddad, 1993; Tschanz, 2003). He also trained his son Ishaq and his nephew Hubaysh to continue his work. He is credited with translation of 116 manuscripts, including the Old Testament, into Syriac and Arabic. In his many translations, he was assisted by a number of assistants, estimated at ninety, including his son Ishaq and his nephew Hubaysh. In his translations, Hunayn attempted to convey the meaning of the translated text instead of word-byword translations, which other translators did (http://en.wikipedia.org/wik/hunayn_bin_Ishaq; Haddad, 2003). Because of his multilingual knowledge and accurate translations, he was also referred to as "Ya Rabin Hunayn," which translates into "the learned teacher" (Al-Samerrai, 1990). He also returned to the company of his previous teacher Ibn Masaweh to help him translate Galen's Books (Al-Samerra'i, 1989; Haddad, 1993).

Because of his mastery of the Greek language, he was the most productive of translators of Greek medicine into Arabic. Seven of the ten Hippocratic writings (including his Aphorisms) existing in Arabic were his translation; the other three were translations by his student Isa Ibn Yahya (Afnan, 1958; Brown, 1962; Haddad, 2003).

Hunayn was particularly interested in translating Galen's books. It is reported that almost all, if not all, the books of Galen (140 books) have been translated by Hunayn (Afnan, 1958; Campbell, 2011) or are the translation by others corrected by Hunayn. He was only seventeen years old when he translated Galen's "On the Natural Faculties" and went on to translate such important works of Galen as "On the Anatomy of Veins and Arteries" and "On the Anatomy of Nerves" (Al-Khalili, 2011).

One of the most important manuscripts of Hunayn Ibn Ishaq, found in St Sophia Church in Istanbul, contains a record of 129 of Galen's books. In it, he detailed who wrote each book and by whom and to what language each was translated. He said one of the books was not authored by Galen, twenty books were not found in the Greek original, and one was not translated. Eleven were translated into Syriac, and ninety-six were translated into Syriac and Arabic by either him or his pupil and nephew Hubaysh (Brown, 1962; Haddad, 1975; Haddad, 2003; Freely, 2011).

Ibn Ishaq went beyond the expected to search and find old Greek manuscripts. In searching for Galen's "De Demonstratione," he traveled in search for it in Mesopotamia, Syria, Palestine, and Egypt, only to find only half of it in Damascus (Brown, 2010; Freely, 2011).

In addition to translations of Hippocrates's and Galen's works, Ibn Hunayn and his coworkers translated Euclid's "Elements" and Dioscorides's "De Materia Medica," which was the basis for Islamic pharmacology (Freely, 2011).

Of all his translations, it is his translation of the medical work of Galen that is his most important legacy, for opening up the Islamic world to this great treasure, and through those Arabic translations much of Galen's work reached us (Al-Khalili, 2011).

His keen interest in finding and translating Greek books was triggered by Caliph Al-Mamoun, who had a dream about an old man calling himself Aristotle, lecturing from a podium. When he found out who Aristotle was, he urged Ibn Ishaq to search for Greek texts and translate them into Arabic (Ibn Abi Usaibiah, 1245/46).

Because of his reputation as a translator, he was appointed by Caliph Al-Mamoun to head the House of Wisdom (Bayt Al-Hikma) in Baghdad (Al-Samerra'i, 1989; Tschanz, 2003; Tarabay, 2011). It is reported that, in his translation of manuscripts, Hunayn was known to use large letters, triple or quadruple spacing, and heavyweight paper in order to increase the weight of the translated manuscript to get more gold for it. The caliph paid translators the weight of their translated manuscripts in gold (Al-Samerra'i, 1989).

SCHOLARSHIP

Ibn Ishaq is known as a translator more than an author of books, although he was also a prolific writer (Tschanz, 2003). His total scholarly output is estimated at 140 books, most are translations (Al-Samerra'i, 1989). He is credited with writing thirty-six books, twelve of which were about medicine. Of his most notable works were his "Ten Treatises on the Eye" and "Questions on Medicine."

Ten Treatises on the Eye (kitab Al Ashr Maqalat Fi Al Ayn):

Covering the anatomy, physiology, and disease of the eye and the nature of sight, this book is considered to be the earliest existing systematic textbook of ophthalmology and the first by an Arab. It was also the earliest work to include anatomical charts of the eye. It showed considerable advancement in knowledge over that in the Greco-Roman treatises (Al-Mahi, 1959; Siraisi, 1990; Haddad, 1993; Tschanz, 2003; Al-Kurdi, 2004). It was a compilation of articles written by Ibn Ishaq over a thirty-year period. The book started as a series of nine articles of different lengths on different issues related to the eye. The different articles were collated at the suggestion of his nephew and student Hubaysh and a tenth chapter added to complete the book (Ibn Abi Usaibiah, 1245/46; Al-Samerra'i, 1989). In the book, Ibn Ishaq adopted Galen's view that vision occurred by means of an extra mission of rays from the eye (Siraisi, 1990).

The influence of the book on the development of ophthalmology was profound, not only in the Islamic world, but in Europe as well. Oculists quoted and consulted the book through the fifteenth century (Tschanz, 2003).

The ten chapters address the following topics (Ibn Abi Usaibiah, 1245/46; Al-Samerra'i, 1989):

Chapter 1: The structure of the eye

Chapter 2: The nature of the brain and its benefits

Chapter 3: The optic nerve

Chapter 4: Essentials to preserve health and well-being

Chapter 5: Etiology of eye problems

Chapter 6: Signs of diseases of the eye

Chapter 7: General medicines and their uses

Chapter 8: Specific medicines used to treat eye diseases and their categories

Chapter 9: Treatment of diseases of the eye

Chapter 10: Compound drugs used in treating eye diseases and their availability

The book was translated in 1087 AD into Latin by Constantine the African under the title "Diseases of the Eye," who claimed its authorship. It was this translation that made Ibn Ishaq's book known and used in European medical schools (Al-Samerra'i, 1989).

Several copies of the original manuscript are still available:

The first, in the Leningrad library, was in the possession of Gregory the First, the Greek orthodox Patriarch of Antioch, who passed it on, in 1911, to the Tzar of Russia.

The second copy is in the private library of Timur Pasha in Cairo, Egypt.

Other copies are in Athens, British museum, Leydin, and Tubingen.

The original manuscript was translated, in 1928, into English by M. Meyerhoff (Haddad, 1975; Al-Samerra'i, 1989; Haddad, 2003).

Kitab Masa'il Hunayn , al-Masa'il fil Tibb (Questions in Medicine, Introduction to the Healing Art):

The book was designed and started by Hunayn and completed after Hynayn's death by his nephew Hubaysh, who added two chapters based on Galen's work. Because of these added chapters, the book is at times referred to as "Masa'el Hunayn Ma' Ziyadat Li Hubaysh" (Questions of Hunayn with Additions by Hubaysh). The book was quickly adopted as the principal manual used by examiners in testing physicians seeking li-censure. Presented in the form of questions and answers, the book was extremely beneficial to medical students as a guide to their studies, espe-cially to beginners to acquaint them with the fundamentals of the subject (Al-Mahi, 1959; Al-Samerra'i, 1989; Tschanz, 2003; al-kurdi, 2004; Freely, 2011; Hunayn ibn Ishaq; http://en.wikipedia.org/wiki/hunayn_bin_Ishaq; http://http:www.nlm.nih.gov/exhibition/islamic_medical/islamic_09.html).

The book was commented on, summarized, and interpreted by authors from the tenth through the fourteenth centuries. Translated into Latin, it was a widely consulted medical reference work for Western physicians throughout the Renaissance (Tschanz, 2003). The book was most popu-lar among practicing physicians and students prior to the publication of Avicenna's "The Canon of Medicine" (Al-Samerra'i, 1989). It influenced the discipline along with Tabari and Al-Razi in the second half of the ninth century (Tarabay, 2011).

Because of its popularity, abridged forms of the book were written under the titles of "Ikhtisar Kitab Al Masa'el" (Summary of Masa'el) and "Kitab Hasil Al-Mahsoul" (The Cream of the Cream) (Al-Samerra'i, 1989).

Other contributions of Ibn Ishaq include (Ullmann, 1997, Freely, 2011):

Kitab al Mudkhal fil Tibb (Entry Book into Medicine)

This is the same book as the "Kitab Masa'il Hunayn" discussed above. This title of the book was used by late authors to refer to "Kitab Masa'il of Hunayn" (Al-Samerra'i, 1989).

Qawl fi Hifz al-Asnan (How to Preserve Teeth and Repair Them)

This book is a treatise on dentistry, the first comprehensive presentation in the field of dentistry. It was referred to by Al- Razi in his book "Al-Hawi" (Al-Samerra'i, 1989; Ullmann, 1997; Freely, 2011).

Kitab al-Agthiyah (Book on Nutrition)

This is a book on diet, largely based on Galen and other Greek writers. It was used by Al-Razi as a source for his book "Al-Hawi" (Samerra'I, 1989; Ullmann, 1997; Freely, 2011).

Kitab fi Tadbeer al-Sihha bil-Ma'kal wal-Mashrab (Healthy Diets and Drinks)

This book was used by Al-Razi as a source for his book "Al-Hawi." Original manuscripts are kept in Tehran and Aleppo (Al-Samerra'i, 1989).

A book on neurology in which he discussed pediatric epilepsy, muscle, and nerve (Al-Mahi, 1959)

Kitab al-Fawa'id fi Tanwi' al-Mawai'd (Benefits of Food Variations) (Al-Samerra'i, 1989)

Book on Misfortunes and Hardships which Befell Him at the Hands of his Adversaries, Those Renowned and Wicked Physicians of His Time

It reflects on the suffering he endured from his rivals, who complained that his medical knowledge came solely from his translations (Freely, 2011).

Besides his medical treatises, Ibn Ishaq wrote on other subjects, which include (Goodman, 2003; Freely, 2011):

"Book on Meteors"

"Book on Colors"

"Treaties on Comets"

"Book on Rainbows"

"Book on Ebb and Flow of Tides"

"Truth of Religious Creeds"

"Book on the Cause of Sea Water Becoming Salty"

"Book on Alchemy"

"A Paraphrase of Aristotle's 'On the Heavens'"

"Book on History of the World"

Hunayn's books were still required reading by the medical students in 1530 at Montpellier (Haddad, 1993).

In addition to his scholarly scientific contributions, Hunayn Ibn Ishaq was well versed in Arabic grammar and collaborated in this discipline with the famous Arabic grammarian Sibaweyh (Ibn Abi Usainiah, 1245/46).

Hunayn Ibn Ishaq died in Baghdad on December first, following a stroke at the age of seventy. His year of death is variably reported in 873, 877, and 879 AD. Afnan (1958) attributed his death to suicide as a result of the displeasure of the church and his excommunication (Afnan, 1958).

Leclerc said about him, "He is the greatest figure of the 9ᵗʰ century. He possessed one of the most excellent intellects and one of the most beautiful personalities that one can ever meet in history" (Haddad, 1993).

IBN HUNAYN, ISHAQ AL-IBADI (ABU YAQUB) (854–911 AD)

Ishaq was the son of the famous Greek-to-Arabic translator and physician Hunayn Ibn Ishaq. He was a student of his father and assisted his father in the translation of a number of texts, particularly of a mathematical and philosophical nature. His translations included Ptolemy's "Almagest." His translation of Aristotle's "Physics" was considered the best of the work in Arabic (Freely, 2011). He had a better command of Arabic than his father and came to write much better, which endeared him to the Arabs (Afnan, 1958; Al-Samerra'i, 1989).

Ibn Hunayn composed a number of medical treatises. Among his scholarly contributions are:

Kitab al Adwiyah al Mufrada (Book on Simple Drugs)

This book was translated into Latin by Niqula al-Dimashqi and printed in 1841 AD (Ibn Abi Usaibiah, 1245/46; Al-Samerra'i, 1989).

Tarikh al-Attiba (History of Physicians)

This book is considered the earliest book to reflect the views of ninth-century physicians and their predecessors. It was used as a source on the subject by Ibn Al-Nadim in his book "Al Fahrest" and Ibn Juljul in his book "Tabaqat Al-Attiba." The book was translated into English by France Rosenthal and published in volume 7 of the journal "Oriens" (Ibn Abi Usaibiah, 1245/46; Al-Samerra'i, 1989).

Kitab al-Tiryaq (Book on Cures)

This book was used as a source by Al-Razi in his book "Al-Hawi" in the sections on colitis and treatment of measles and chicken pox (Al-Samerra'i, 1989).

Kitab Ma'rifat al-Boul (Book on Urine)

A copy of the original of the book is kept in Tehran (Ibn Abi Usaibiah, 1245/46; Al-Samerra'i, 1989).

Kitab al-Muhktasar fil-Tibb (Summary of Medicine)

A copy of the book is kept in Cambridge University Library (Al-Samerra'i, 1989).

Al-Risala al-Safiyah fi Adwiyat al Nisyan (Clear Message on Drugs for Forgetfullness)

This book was dedicated to Abdullah Ibn Sham'oun (Ibn Abi Usaibiah, 1245/46; Al-Samerra'i, 1989).

Kitab al-Adwiyah al Mawjuda fi Kull Makan (Book on Drugs Available Everywhere)

A copy of the book is available in the Nahhas Library in Allepo, Syria (Ibn Abi Usaibiah, 1245/46; Al-Samerra'i, 1989).

Kitab al-Adwiyah al Mushilah (Book on Laxative Drugs) (Ibn Abi Usaibiah, 1245/46; Al-Samerra'i, 1989),

Kitab fil-Nabd (Book on Pulse) (Al-Samerra'i, 1989)

Kitab Sina'at al-Ilaj bil-Hadeed (Book on Treatment with Iron) (Al-Samerra'i, 1989)

Kitab Adab al-Falasifah Wa Nawadirahum (Book on Work of Philosophers and Their Anecdotes).

This book was printed in Kuwait in 1985 by the Kuwaiti Center of Arabic Manuscripts (Ibn Abi Usaibiah, 1245/46; Al-Samerra'i, 1989).

In addition to the above books, Ishaq Ibn Hunayn either participated in translation or himself translated a large number of books by Hippocrates, Galen, Euclides (Al-Samerra', 1989).

Ibn Hunayn's translation of Paul of Aegina's book on obstetrics is considered the chief source of obstetrical knowledge in Arabic language (Khairallah, 1942).

Ibn Hunayn enjoyed reading and composing poetry. He died in Baghdad on December 1st, 911, following a stroke. It was rumored that he converted to Islam in his old age (Al-Samerra'i, 1989).

IBN QURRA AL-HARRANI, THABET, ABU AL-HASAN (836–901 AD)

Ibn Qurra was born in the city of Harran, in northwest Mesopotamia (now in Turkey). Harran was the center of the Sabeans, a cult of astral religion who worshipped the sun and moon and five planets (Al-Khalili, 2011; Freely, 2011).

He started his career as a money changer in Harran before developing interest in natural sciences, mathematics, philosophy, astronomy, and medicine (Al-Samerra'i, 1989; Al-Khalili, 2011). He is better known as a philosopher and astronomer (Al-Samerra'i, 1989).

Ibn Qurra served Calioh Al-Mutawakkil Billah as astronomer (Al-Samerra'i, 1989; Haddad, 2003). He was very close to Abi Al Abbas al-Mu'tadid bi-Allah when the latter was imprisoned by his father. When Al Abbas became caliph, he gave Ibn Qurra a number of villages and kept him close in his court. Ibn al Abbas had a high respect for scholars and considered scholarship above royalty. He is known to have said "Al-Ulama' Ya'loun wa la Yu'loun" (Scientists are above all others) (Ibn Abi Usaibiah, 1245/46; Al-Samerra'i, 1989).

TRANSLATOR

Thabet was a celebrated translator from a family of translators, including his sons Ibrahim and Sinan, grandsons Thabet and Ibrahim, and great-grandson Sinan. His translations were known for accuracy and were of quality close to that of the "sheikh" of translators, Hunayn Ibn Ishaq (Myers, 1964; Haddad, 2003). He is considered one of the four top translators in Islam, the others being Hunayn Ibn Ishaq, Yaqoub Ibn Ishaq Al-Kindi, and Omar Ibn Al-Farkhan Al-Tabari (Al-Samerra'i, 1989).

Fluent in three languages, Greek, Syriac and Arabic, he is credited with composing 150 books in Arabic and 15 books in Syriac on medicine, mathematics, and astronomy and was among those who translated Galen's books. He was also involved in original research and showed how algebraic and geometrical proofs were related to each other (Brown, 2010).

Along with Ishaq Ibn Hunayn's, Ibn Qurra's abilities as translator were discovered by Muhammad Ibn Musa, one of the Bani Musa brothers, who contracted translations for the caliphs (Freely, 2011).

SCHOLARLY OUTPUT:

Of his manuscripts, only eighty survive, including thirty in astronomy, twenty-nine in mathematics, two in medicine, two in mineralogy, two in music, one in physics, and one in zoology (Freely, 2011).

Among his books are:

"Al-Zakira" (On Memory), a thirty-chapter book, which describes diseases of memory and their treatments, including his own experience on the subject (Haddad, 2003)

"Kitab fi Shakl al-Qatta"

This is a book of anatomy. It was translated from Arabic to Hebrew by Qalonymos Bin Qalonymos.

Kitab fi Ajnas al-Amrad (Book on Types of Illnesses) (Al-Samerra'i, 1989)

Jawam'i Kitab Galinos fil Adwiyah al-Manqiyyah (Translation of Galen's Book on Simple Drugs) (Ibn Abi Usalbiah, 1245/46; Al-Samerra'i, 1989)

Jawam'i Kitab Galinos fil Mawludeen Sab'at Ashhur (Translation of Galen's Book on Seven Months Births) (Ibn Abi Usaibiah, 1245/46; Al-Samerra'i, 1989).

Kitab fil Hasa al Mutawallida fil Kila wal-Mathana (Book on Stones in the Kidney and Bladder) (Ibn Abi Usaibiah, 1245/46; Al-Samerra'i, 1989).

Kitab fil Nabd (Book on Pulse) (Ibn Abi Usaibiah, 1245/46; Al-Samerra'i, 1989).

Kitab al-Basar wal-Basirah (Book on the eye and its Diseases) (Ibn Abi Usaibiah, 1245/46; Al-Samerra'i, 1989)

Kitab fima Tanqasim Elayhi al-Adwiyah (Book on Categories of Drugs) (Ibn Abi Usaibiah, 1245/46; Al-Samerra'i, 1989).

Kitab fi Waja' al-Mafasil wal Nocros (Book on Joint Pains and Gout) (Ibn Abi Usaibiah, 1245/46; Al-Samerra'i, 1989).

Kitab Tashrih al-Rahm (Book on Dissection of the Uterus (Al-Samerra'i, 1989)

Kitab fi Mas'alat al Tabib al 'Alil (Book on the Sick Physician) (Al-Samerra'i, 1989)

Kitab fi Sifat Kawn al-Janeen (Book on Formation of the Embryo) (Al-Samerra'i, 1989)

His books were of the same high quality as those of Hunayn Ibn Ishaq (Myers, 1964).

Ibn Qurra's original works in mathematics, physics, astronomy, and medicine, which were translated from Arabic to Latin, highly influenced the early development of European science. That Ibn Qurra was so revered by European scientists is evident from reference to him by Roger Bacon as the "supreme philosopher among all Christians (although Ibn Qurra never converted from Sabean to Christianity), who added in many respects, speculative as well as practical information, to the work of Ptolemy" (Freely, 2011).

Ibn Qurra was one of few, including Al-kindy, Al-Farabi, Al-Mosuli, and Ibn Khaldoun, who paid attention to music as a science, tune, instrumentation, singing, and performing. As such, Ibn Qurra contributed to the development of Arabic musical notation, using Arabic letters and numbers that were read from right to left (Geha, 2011).

QUOTES FROM IBN QURRA (Ibn Abi Usaibiah, 1245/46: Al-Samerra'i. 1989).

The following quotes are attributed to Ibn Qurra:

"The worst for the elderly are a gourmet cook and a beautiful girlfriend, for he will eat much and get sick, and engage excessively in sex and will age."

"The body will rest with less food, the heart will rest with less worry, and the tongue will rest with less gossip."

Ibn Qurra died at the age of seventy -seven years (Ibn Abi Usaibiah, 1245/46).

AL-A'SAM, HUBAYSH

Al-A'sam was among the best translators. He is considered to have been one of the three famous translators, along with Hunayn Ibn Ishaq and Thabit Ibn Qurra (Khairallah, 1946). A prolific translator, he was the right hand to Hunayn Ibn Ishaq, his uncle. Most of his translations have been credited to Hunayn Ibn Ishaq (Khairallah, 1946). He translated most of Galen's books including the following (Khairallah, 1942):

Dissection of Live Animals

Dissection of Dead Animals

Hippocratic Anatomy

Anatomy of Erasistratus

Anatomy of the Womb

Differences of Opinions in Anatomy

The original texts of these books are lost and are only known through their Arabic translation (Khairallah, 1942).

Besides being a famous translator, Al-As'am was a good physician who served the court of Caliph Al-Mutawakkil (Khairallah, 1946).

IBN ABI AL-ASH'ATH, AHMAD IBN MOHAMMAD (ABU JA'FAR) (d. 970 AD)

Not much is known about the early life of Ibn Al-Ash'ath, except that he was a Persian scientist and physician who fled Persia when it was attacked by the Mongols. He first went to Armenia, and in 959 AD, he moved to Mosul in Iraq. While in Mosul, he attended to the son of Nasir Al-Dawla, who suffered from an intractable disease, and cured him. He was well compensated, became close to the ruler, and lived the rest of his life in Mosul (Ibn Abi Usaibiah, 1245/46; Al-Samerra'i, 1989). He died in Mosul in 970 AD, leaving many children, one of whom, Mohammad, became well- known as a physician (Ibn Abi Usaibiah, 1245/46; Al-Samerra'i, 1989).

Ibn Abi Al-Ash'ath was well versed in the writings of Galen and Aristotle. He is credited with classifying the materials in Galen's and Aristotle's books to make it easier for the reader (Ibn Abi Usaibiah, 1245/46; Al-Samerra'i, 1989).

SCHOLARSHIP

Beside his classifications of Galen and Aristotle's books, Ibn Abi Al-Ash'ath wrote the following books):

Kitab al Adwiyah al Mufradah (Book on Simple Drugs),

This book was written at the urging of several of his students who were about to graduate from medical school. It was intended for those physicians who had finished their basic training and were launching their careers in medicine. Its purpose was to make the information about simple drugs readily available to young physicians. Copies of the original manuscript are in the British Museum, Al-Awqaf Library in Rabat, and the Zubaidi Library in Aleppo (Ibn Abi Usaibiah, 1245/46; Al-Samerra'i, 1989).

Kitab fil Judari wal-Hasbah (Book on Smallpox and Measles) (Ibn Abi Usaibiah, 1245/46; Al-Samerra'i, 1989)

Kitab fil Sara'a (Book on Epilepsy) (Ibn Abi Usaibiah, 1245/46)

Kitab fil Baras wal Bahaq (Book on Leprosy and Vitiligo) (Ibn Abi Usaibiah, 1245/46; Al-Samerra'i, 1989)

Kitab fil Istisqa (Book on Dropsy) (Ibn Abi Usaibiah, 1245/46; Al-Samerra'i, 1989)

Kitab fil Malinkholia (Book on Malincholy) (Ibn Abi Usaibiah, 1245/46; Al-Samerra'i, 1989)

Kitab Amrad al Ma'idah wa Mudawtuha (Book on Diseases of the Stomach and Their Treatment) (Ibn Abi Usaibiah, 1245/46; Al-Samerra'i, 1989).

Kitab fil Qoulange wa Asnafihi wa Mudawatihi (Book on Colitis, Types and Treatment) (Al-Samerra'i, 1989)

Kitab al-Hayawan (Book on Animals)

An original manuscript of the book is in Oxford University Library (Al-Samerrai, 1989).

Kitab fi Tarkib al-Adwiyah (Book on Formulation of Drugs) (Al-Samerra'i, 1989)

AL-MUSALI, ABU ABDALLAH MOHAMMAD IBN THAWAB (IBN AL-THALLAJ)

Al-Musali, from Musol in Iraq, was a student of Ahmad Ibn Abi Al-Ash'ath. He was well versed in the art and science of medicine and wrote several books on the subject (Ibn Abi Usaibiah, 1245/46).

AL-BALADI, ABUL-ABBAS AHMAD IBN MOHAMMAD IBN YAHYA

Al-Baladi was one of the best students of Ibn Al-Ash'ath, with whom he worked for several years (Ibn Abi Usaibiah, 1245/46).

SCHOLARSHIP

Kitab Tadbir al-Habala wal Atfal wal Subian (Book on Pregnancy, Babies and the Young)

This is a book that addresses preventions from diseases and treatment of diseases that affect pregnant women, their babies, and the young children. The book was written in honor of Vezier Abul Faraj Ya'qoub Ibn Yousef who served in the court of AL-Aziz Bi Allah in Egypt (Ibn Abi Usaibiah, 1245/46).

IBN QAWSAYN

Ibn Qawsayn was a famous Jewish physician in Mosul, Iraq. He converted to Islam (Ibn Abi Usaibiah, 1245/46).

SCHOLARSHIP

Kitab Maqala fil Radd ala al Yahoud (Book of response to Jews) (Ibn Abi Usaibiah, 1245/46)

IBN RADWAN AL-MASRI, ABU AL-HASAN ALI (d. 1067)

Ibn Radwan was born and raised in the al-Jeeza district of Cairo, Egypt, where he also studied medicine. In his writings, he stated that by astrological signs at his birth, he was destined to become a physician. He started the study of medicine and philosophy at the age of fifteen. He considered medicine and philosophy as disciplines that bring humans closer in the service of God. He was a man of few financial means. His father, a bread maker, died young at the age of thirty-one, when his son, Ali, was at age of fourteen (Al-Samerra'i, 1990). He worked as an astrologist and teacher to raise money to be able to pursue his studies. He worked enough to earn a living. In his memoirs, he described his daily routine as follows: "Working as a physician enough hours to earn a living, exercise enough to stay healthy, take a rest at the end of exercise before eating a nutritious meal. The rest of the day was spent in reading Aristotle's writings and in prayers and admiration of God's creations. At the end of the day, review the days achievements, enjoy what good I did, and regret what was not good or useful in order to avoid it in the future" (Ibn Abi Usaibiah, 1245/46; Al-Samirra'i, 1990).

Ibn Radwan lived in Egypt at a time of drought, inflation, and difficulty obtaining food. He took care of an orphan girl who stole his valuables, including his savings in gold, and disappeared from the town. This incident has been blamed for his mental depression late in his life (Ibn Abi Usaibiah, 1245/46).

Ibn Radwan was known to be disrespectful in dealings with his colleagues, such as Al-Razi and Hunayn Ibn Ishaq (Ibn Abi Usaibiah, 1245/46).

In learning medicine, Ibn Radwan depended mostly on the books he read, and he documented this in the book he wrote, "The Useful Ways in Learning the Profession of Medicine." He was not affiliated with any medical luminary teacher, partly because, as he said in his memoirs, of the high fees charged by the luminaries and because he felt that those teachers did not take the time to discuss what they read in the books to students (Samerra'i, 1990). He promoted the idea that learning medicine from books is far superior to learning it from famous physicians. This concept did not go well with his contemporaries, among them Ibn Botlan, who wrote a book on the subject challenging Ibn Radwan's concept (Ibn Abi Usaibiah, 1245/46; Al-Samerra'i, 1990).

Although he promoted learning medicine from books, he did not keep a large library. He disposed of the books he read except those by Al-Razi ("Al-Hawi fil Tibb"), Avicenna ("The Canon"), Galen, Hippocrates, and Rufus (Al-Samerra'i, 1990).

Ibn Radwan is quoted to have defined the good physician in line with Hippocratic principles as one who:

Was healthy and well mannered

Was well dressed

Kept patients' information in confidence

Focused on curing patients more than earning money

Attended to the poor as much if not more than the rich

Kept up with new knowledge for the benefit of his clients

Did not use harmful medicines and did not practice abortions

Treated his enemy the same as he would treat his friend

Treated families he visited at home with dignity and avoided flirting with womenfolk.

He also wrote about the desirable qualifications in the teacher of medicine. Those included (Ibn Abi Usaibiah, 1245/46):

Being well versed in the literature and kept updating his knowledge

Having interest and proficiency in teaching

Having good memory of what he learned

Having good manners with his students

He is also quoted to have said, "If you are called to attend to a sick person, do not give him a medicine until you make the diagnosis" (Ibn Abi Usaibiah, 1245/46; Al-Samerra'i, 1990).

SCHOLARSHIP (Ibn Abi Usaibiah, 1245/46; Al-Samerra'i, 1990)
Ibn Radwan wrote over seventy books. Among them are:

Sharh Kitab al-Sina'a al-Saghira li Galinos (Commentary on Galen's Book on the Smaller Profession)

Sharh Kitab al-Nabd al-Saghir li Galinos (Commentary on Galen's Book on Pulse) of which only the Hebrew translation is available

Kitab al-Usoul fil Tibb (Book on Basics in Medicine)

Risala fi Ilaj al Juzam (Message on Treatment of Leprosy)

Kitab al-Nafi' fi Kayfiyat Ta'alum Sina'at al-Tibb (Book on the Useful Ways to Learn Medicin) in which he promoted learning from books rather than matriculating with teachers; two incomplete copies of the book are available, one in Egypt (House of Books) and another in the library of Jester Baiti (Al-Samerra'i, 1990)

Kitab fi Hall Shukuk Al Razi li Kutub Galinos (Book on Doubts of Al-Razi about Galen's Books),

Kitab fil Adwiyah al Mufrada (Book on Simple Drugs)

Kitab fi ma Yanbaghi an Yakun fi Hanut al-Tabib (Book on What Needs to be in a Doctor's Clinic)

Jawab 'An Halat Illat al-Faleg fil Shaq al Aysar (response on cases of left sided hemiplegia)

When he became known as a good physician, he was invited by Caliph Al-Hakim bi Amr Allah to be his court physician and appointed chief physician of Egypt (Al-Samerra'i, 1990).

Ibn Radwan was married and had two children; both died young. He died in Cairo in 1067 AD in his sixties (Al-Samerra'i, 1990).

IBN AL-NAQQASH, MUHAZZAB AL DIN ABU AL-HASAN ALI (d. 1187/1202 AD)

Ibn Al-Naqqash was born and studied medicine in Baghdad. He was a student of Amin Al-Dawlah Hibat Allah Ibn Al-Tilmidh. He was recognized as a physician and literary man (Ibn Abi Usaibiah, 1245/46; Al-Samerra'i, 1990).

From Baghdad, he moved to Damascus and served in the court of Al-Malik Al-Adil Nur Al-Din Al-Zinki and became his secretary (Katib), in addition to practicing medicine and teaching at the Al-Nuri Hospital in Damascus (Ibn Abi Usaibiah, 1245/46; Jadon, 1970; Al-Samerra'i, 1990).

He left for Egypt for a higher pay and returned to Damascus when Saladin took over Syria. He became very close to Saladin, to the extent that Saladin employed one of Ibn al-Naqqash students in his court simply based on Ibn al-Naqqash recommendation (Ibn Abi Usaibiah, 1245/46; Jadon, 1970; Al-Samerra'i, 1990).

Among his students were As'ad Ibn Al Mutran, Yahya Al-Bayyasi, Radiy Al-Din Al-Rahbi, and Ibn Al-Hajib (Jadon, 1970; Al-Samerra'i, 1990).

He remained bachelor all his life and died in Damascus in 1187/1202 AD (Ibn Abi Usaibiah, 1245/46; Al-Samerra'i, 1990).

AL-BAYYASI, AMIN AL-DIN ZAKARIA YAHYA

Al-Bayyasi was a Muslim physician and mathematician. He went to Egypt from the Maghrib (Arab North Africa) and stayed in Cairo several years before moving to live in Damascus (Ibn Abi Usaibiah, 1245/46).

He matriculated with Muhazzab Al-Din Al-Naqqash and served in Saladin's Court when in Diyarbakr but resigned from his services for unknown reasons and lived in Damascus. In spite of the resignation, Saladin continued to pay his salary until his death (Ibn Abi Usaibiah, 1245/46; Jadon, 1970).

In addition to being a physician and mathematician, Al-Bayyasi was a musician and teacher of music. He played the oud and the organ. He was interested in handicraft and built several engineering instruments for his teacher, Al-Naqqash (Ibn Abi Usaibiah, 1245/46; Jadon, 1970).

He wrote several books in medicine as well as other disciplines (Ibn Abi Usaibiah, 1245/46; Jadon, 1970).

IBN AL-HAJIB, MUHAZZAB AL-DIN

Ibn Al-Hajib was born and raised in Damascus. He was a physician, mathematician, and literary grammarian. He matriculated in medicine with Muhazzab Al-Din Ibn Al-Naqqash and worked with him for some time before moving to Mosul and Irbil in Iraq in pursuit of the philosopher and mathematician Sharaf Al-Din Al-Tusi, who had by then had moved to Al-Tus where Ibn Al-Hajib went to study with him (Ibn Abi Usaibiah, 1245/46; Jadon, 1970).

Ibn Al-Hajib returned to Damascus where he served at the Nuri Hospital. He then moved to Hamat in Syria to serve in the court of the ruler of Hamat, Takki Al-Din Omar. Following the death of the ruler, he returned to Damascus and moved to Egypt to serve in the court of Saladin. Following Saladin's death, Ibn Al-Hajib returned to Hamat to serve in the court of the then ruler Al-Malik Al-Mansour. He died in Hamat from dropsy (Ibn Abi Usaibiah, 1245/46; Jadon, 1970).

Before studying medicine, Ibn Al-Hajib worked in the Ummayad Mosque in Damascus setting its clocks (Ibn Abi Usaibiah 1245/46; Jadon, 1970).

SINAN IBN THABET IBN QURRA (ABU SAID) (d. 942 AD)

Sinan was the son of Thabet Ibn Qurra, and like his father, he was a noted physician and scholar. He matriculated in medicine under his father (Al-Samerra'i, 1989). Ethnically, he was Mandean, Aramic speaking. He believed that John the Babtist was the true Messiah (http://en.wikipedia.org/wiki/sinan_ibn_thabit).

He served three Abbasid caliphs: Al-Muqtadir Bi Allah, Al-Qahir, and Al-Radi Bi Allah (Al-Samerra'i, 1989). Al Qahir wanted him to convert to Islam. Sinan ran away to Khorasan but then returned fearing Al-Qahir and converted. He died in Baghdad (Al-Samerra'i, 1989).

Sinan proposed to the caliph Al-Muqtadir to build the Muqtadiri Hospital in Baghdad, which he later directed (Ibn Abi Usaibiah, 1245/46; Haddad, 1975; Al-Samerra'i, 1989; Haddad, 2003). During his management of the hospital, a patient died from a physician's error. Subsequently, the caliph decreed that no physician was to be allowed to practice at Baghdad hospitals unless examined and certified by Sinan. The number of such physicians was reported to have exceeded eighty. Exempted from the examination were physicians who had already established their reputation and those who were in the service of the caliph (Ibn Abi Usaibiah, 1245/46; Al-Mahi, 1959; Haddad, 1975; Al-Samerra'i, 1989). Sinan also is credited with suggesting to Sayidda Shaghab, mother of the caliph, to build a hospital in her name in Baghdad. The hospital was built and named after her (Al-Sayidda Hospital) (Al-Samerra'i, 1989).

Sinan is also credited with initiating the concept of "traveling clinics," for at the order of Vezier Ali Ibn Isa Al-Jarrah, he led a team of physicians to villages to treat and provide needed medicines (Al-Samerra'i, 1989).

Sinan died in Baghdad in 942 AD, leaving two children who became physicians: Thabet Ibn Sinan and Ibrahim Ibn Sinan (Al-Samerra'i, 1989).

Sinan made contributions in medicine, philosophy, astronomy, and engineering. Mathematics was his hobby. He translated five books of Euclid (Al-Mahi, 1959; Haddad, 1975).

Other nonmedical contributions include the following (Ibn Abi Usaibiah, 1245/46):

History of the Syriac Kings

Kitab al-Sira, also known as Kitab al-Naji, in which he described the nobility of the Adud Al Dawla's family

Risala fil Nujum (On Stars)

Risala on Sabeans sect

In medicine, he authored the book "Al-Thakira fi-Tibb" (The memory in Medicine) (Al-Mahi, 1959; Haddad, 1975).

Not much is available in the literature about Sinan compared to other luminaries.

AL-TABARI, ALI IBN SAHL RABBANI (RABN), ABU AL-HASAN (838–870 AD)

Al-Tabari was Christian or Jewish and from Tabaristan (a Persian province south of the Caspian Sea), where the name Al-Tabari comes from. The "rabbani," master, teacher, was his title (Browne, 1962; Al-Samerra'i,

1989). He studied medicine, astrology, and engineering under his father, Sahl Rabban Al-Tabari (786–845), and like his father, he was interested in learning about science. He learned Arabic, Syriac, Persian, and some Greek, Indian, and Hebrew languages and was involved in translation of books from these languages (Al-Samerra'i, 1989).

Attracted by the scientific and cultural activities in Baghdad, he left Tabaristan for Baghdad, where he started the writing of his book "Firdaws Al-Hikma" but left Baghdad before completing the book. He returned to Tabaristan, where he practiced medicine and taught it (Al-Samerra'i, 1989). Among his students was Al-Razi (Haddad, 1975; Al-Samerra'i, 1989; Al-Khalili, 2011). Al-Tabari was considered the first Muslim doctor, before Al-Razi, who eclipsed his contributions in the field (Tarabay, 2011).

Al-Tabari converted to Islam, probably at the request of Caliph Al-Mu'tasim, and wrote the following to justify his conversion: "Among the prophet's miracles is this Quran. It is a miracle for reasons I have not seen discussed fully by any author in this genre, but merely in broad and general terms or claims. While still a Christian I would argue about the Quran and an uncle of mine, a learned and eloquent Christian scholar, would argue back that ornaments of rhetoric do not constitute proofs of prophecy since these are common among all nations. But when I rejected imitations and force of custom and upbringing, and carefully considered the theses of the Quran, I found the matter to be as asserted by Muslims. For I have not found any book, whether written by Arab, Persian, Indian or Byzantine, that joins the unicity of God and His praise and thanks, to firm belief in Prophets, the urging to virtue, command of good and forbidding of evil, and exhortation of Paradise and censure of Hell-like the Quran, since the world began. He who brought us such a book, with such a place in the hearts by reason of both its integrity and greatness, and endorsed with such good fortune and triumph, while the person bringing it was an illiterate who could neither write nor have any knowledge of rhetoric-such a book must beyond any doubt constitute proof of his prophecy" (Khalidi 2009). His conversion took place during the caliphate of Al-Mu'tasim (Ibn Abi Usaibiah, 1245/46).

SCHOLARLSHIP:

Having lived in Tabaristan (modern-time Iran), Al-Tabari was greatly influenced by Indian medicine as evident in his "Firdaws al-Hikma" (Tarabay, 2011).

Firdaws Al-Hikma fil Tibb (Paradise of Wisdom in Medicine)

Al-Tabari wrote only four books, of which "Firdaws Al-Hikma'"(Paradise of Wisdom) is the most important. In it, Al-Tabari presented a thorough description of Indian medicine (Tarabay, 2011). It is considered the first medical encyclopedia written in Arabic (not translated from other languages). It represented a new trend in Islamic science in which books were not purely translations from other languages. It was the first reference that included all branches of medicine, including a theoretical part, a detailed description of human anatomy, preemptive medicine, description of color, taste, and flavor, and the importance of diet on health (Tarabay, 2011). It was written in two languages, Arabic and Syriac (Browne, 1962; Al-Samerra'i 1989; Al-Khalili, 2011). The author justified writing in two languages to ensure that no other author would claim authorship (Al-Samerra'i, 1989). It is a book on medicine and natural philosophy. Although it dealt mainly with medicine, it also addressed philosophy, meteorology, zoology, embryology, psychology, and astronomy. It also contained sections on treatment with prayers (Browne, 1962; Al-Samerra'i, 1989). Al-Tabari stated that among the sources for the information in the book were the writings of Hippocrates, Aristotle, Galen, Yuhanna Ibn Masaweh, and Hunayn Ibn Ishaq (Keys, 1953; Brown, 1962; Al-Samerra'i, 1989). It is considered the oldest existing book on Arab medicine (Keys, 1953; Haddad, 1975). Two copies of the book still exist, one (intact copy) in the British Museum, the other, an abbreviated (mutilated) copy, is in the Berlin Museum (Al-Mahi, 1959; Haddad, 1975).

The book consists of 550 pages, seven parts, thirty discourses, and 360 chapters. Discourse in two of the fourteen chapters deals with diseases and injuries of the head, diseases of the brain (including epilepsy), various types of headaches (differentiated migraine "Shaqiqa" from other headache types), tinnitus, vertigo, amnesia, and nightmares. He divided the brain into three functional areas: anterior area for imagination; middle area for rationality; and posterior area for memory. Discourse four (in seven chapters) deals with nervous system disease, including spasms, paralysis, tetanus, facial palsy. The last discourse of the seventh part is a summary of Indian medicine in thirty chapters (Brown, 1962; Al-Samerra'i, 1989). Al-Tabari completed writing the book in 235 HA (849 AD) (Haddad, 2003).

Other scholarly outputs include:

Kitab Tuhfat al-Muluk (Book of Kings Gifts) (Ibn Abi Usaibiah, 1245/46; Al-Samerra'i, 1989)

Kitab Manaf'i al At'imah wal-Ashribah wal-Aqaqir (Book on Benefits of Foods, Drinks and Drugs) (Ibn Abi Usaibiah, 1245/46; Al-Samerra'i, 1989)

Kitab Hifz al-Sihha (Book on Maintenance of Health) (Ibn Abi Usaibiah, 1245/46; Al-Samerra'i, 1989)

Kitab fi Tartib al-Aghthiya (Book on Organization of Nutrition) (Ibn Abi Usaibiah, 1245/46)

Kitab fil Hajama (Book on Cupping (Ibn Abi Usaibiah, 1245/46; Al-Samerra'i, 1989)

Kitab al-Hadra
This was another name for Firdaws Al-Hikma (Al-Samerra'i, 1989).

Kitab al-Lu'Luah (Book of Pearl)

It is believed that this is the same book as Firdaws Al-Hikma (Al-Samerra'i, 1989).

Kitab fil Ruqi (Book of Treatment with Prayers) Al-Samerra'i, 1989)

Kitab al-Idah fil Sumn wal-Hizal (Book Explaining Obesity and Loss of Weight (Al-Samerra'i. 1989)

Nonmedical books include:

Kitab al-Din wal-Dawla (Book on Religion and State)

This book was republished by Adel Nuwayhid in 1977 (Al-Samerra'i, 1989).

Kitab al-Amthal wal -Adab ala Mathhab al-Furs wal-Rum wal-Arab (Book of Literary Quotes Used by the Persians, Romans, and Arabs (Al-Samerra'i, 1989)

Al-Tabari quotes:

The following quotes are attributed to Al-Tabari (Al-Samerra'i, 1989):

"The ignorant doctor brings death."

"Experience translates into wisdom."

"The worst talk is that which contradicts itself."

AL-RAHAWI, ISHAQ IBN ALI (854–931 AD)

Al-Rahawi was a well-known and respected physician and scholar, well versed in the work of Galen (Ibn Abi Usaibiah, 1245/46).

Al-Rahawi is known for his book "Adab Al-Tabib" (the Conduct of a Physician), the earliest known Arabic treatise dedicated to medical ethics (Al-Khalili, 2011). It contains the first description of the peer review process (Spier, 2003). In the book, Al-Rahawi stated that it is the duty of a visiting physician to make duplicate notes of the condition of the patient on each visit. At the patient's discharge, cured or if he died, the notes of the physician were examined by a peer council of physicians who would decide whether the physician acted in accordance with prevailing standards of care. Based on their ruling, the physician may be sued for negligence (Spier, 2002).

Al-Rahawi is also known for collating Galen's ten articles in which medicines are organized according to organs they are used for, from the head to the foot (Ibn Abi Usaibiah, 1245/46).

IBN SARAFYUN, YAHYA (JOHANNES SERAPION, SERPION THE ELDER)

Ibn Sarafyun was a Christian Syrian physician who lived in the second half of the ninth century. Serapion the Elder was used to differentiate him from Serapion the Younger, with whom he was confused (http://en.wikipedia.org/wiki/yahya_ ibn_sarafyun).

Of his scholarly output, the following two are known (http://en.wikipedia.org/wiki/yahya_ibn_sarfyun):

Aphorismi Magni Momenti de Medicina Practica

Al-Kunnash (Pandectae, Aggregator, Breviarium, Practica, Therapeutica Methodus)

LATE ABBASID PERIOD (900–1300 AD)

AL-RAZI (RHAZES), ABU BAKR (BEKR) MUHAMMED IBN ZAKKARIYA (832/840/841/850/854/865/885 to 923/925/926/930/932/935 AD)

Known among medieval Latinists as Albubater, Al-Razi was born in Rayy (Rhages) in Khurasan, from which came the name Al-Razi. He moved to Baghdad when he was over the age of thirty (Ibn Abi Usaibiah, 1245/46; Al-Samerra'i, 1989; Campbell, 2011; Tarabay, 2011) and stayed there long enough to become the head of the famous Al-Muqtadiri Hospital (Afnan, 1958; http://wzzz.tripod.com/RAZI.html). He then returned to Persia, where he won fame and notoriety (Afnan, 1958).

His date of birth is variably reported to have been in 832, 840, 841,850, 854, 864, 865, and 885 AD. Similarly, the date of his death is variably reported to have been in 923, 925, 926, 930, 932, and 935 AD.

His city of birth (Al-Rayy) was one of the ancient Persian cities, a few miles from the current capital of Iran, Tehran (Wakim, 1944; Browne, 1962; Turner, 1995; Ligon, 2001; Tarabay, 2011; Campbell, 2011). Currently, it is a densely populated suburb of Tehran (Al-Khalili, 2011).

Al-Razi was a polymath who made contributions in a wide range of disciplines including philosophy, mathematics, astronomy, literature, and music, but all those pale in significance when compared to his contributions in medicine (Otri, 2008; Al-Khalili, 2011).

He began his life as a money changer and, some say, jeweler (Al-Samerra'i, 1989). He was a poet, singer, and musician who played the lute and wrote a treatise on musical theory in his early youth (Afnan, 1958; Goodman, 2003). He abandoned music, saying, "Music proceeding from between mustachios and beard had no charms to recommend it." Instead, he immersed himself in the study of alchemy and chemistry, philosophy, mathematics, and physics (Ather, 1993; Ligon, 2001; Freely, 2011). Some doubt his work in alchemy and suggest that his interest was limited to the science of chemistry, in which he published about twenty books (Al-Samerra'i, 1989). In chemistry, he took the classification of chemicals further than anyone before him based on laboratory experiments (Al-Khalili, 2011).

Problems with his vision led him to seek medical treatment before devoting his energies to the practice of medicine (Ramen, 2006).

He began the study of medicine late in his life, in his thirties or forties (Ibn Abi Usaibiah, 1245/46; Al-Mahi, 1959; Al-Samerrai, 1989; Haddad, 2003; Souayah, 2005; Campbell, 2011). His interest in medicine is attributed to a visit he made to a hospital in Baghdad where he saw interesting cases that endeared the study of medicine to him (Ibn Abi Usaibiah, 1245/46). He was under the tutelage of the renowned teacher and physician Ali Ibn

Rabban Al-Tabari in Al Muqtadiri Hospital (the main hospital in Baghdad), where he later became its head, between 902 and 907 AD (Ligon, 2001; Souayah, 2005; Al-Khalili, 2011; Campbell, 2011). Some doubt this relationship to Al-Tabari because of the different time span in which the two lived (Al-Samerra'i, 1989).

Al-Razi was an obsessive scholar who read all the books he could lay his hands on. A regular visitor to him described those visits: "I never went in to him without finding him reading or transcribing, whether to make a rough draft or a revised text" (Al-Khalili, 2011).

Al-RAZI, THE PHYSICIAN:

Al- Razi, along with Ibn Sina (Avicenna), is considered one of the two greatest physicians in medieval medicine. While Avicenna contributed to the theory of medicine, Al-Razi contributed to its practice (Souayah, 2005). Some consider him the greatest clinician of all time (Haddad, 1993).

Al-Razi represented a trend in Muslim medicine where the theoretical and practical knowledge intersected. The trend expanded empirical medical knowledge and practical procedures for treatment as opposed to making theoretical reflections on illness (Dallal, 2010). He was considered the greatest clinical genius among all physicians in the Islamic world (Afnan, 1958). He was also an independent thinker fond of speculation and fearless to express his views (Afnan, 1958). He was original in his belief that fever in itself was not a disease but a natural means for combating an infection. He did not agree with his contemporaries in giving great diagnostic importance to the urine (Wakim, 1944).

As a physician, he was famous in the East, where he was known as the "unsurpassed physician," and in the West, where he was known as "the second Galen" (Freely, 2011). He is ranked, along with Hippocrates and Galen, as a founder of clinical medicine (Morton, 1997; Campbell, 2011).

He was court physician for the caliph in Baghdad, who appointed him to head the main hospital (Al Maristan Al-Udadi) in Baghdad. Consulted by Caliph Al-Muhtadi on the best locale for a new hospital in Baghdad, he hung pieces of fresh meat in various districts of Baghdad and recommended the location in which, after few days, the meat was least disintegrated, stating that the air in that location was cleaner and healthier (Al-Mahi, 1959; Haddad, 2003; Souayah, 2005; Al-Khalili, 2011).

As a physician, his skills were unparalleled in his time. He was both competent and conscientious. Both the rich and poor sought his counsel. He never forced fees from the poor. Despite his renown, he was not wealthy and lived and died in comparative penury (Ligon, 2001; Campbell, 2011). He is quoted to have said, "The physician should aspire to cure his patient not to take his money, furthermore he should prefer the treatment of the poor rather than the treatment of the rich" (Haddad, 1993).

In his practice, he emphasized proper nutrition along with proper treatment. He is quoted to have said, "If a physician can treat a patient through nutrition rather than medicine, he has done the best thing" (Al-Samerra'i, 1989; Haddad, 1993; Ligon, 2001).

He was keen on the importance of anatomy in the practice of good medicine, so much that he refused to allow a cataract surgeon to operate on him when the surgeon failed to enumerate the number of the membranes in the eye. He remained blind the rest of his life, saying, "He had seen enough of the world" (Al-Mahi, 1959; Brown, 1962; Al-Samerra'i, 1989; Ligon, 2001; Souayah, 2005; Freely, 2011).

Al-Razi was well versed in the Hippocratic approach and challenged some of Galen's dogmas. He disagreed with Galen's course of fevers and argued that cases of fever he encountered in Rayy and Baghdad show that the number of cases that did not follow Galen's description of fevers was as high as cases that did. He also argued that while Galen had seen only three cases of a certain urinary ailment, he himself had seen hundreds and, thus, was better informed (Ligon, 2001; Taylor, 2008).

Al-Razi had a deep admiration for Socrates's life and teaching, calling him "our Imam." When people criticized him for his worldly style of life, he answered that Socrates had been no ascetic, and he saw no reason why he should be one (Afnan, 1958).

In spite of his experience and reputation as a clinician, Al-Razi did not hesitate to seek a second opinion and to consult colleagues in difficult cases (Al-Samerra'i, 1989).

QUOTES ATTRIBUTED TO AL-RAZI

The following quotes are attributed to Al-Razi:

"Truth in medicine is an attainable goal, and the art as described in books is far beneath the knowledge of an experienced and thoughtful physician" (Al-Samerra'i, 1989; Taylor, 2008).

"A patient should limit himself to only one physician in whom he has confidence, because he is more than often right than wrong; but he who consults a great many physicians may have a very confused state of mind" (Taylor, 2008). In another version (Ibn Abi Usaibiah, 1245/46; Al-Samerra'i, 1989; Haddad, 1993): "The patient who consults a great many physicians is likely to fall in the error of each of them" (Haddad, 1993; Otri, 2008).

"Surgery is a handcraft unworthy of medical honor" (Al-Mahi, 1959; Taylor, 2008).

"Some diseases form in days and are cured in an hour" (Al-Mahi, 1959; Taylor, 2008).

"Illness last least when the physician is learned and the patient compliant" (Al-Mahi, 1959; Al-Samerra'i, 1989; Taylor, 2008).

"When possible treat with nutrition, not drugs" (Al-Mahi, 1959; Al-Samerra'i, 1989; Taylor, 2008).

"Stick with monotherapy when you have to use drugs" (Al- Mahi, 1959; Taylor, 2008).

"Physicians ought to console their patients even if the signs of impending death seem to be present" (Ibn Abi Usaibiah, 1245/46; Scott, 1933; Al-Samerra'i, 1989).

SCHOLARSHIP

Al-Razi is credited with 200–250 major written works and treatises. Ibn Abi Usaibiah (1245/46) mentioned 232. The Fihrist enumerated 113 major and 28 minor works and two poems (Campbell, 2011), most of which have been collated by the historian and natural scientist Abu Al-Rihan Al-Biruni and published by the orientalist Paul Kraws in 1936 (Wakim, 1944; Al-Samerra'i, 1989). Most of his publications are in medicine; the rest cover a variety of subjects including theology, philosophy, mathematics, physics, astronomy, music, the natural sciences, and alchemy (Al-Khalili, 2011; Tarabay, 2011). Al-Biruni credited Al-Razi with eighty works on philosophy, of which only few survive (Freely, 2011).

Al-Razi's medical contributions are characterized by emphasis on diagnosis and treatment and less on theory of illnesses and their cure (Freely, 2011). Titles of some of his works reveal a sense of humor on the limitations and misuse of the medical profession such as in his treatises:

"The fact that even the most skillful physicians cannot heal all diseases" (Freely, 2011), in which he made a distinction between curable and incurable diseases, and the physician should not be blamed for not curing the incurable diseases (Al-Khalili, 2011).

"Why people prefer quacks and charlatans to skilled physicians" (Turner, 1995; Ligon, 2001; Freely, 2011), in which he attacked those without medical training who roamed the cities and countryside selling their "cures" (Al-Khalili, 2011).

"Why some people leave a physician if he is intelligent" (Freely, 2011)

"Why ignorant physicians, common folks, and women in the cities are more successful than scientists treating certain diseases and the physician's excuse for this" (Freely, 2011)

Kitab al-Judari Wal-Hasba (On Small Pox and Measles) (De Variolis et Morbiliis; de Peste, de Pestilentia)

This book, first published in 1766, is considered the best contribution of Al-Razi. It is believed to be the oldest and most original work in Arabic and Latin differentiating smallpox from measles and chicken pox (Wakim, 1944; Keys, 1953; Haddad, 1993; Morton, 1997; Souayah, 2005; Otri, 2008; Al-Khalili, 2011; Tarabay, 2011; Campbell, 2011). Smallpox had been unknown to Greek medicine (Afnan, 1958). The book is considered an ornament to the medical literature of the Arabs and the ultimate masterpiece of Muslim medicine (Keys, 1953; Browne, 1962; Ligon, 2001; Al-Khalili, 2011; Campbell, 2011). Some attribute the first description of smallpox to a priest physician who lived in pre-Islamic Alexandria (Al-Mahi, 1959; Souayah, 2005). Other sources credit Thabit Ibn Qurrah, a ninth-century Sabian, Syriac-speaking translator and scholar, with description of smallpox (Ligon, 2001). In any case, Al-Razi's book was the first to describe measles as a clinical entity and differentiate it from smallpox (Al-Mahi, 1959; Ather, 1993; Souayah, 2005). This is the first work in which the illness is fully treated, dealing with the causes, diagnosis, and treatment, universal occurrence, precautions that should be taken against its spread, and the characteristics that differentiate it from smallpox (Ullmann, 1997; Tarabay, 2011; Campbell, 2011). It was by far the more influential work than that of Thabet Ibn Qurra (Ligon, 2001). It ranks high in importance in the history of epidemiology (Browne, 1962; Ligon, 2001).

The book consists of fourteen chapters (Al-Samerra'i, 1989). In one of the chapters, Al-Razi attributed the motive for writing the book to a request by a patron of science who could not find anything on the subject in the literature and asked Al-Razi to compile an exhaustive treatise on the subject (Ligon, 2001).

The book notes the higher incidence of smallpox in children, and during spring and autumn months, it differentiated discrete from confluent types of smallpox lesions and the grave prognosis with green or black pustules (Ligon, 2001).

In the book, he showed particular concern with protecting the eye, for corneal damage from smallpox was a major cause of blindness in the Middle East until relatively modern times (Al-Khalili, 2011). His description of treatment for the condition is stated as: "As soon as symptoms of small pox appear, drop rose water into the eyes from time to time, and wash the face with cold water. For if the disease be favorable and the pustules few in number, you find that this mode of treatment prevents their breaking out in the eyes" (Al-Khalili, 2011).

The book was translated into Greek in Paris in 1548. Latin editions were published in Venice in 1498 and 1555, Basle in 1529 and 1544, Strasburg in 1549, London in 1747, and Gottingen in 1781. A French translation was published in Paris in 1762, an English translation in 1847, and a German translation in 1911 (Afnan, 1958; Turner, 1959; Al-Samerrai, 1989; Athar, 1993; Ligon, 2001; Campbell, 2011; Freely, 2011; Ather, 1993).

Copies of the book are in Leydin Library, Al Azhar University Library, and the Tehran Library, among other libraries (Al-Samerra'i, 1989).

Al-Hawi fil Tibb (The Comprehensive Book on Medicine), Liber Continens

The best known and most widely used of his books is "Al-Hawi fil Tibb", known in Latin as "Liber Continens"; it is an enormous comprehensive work giving the results of a lifetime of medical practice (Wakim, 1944; Afnan, 1958; Campbell, 2011). It is a twenty-five-volume medical encyclopedia kept in the Paris Faculty of Medicine library (Al-Kurdi, 2004; Souayah, 2005; Otri, 2008; Dallal, 2010). In 1395, Al-Hawi was one of nine volumes constituting the entire library of the Paris Faculty of Medicine (Wakim, 1944; Ligon, 2001; Al-Khalili, 2011; Campbell, 2011). It is considered the most extensive medical text written by a physician prior to the nineteenth century. It was the largest and heaviest of all books written prior to 1501 (Otri, 2008). It is a compilation of works of Greek, Syriac, Indian, and Arabic medical knowledge. In the text, the author added his own experience to those of previous authors (Ibn Abi Usaibiah, 1245/46; Afnan, 1958; Al- Samerra'l, 1989; Turner, 1995; Ligon, 2001; Souayah, 2005; Al-Khalili, 2011; Ead, http://www.levity.com/alchemy/islam 14.html). In the book, Al-Razi listed medical theories for each disease entry from Greek, Syriac, Indian, Persian, and Arabic medicine; these theories were followed by then-current ideas and by his own observations and opinions (Otri, 2008). In several places, Al-Razi criticized Galen, pointing out that his own clinical observations did not conform to those of Galen (Dallal, 2010; Tarabay, 2011).

The book was published posthumously by Mohammad Ibn Al-Amid, a scholar friend of Al-Razi who paid Al-Razi's sister a price for a draft of the book. He then paid Razi's students to edit and organize the draft and had it published (Afnan, 1958; Al-Mahi, 1959; Al-Samerra'i, 1989; Ligon, 2001; Campbell, 2011). The draft must have been a private notebook in which Al-Razi inserted extracts from medical works of Greek, Syriac, Arab, and Persian, along with notes about his own patients.

Only ten out of the original twenty-three volumes are extant today (Afnan, 1958; Al-Samerra'i, 1989; Al-Kurdi, 2004; Souayah, 2005):

Volume one contains eleven chapters and is devoted to organic and psychological disorders of the brain.

Volume two deals with eye diseases and treatments.

Volume three deals with disorders of the ear, nose, and throat.

Volume four is devoted to diseases of lungs and their treatment.

Volume five deals with stomach and intestines, their diseases and treatments.

Volume six deals with debilitation, causes, and treatment.

Volume seven deals with disorders of the heart, liver, spleen, and breast and their treatments.

Volume eight is about stomach ulcers and their treatments.

Volume nine is devoted to disease of women and obstetrical delivery.

Volume ten is about kidney and bladder disorders and their treatment.

Volume eleven deals with hemorrhoids and intestinal worms and their treatments.

Volume twelve is about tumors and boils and their treatment.

Volume thirteen deals with contusions, tissue tears, and joint dislocations.

Volume fourteen deals with fever, vomiting, stools, and treatments.

Volume fifteen is about febrile acute diseases and their treatments.

Volume sixteen deals with loss of weight, causes and treatments.

Volume seventeen deals with chicken pox and smallpox.

Volume eighteen is on halitosis.

Volume nineteen deals with urine and signs of diseases from examining it.

Volume twenty is about simple drugs, part one.

Volume twenty-one is about simple drugs, part two.

Volume twenty-two is about pharmaceuticals.

Volume twenty-three deals with regulations for prescribing drugs.

The ninth volume deals with pharmacology and was a source of therapeutic knowledge in Europe long after the Renaissance. It was used as the main textbook in the medical school in Paris (Ather, 1993; Campbell, 2011).

It is to Al-Hawi's book that the origins of disciplines like gynecology, obstetrics, and ophthalmic surgery be traced (Al-Khalili, 2011).

The book was translated, under the patronage of King Charles the first of Anjou, into Latin in 1278 (according to Ligon, 2001), and in 1270 (according to Freely, 2011) by a Jewish Sicilian, Faraj Ibn Salim (Farragut), under the title "Liber Continens." The Farragut translation was printed in Brescia, Italy, in 1486 (Ligon, 2011; Campbell, 2011) and Venice in 1500, 1506, 1509, and 1542 (Freely, 2011; Campbell, 2011). The Latin translation by Farragut was also printed in Venice in 1905 (Al-Samerra'i, 1989).

Parts of the original manuscript are in Munich, the Egyptian Book Repository, the British Museum, the Bodleian Library in Oxford, the Zahiriyya Library in Damascus, Petersburg, Mosul, Princeton, the Sulaymanieh Library in Istanbul, and in Madrid (Al-Samerra'i, 1989).

These different parts were collected in twenty-three chapters and printed in Pakistan in 1960 (Al-Samerra'i, 1989).

Kitab al-Mansuri (Liber al-Mansuri; Liber al-Mansoris)

A smaller compilation than Kitab al-Hawi, it is primarily based on Greco-Arab medicine (Souayah, 2005; Campbell, 2011 (http://www.levity.com/alchemy/islam 14.html). In addition to its medical contents, the book contains a scathing commentary on medical quacks and charlatans (Ligon, 2001).

The ten-volume book was dedicated, in 903 AD, to Amir Abu Salim Al-Mansur, Governor of Rayy, and ruler of Khorasan (Al-Samerra'i, 1989; Campbell, 2011).

The book discusses general medical theories and definitions, diets, drugs and their effects on the body, mother and child, skin diseases, mouth hygiene, epidemiology, toxicology, and the effects of the environment on health (Tarabay, 2011).

An entire first volume in the book is devoted to anatomy and physiology, including neuroanatomy (Al-Samerra'i, 1989; Ather, 1993; Souayah, 2005; Majeed, 2005; Campbell, 2011), and is taken mostly from Hippocrates, Galen, and Oribasius (Campbell, 2011).

The second volume deals with temperament and has a section on slavery (Campbell, 2011).

The third vlume deals with simple remedies (Campbell, 2011).

The fourth volume discusses means of preserving health (Campbell, 2011).

The fifth volume deals with skin diseases and cosmetology (Campbell, 2011).

The sixth volume is on diet for the traveler (Campbell, 2011).

The seventh volume is on surgery (Campbell, 2011).

The eighth volume is on poisons (Campbell, 2011).

The ninth volume (Nonus Almansoris), the most influential in the Latin West, is devoted to a consideration of various organs of the body from "top to toe." It was a famous book in the Middle Ages, and was subject of many commentaries. It formed a portion of the medical curriculum of the University of Tubingen at the end of the fifteenth century and was publicly read in medical schools of Western Europe for some hundreds of years (Campbell, 2011). It was also published in Italian, and an Arabic-Latin edition was published at Halle in 1776 (Campbell, 2011).

The tenth and last volume deals with fevers.

The first Latin translation was by Gerard of Cremona in Toledo, Spain and printed in Milan in 1481 (Al-Samerra'i, 1989; Campbell, 2011). Other Latin translations were published in Venice in 1497, Lyon in 1510, and Basle in 1544 (Campbell, 2011). The Nonus Almansoris with commentaries was published separately in Venice in 1483, 1490, 1493, and 1497 and at Padua in 1480.

The original Arabic manuscript was published by the German orientalist Reiske in 1776 (Al-Samerra'i, 1989). In the book, Al-Razi defined medicine as "the art concerned in preserving healthy bodies, the combating of disease, and in restoring health to the sick." Al Razi then outlined three domains of medicine: public health, preventive medicine, and treatment of specific diseases (Ather, 1993).

One of the earlier editions of the book stated the name of the author as "Mohammad Ibn Zakaria Al-Razi Al-Sairafi," referring to the author's early involvement in Sairafa (money changing) (Ibn Abi Usaibiah, 1245/46).

The book was still part of the medical curriculum in 1588 at the University of Frankfurt (Haddad, 1993).

Practica Puerorum

Dated to 900 AD, the Practica is considered the first treaties on pediatrics. Prior to the Practica, the subject of pediatrics was treated incidentally in the works of Hippocrates, Galen, and Soranus (Radbill, 1971). The Practica first appeared in print in 1481 (Radbill, 1971). The first published pediatric book, Bagellardus's De Egritudinibus Infantum, published in 1472, was largely based on the Practica (Radbill, 1971).

The book addresses the following childhood disorders (Radbill, 1971):

Enlargement of the head, abdominal distention, sneezing, sleeplessness, epilepsy, eye diseases, teeth disorders, mouth pustules, vomiting, diarrhea, constipation, cough, pruritus and vesicles, worms, hernia, bladder stones, paralysis.

The book also includes descriptions of what could be called today "night terror" and febrile seizures (Ligon, 2001).

Al-Murshid (Al-Fusul):

Al-Razi wrote this book in criticism of the book by Hippocrates of the same name (Al-Fusul). He considered Hippocrates's "Al-Fusul" "vague, and incomplete" (Al-Samerra'i, 1989).

In the book, Al-Razi pointed out seven principles that students should adhere to in the practice of medicine (Ajlouni, 2003):

Define diseases according to history and findings on physical examinations.

Identify the cause of the illness.

Based on one and two, decide whether the patient harbors a single or multiple disease entities.

Distinguish one disease type from another.

Recommend treatment whether by diet, drugs, or both.

Gain patient confidence to ensure that he/she will follow your advice, and raise patient's morale.

Be familiar with complications and prognosis and alert the patient about them.

The book addressed several topics, including causes of diseases and treatment, pulse, breathing, fevers, stomach, intestines, liver, kidneys, nutrition, sleep, water, exercise, bathing, laxatives, intercourse, among many others (Al-Samerrai, 1989).

The book was edited by Albert Lexander and published in 1961 by the Arab League Center for Arabic Manuscripts in Cairo (Al-Samerrai, 1989).

On Sexual Intercourse. Its Harmful and Beneficial Effects and Treatment

This is one of the least publicized books of Al-Razi. In it he proposed that intercourse was among the things to be avoided because "it weakens the eyesight, wrecks and exhausts the body, speeds up aging, senility, damages the brain and nerves, and renders the body strength weak and feeble" (Ajlouni, 2003).

Mujjarabat (Al-Tajarub)

This is a collection of medicines used and deemed effective by Al-Razi in 650 cases of men, women, and children that Al-Razi treated (Rosenthal, 1978; Al-Samerra'i, 1989).

Al-Fakhir (The Splendid)

This is a description of diseases from head to toe as reported by other scholars. The manuscript was never published; written copies of the manuscript are few (Haddad, 2003). Copies are in the libraries of Leydin, Petersburg, Alexandria, and Paris (Al-Samerra'i, 1989).

Kitab al Tibb al Ruhani (Book of Spiritual Physique)

This is a treatise on ethics based on Plato's concept of the soul in "The Republic." It was a companion book to Al-Razi's "Kitab al-Mansuri, Liber al-Mansoris."

The book reflected Al-Razi as a thoughtful physician. In the book, he promoted the principles of mutual helpfulness, division of labor, that a healthy and effective social organization is possible only on the basis of cooperation and mutual support. The ideas promoted in this book had a revival in 1902 in the publication of "Mutual Aid" by Peter Kropotkin as a refutation of Darwin's theory of the survival of the fittest (Myers, 1964).

The book is divided into twenty chapters (Ibn Abi Usaibiah, 1245/46; Freely, 2011):

On the excellence and praise of reason

On supporting the passion

On how a man may discover his own vices

On repelling carnal love and familiarity

On repelling conceit

On repelling envy

On repelling excessive and hurtful anger

On casting away mendacity

On casting away miserliness

On repelling excessive and hurtful anxiety and worry

On dismissing grief

On repelling greed

On repelling habitual drunkenness

On repelling addiction to sexual intercourse

On repelling excessive fondness, trifling, and ritual

On the amount of earning, acquiring, and expending

On repelling the strife and struggle in quest of worldly rank and station

On the difference between the counsel of passion and reason of the virtuous life

On the fear of death

In the chapter on drunkenness, Al-Razi addressed a poem to those addicted to drinks (Freely, 2011):

"When will it be within the Power

To grasp the good things God does shower

Though they may be but a span from thee,

If all thy night in revelry

Be passed, and in the morn thy rise

With fumes of drinking in thine eyes

And heavy with its wind, ere noon

Return to thy drunkard's boon."

The Philosophical Way of Life:

In this book, Al-Razi described his own lifestyle. A contemporary of Al-Razi described that lifestyle as: "He (Al-Razi) used to sit in his reception room surrounded by his students. A patient would come in and present his complaint to the first one he meets. If the first one did not know what was wrong, the patient would proceed to the next circle of students. If this group did not make a diagnosis, Al-Razi would then discuss the case. He was generous, dignified, and honest. He was so compassionate with the poor and the sick that he would supply them with ample food and provide them with nursing care" (Freely, 2011).

Copies of the book are in the Vatican and the British Museum. The book was published (undated) by the College of Arts in Fuad the First University in Egypt (Al-Samerra'i, 1989).

Kitab al-Asrar (Book of Secrets)

In this book on alchemy, Al-Razi discussed chemical processes and substances, including Naft (petroleum), and laboratory equipment involved, and less on philosophical aspects of alchemy.

In the book, he divided Naft into white (distillate oil) and black (crude oil) Naft (Freely, 2011). There is very little trace of alchemical mysticism and symbolism despite the evocative title (Al-Khalili, 2011). Al-Razi was not impressed by anything that could not be confirmed experimentally (Al-Khalili, 2011). The book was not a text on alchemical magic but a real chemical laboratory manual (Al-Khalili, 2011). Some doubt that the book was written by Al-Razi (Al-Samerra'i, 1989).

As chemist, Al-Razi was the first to produce sulfuric acid together with some other acids and to prepare alcohol by fermenting sweet products (http://wzzz.tripod.com/Razi.html).

Book of Exorcism, Fascination, and Incantations

In this book, Al-Razi discussed the use of those practices in causing and curing disease (Freely, 2011).

Birr al Sa'a (One-Hour Cure)

This is a small book about diseases that are cured within the hour, written at the request of Vezier Hussein Abi Al-Kassem Ibn Ubaydullah (Al-Samerra'i, 1989; Haddad, 2003). The book was translated into Persian, Indian, and French languages (Al-Samerra'i, 1989). Copies of the book are in Berlin, Paris, Cambridge, Leyden, Petersburg, Al-Khalidiyya Library in Jerusalem, Munich, and Beirut (Al-Samerra'i, 1989). The original Arabic text was published in Cairo in 1936 (Al-Samerra'i, 1989).

Al-Jami' (Compendium)

This book is also known as "Al-Jami' fil Tibb" (Compendium in Medicine).

The contents are collections from Al-Razi's other books and books authored by other scholars. It took him fifteen years to complete, during which he suffered poor vision and a weak hand (Al-Samerra'i, 1989).

According to Ibn Abi Usaibiah (Ibn Abi Usaibiah, 1245/46; Al-Samerra'i, 1989), the book contains twelve sections:

Section one deals with preservation of health.

Section two deals with nutrition and compound drugs.

Section three deals with pharmacology of compound drugs.

Section four deals with the pharmacist work in preparation and presentation of drugs.

Section five deals with qualities of pharmaceutical drugs (color, taste, smell) and the difference between the good and bad drugs.

Section six deals with drug replacement when the required drugs are not available.

Section seven deals with explanation of names, weights of drugs, and names of organs in Greek, Syriac, Persian, Indian, and Arabic.

Section eight deals with anatomy and physiology of organs.

Section nine deals with natural causation of disease.

Section ten deals with introduction to the study of medicine.

Section eleven deals with a group of prescriptions for treatments of diseases.

Section twelve deals with parts of Galen's books not included in Hunayn Ibn Ishaq books.

Some believe that the book was put together posthumously from notes left by Al-Razi. Ibn Abi Usaibiah, however, disagreed with this notion and believed that the book was written during Al-Razi's life (Al-Samerra'i, 1989; Al-Khalili, 2011).

Kitab fi Kayfiyyat al Ibsar (Book on Theory of Vision)

In this book, Al-Razi challenged the concept of Euclides, which suggested that vision is the result of rays that originate within the eye (Ibn Abi Usaibiah, 1245/46; Al-Samerra'i, 1989).

Kitab Taqseem al-Ilal (Book of Classification of Diseases)

The title of the book reflects its contents. It was translated into Latin by Gerard of Cremona. The original Arabic manuscript is in the British Museum (Al-Samerra'i, 1989)

Kitab al-Madkhal al-Sagheer Ila Ilm Al-Tibb (Small Book of Entry into the Science of Medicine)

This book combines discussions of medicine, philosophy, and natural events. The original manuscript is in the Egyptian Book Repository. The book was published in Cairo in 1977.

Kitab al-Fuqara' (Book for the Poor)

The book is also known by the name "Kitab Man La Yahduruh Tabib" (Book for Who Has No Access to a Doctor). It is basically a book on first aid. Copies of the book are in Leydin and the Iraqi Museum (Ibn Abi Usaibiah, 1245/46).

OTHER BOOKS (Ibn Abi Usaibiah, 1245/46; Keys, 1953; Afnan, 1958; Al-Mahi, 1959; Al-Samerra'i, 1989; Souayah, 2005; Al-Khalili, 2011):

On the Fact that Even Skillful Physicians Cannot Heal Disease (see above)

Why People Prefer Quacks and Charlatans to Skillful Physicians (see above)

Al-Madkhal (The Introduction)

The book was published in Spain in 1875.

Kitab al-Laqwah (Book on Facial Palsy)

Al-Kafi (The Sufficient)

Kitab al-Farq Bayna al-Amrad (Book of Differences Between Diseases)

Copies of the book are in Welcome Library in London and in Najm Adadi Library in Tehran.

Kitab fi Hay'at al-Kabid (Book on the Structure of the Liver)

Kitab fi Hay'at al Kila (Book on Structure of the Kidney)

Kitab fi Hay'at al 'Ayn (Book on the Structure of the Eye)

Kitab fil Hasa fil Mathana (Book on Bladder Stones)

Copies of the book are in Leydin Library and the Iqab Library in Aleppo. The book was translated into German.

Kitab fil Falig (Book on Paralysis)

Kitab fil Jabr wa Kayfa Yusakin Alamuhu (Book on Fractures and How to Reduce its Pain)

Kitab fi Mihnat al-Tabib (Book on the Medical Profession)

This book described what the physician should be in his character, body, appearance, and knowledge. Copies of the book are in Cambridge, Oxford, and Najm Abadi Library in Tehran.

Kitab al-Tibb al-Malaki (The Royal Book of Medicine)

Copies of the book are in the Egyptian Book Repository and Princeton.

Of Habits Which Become Natural, in which he anticipated Sherrington's conditioned reflex theory

One of his books on the wisdom of creation, in which he listed the anatomy of organs and their benefits to the survival of the organism, as proof of the theory of creation

Al-Razi is also credited with writing a twenty-two-chapter book on rheumatology, gout, and sciatica (Ibn Abi Usaibiah, 1245/46).

AL-RAZI'S CONTRIBUTIONS TO NEUROLOGY:

In his book "kitab al Hawi fil Tibb," "Liber Continens," Al-Razi described seven cranial nerves and thirty-one spinal nerves originating in pairs from the brain and spinal cord and arranged them in the order used by Galen, a classification that lasted until Vesalius. Successive anatomists refined the classification until Soemmerring formulated the classification of twelve cranial nerves, which is still in use (Souayah, 2005).

According to Galen and Al-Razi, the seven cranial nerves were as follows (Souayah, 2005; Shoja, 2009):

CN I, Optic Nerve. The current first cranial nerve, the olfactory, was then considered part of the brain.

CN II, Oculomotor Nerve

CN III and CN IV corresponded partly to the current trigeminal nerve.

CN V corresponded to the current facial and acoustic nerves.

CN VI corresponded to the current glossopharyngeal, vagus, and spinal accessory nerves.

CN VII, corresponded to the hypoglossal nerve.

The spinal nerves and inter-vertebral foramina were elaborately de-scribed. Al-Razi described thirty-one paired spinal nerves and a single caudal nerve originating from the spinal cord. The spinal nerves were classified as eight cervical, twelve thoracic, five lumbar, three sacral, three coccygeal. The single nerve, according to Al-Razi, originated from the middle of the inferior part of the coccyx (Souayah, 2005).

In addition to detailed description of cranial and spinal nerves and their sensory and motor functions, "Kitab "Al-Hawi fil Tibb" included chapters on several neurologic topics. Al-Razi's knowledge of neuroanatomy was evident in correlating etiology of disease to its anatomical locale (Souayah, 2005; Shoja, 2009). There are chapters on sciatic nerve disease, facial pa-ralysis, traumatic nervous system lesions, tremor, epilepsy, headache, meningitis, and hemiplegia (Souayah, 2005; Tubbs, 2007; Al-Khalili, 2011).

In Al-Hawi, Al-Razi discussed facial palsy: "Logveh denotes the paralysis of some facial structures such as the eye, nose, tongue, ear, or lip muscles." He combined both central and peripheral facial palsies in one entity: "The cause of this disease is related to the brain." He made astute observa-tions about involvement of the muscles of facial expression: "In this disease, one side of the face is displaced, a hemiface undergoes flaccid paralysis, the paralyzed side weakens and deviates twards the contralateral side. Occasionally the frontal skin on the weakened side is intensly stretched in a manner that with upward skin motion, the frontal folds on that side disappear, and new skin folds are formed. Such a patient is unable to close the eyelids." Through evaluation of facial sensations, he discerned potential trigeminal nerve involvement: "The patient should be asked about the sen-sation on the same or the other side of the face" (Shoja, 2009).

Al-Razi was the first to use the term "concussion" in its modern usage. He distinguished concussion as an abnormal physiologic state from se-vere brain injury (Souayah, 2005; Tubbs, 2007; Shoja, 2009).

On epilepsy, Al-Razi differentiated acquired from inherited epilepsy, described epileptic auras, and related prognoses to age of onset of epilepsy, with better prognosis in childhood onset and worse prognosis with onset after twenty-five years of age (Al-Kurdi, 2004).

Al-Razi attributed hemorrhagic strokes to a sudden rush of blood (hypertension) to the brain and recommended preventive venisection in susceptible individuals (Al-Kurdi, 2004). He also described the different outcomes associated with nerve cuts, with better outcomes in longitudinal versus transverse cuts (Al-Kurdi, 2004).

In his book "Al-Mansuri," "Liber Mansoris," Al-Razi divided facial palsies into flaccid and spastic, peripheral and central, and stated that they may be complicated with apoplexy that may be fatal or leave the patient with hemiplegia (Souayah, 2005).

Al-Razi advocated surgery for penetrating injuries of the skull (Tubbs, 2007).

Al-Razi is credited with the first description of "Rose Fever, Rose Cold," or allergic rhinitis (Ligon, 2001), the fact that the scent of roses for certain sensitive people produces an allergic rhinitis. Al-Razi described the illness that affected a classical Arabic geographer who, when the roses bloomed every spring, was affected with the condition. Al-Razi attributed the condition to the scent of roses and recommended avoiding smelling the roses. He thus was the first to relate hay fever to the scent of roses. Subsequently, in the sixteenth and seventeenth centuries, cases were reported in Europe. In the nineteenth century, cases were reported by English and American authors. Morill Wyman, in 1872, and Morell Mackenzie, in 1884, described similar cases under the name "rose cold" or "rose fever" (Ullmann, 1997; Ligon, 2001).

AL-RAZI, THE PHILOSOPHER, THE SOUL, AND THE PROPHECY:

On philosophy, Al-Razi was probably the most freethinking scholar of Islam. He believed (as did the Greeks) that a competent physician should also be a philosopher, well versed in the fundamental questions regarding existence. He disagreed with Al-Kindi on the issue of infinity. For him, God did not create the universe from nothing but arranged it out of existing principles (Al-Khalili, 2011).

Al-Razi's belief in the eternity of the soul and its eventual freedom from the body, as well as his rejection of revelation and prophecy, ran counter to Islamic teachings and earned him the title of heretic and infidel (Afnan, 1958; Freely, 2011). Al-Razi was not a lone heretic; he belonged to a group of "freethinkers" of medieval Islam (Khalidi, 2009).

Al-Razi is considered by some the most influential adversary of prophecy and prophets in pre-modern Islamic culture, as clearly shown in "A'lam Al-Nubuwwa" (The Proofs of Prophecy) by Abu Hatem al-Razi, which recorded the debate that took place in the tenth century between the author (Abu Hatem al-Razi), an Ismaili missionary and defender of Islamic orthodoxy, and Abu Bakr Al-Razi, the physician and philosopher (Khalidi, 2011). The debate in Arabic was translated into English by Dr. Tarif Khalidi (Khalidi, 2011).

As for designation of prophets, Al-Razi argued, "Why do you hold it to be necessary that God singled out one particular people for prophecy rather than another, preferred them above all other people, made them to be guides for mankind and caused mankind to need them?...It would have been more worthy of the wisdom of the Wise One, more worthy of the mercy of the Merciful, for Him to have inspired all His creatures with the knowledge of what is to their benefit as well as to their harm in this world and the next" (Khalidi, 2009).

Regarding his belief in the "anti-intellectual thrust of prophecy" and the "perceived fables and absurdities," Al-Razi stated, "Those who adhere to religious laws received their religion from their leaders through imitation. They forbade rational investigation of religious principles, and were very strict in this regard" (Khalidi, 2009).

The third issue raised by Al-Razi dealt with the contradictions that exist among prophets and their teachings: "Jesus claimed he was the son of

God; Moses claimed that God had no son; Mohammad claimed he was a creature like all other humans. Mohammad claimed that Jesus was not crucified. The Jews and Christians deny this and claim that he was killed and crucified" (Khalidi, 2009).

Al-Razi's attitude towards religion is spelled out in the following quotation: "If the people of religion are asked about proof for the soundness of their religion, they flare up, get angry and spell the blood of whoever confronts them with this question. They forbid rational speculation, and strive to kill their adversaries. This is why truth became thoroughly silenced and concealed" (Al-Khalili, 2011).

Although his medical studies were extensive, his philosophy evoked horror, and his nonmedical works have almost entirely disappeared (Afnan, 1958).

FIRSTS ATTRIBUTED TO AL-RAZI (Khairallah, 1942; Al-Mahi, 1959; Ather, 1993; Haddad, 1993; Ullmann, 1997; Ligon, 2001; McCrory, 2001; Al-Kurdi, 2004; Souayah, 2005; Otri, 2008; Campbell, 2011; http: //encyclopedia.the-freedictionary.com/Islamic.medicine):

Account of the method for extraction of cataract

First book on pediatrics

Detailed description of scrotal gangrene (one thousand years before Foumier)

Bladder paralysis in spinal cord tumors

Description of the laryngeal branch of the recurrent laryngeal nerve and the observation that it is sometimes on the right side

Differentiation between smallpox and measles

Effect of light on pupil size, discussion of the pupillary reaction, formed by small muscles that act according to the intensity of light

Recognition of allergic rhinitis

Suggestion of blood-borne diseases (smallpox)

Use of alcohol for medicinal purposes

Use of animal gut for ligation during surgical operations

Introduction of mercurial ointment in medical practice

Use of opium for anesthesia

First to use the term "concussion" in its modern sense and to differentiate it as a transient physiologic state from severe brain damage

First to describe guinea worm disease and a method (still used) to extract the worm

Description of bladder and kidney stones

Thought to have pioneered the method of differential diagnosis and clinical observations, both of which were essential in his differentiation between smallpox and measles

Introduction of controlled experiments into the field of medicine

Al-Razi is considered to be the first to describe what is called now Baker's cyst, attributed to the English surgeon William Baker, who described it in 1877.

AL-RAZI'S LAST DAYS:

Al-Razi went blind at the end of his life and refused to be operated on for cataract because the ophthalmic surgeon was not fully knowledgeable about the anatomy of the eye and "because he had seen enough of the world" (Freely, 2011).

The spirit in which he faced death is illustrated in a poem he wrote in his last days (Freely, 2011):

"Truly I know not—and decay

Has laid his hand upon my heart,

And whispered to me that the day

Approaches, when I must depart—

I know not whither I shall roam,

Or where the Spirit, having sped

From this its

Wasted fleshy home

Will after dwell, when I am dead."

A portrait depicting of Al-Razi writing the title and introductory words of "Al-Hawi fil Tibb" hangs in the chapel of Princeton Unversity (Ligon, 2001).

A stamp in memory of AL-Razi was issued by the Syrian Arab Republic in 1968 (Ligon, 2001).

In Iran, they celebrate Al-Razi's Day (Pharmacy Day) on August 27 of every year (Al-Khalili, 2011).

AL-RAZI ON GALEN AND ARISTOTLE

The following saying by Al-Razi reflects his views about Galen and Aristotle (Campbell, 2011): "When Galen and Aristotle are unanimous in the expression of an opinion there lies absolute truth, but when they are at variance it is hard to decide, and we should arrive at the proper course of conduct by rationalization," and he added, "The skilled and experienced physician will act upon the prompting of his judgement."

IBN AL-JAZZAR (GAZZAR, AL-GIZAR), ABU JA'AFAR AHMAD IBN IBRAHIM IBN ABI KHALID AL-QAYRAWANI (898–980 AD)

He is an almost unknown Muslim physician from a family of physicians, son and nephew of physicians, but he is the best known in his family. Ibn Al-Jazzar was an influential tenth-century Arab Muslim physician, known in Europe by his Latinized name, Al-Gizar. He was born in the city of Qayrawan, in today's Tunisia, hence the name "Al-Qayrawani" (Ibn Abi Usaibiah, 1245/46; Al-Samerra'i, 1989; http://en.wikipedia.org/wiki/Ibn Al_Jazzar).

He matriculated under his father, uncle, Ishaq Ibn Suleiman Al-Israeli, and Ziyad Ibn Khalfun, who were among the best practitioners at that time (Al-Samerra'i, 1989).

Upon his graduation, he practiced in a tent set outside his house. The tent also contained a minipharmacy, from which he dispensed medicines to the needy free of charge (Al-Samerra'i, 1989).

Ibn Al-Jazzar was known to avoid being close to rulers and men of authority and to refuse their gifts, except for descendants of the Fatimid dynasty, who he continued to take care of their health problems. In the summer hot months, he went to the beach to rest and recuperate (Al-Samerra'i, 1989).

SCHOLARSHIP:

Ibn Al-Jazzar wrote on medicine, history, literature, and animals. His scholarly output includes the following:

Zad al-Musafir Wa Qut al-Hadir (Provision for the Traveler and Nourishment of the Settled)

This became influential in Europe, where several translations of it were produced: into Byzantine Greek (in the eleventh century) by Constantine the Protosecretary of Rhegion (Pormann, 2007); Latin (in the twelfth century) by the well-known translator Gerard of Cremona, who titled it "Viaticum Peregrinantis"; and Hebrew and Latin by Moshe Ibn Tibbon (Pormann, 2007) in the thirteenth century. This tome consisted of seven books. The books on "Sexually Transmitted Diseases" and the Book on "Fevers" have been translated into English (http;//www.nlm.nih.gov/hmd/Arabic/boil.html).

The tome contains "a multi-purpose recipe for countering impotency, increased sexual desire, refresh the soul, warm the body, expel gas from the stomach, put an end to coldness of the kidney and bladder, and increase memory. Taken in the winter, it will warm the limbs. Its uses are many, and it is one of the 'royal electuaries', and I have named it 'reliable against calamities' (Ma'mun al-ghaud'il). An amount of the size of walnut is to be taken before and after meals. And it will be efficacious, God willing" (Pormann, 2007).

The recipe contained: Chinese cinnamon, sweet cost, Indian Spikenard, saffron, fennel seeds, ginger, dried mint leaves, wild mountain thyme, cinnamon bark, white and black pepper, plum seeds, caraway, cloves, wild carrot, cardamom, radish seeds, turnip seeds, sesame, walnut, pistachios, almonds, pine nuts, sugar candy, honey of wild thyme (Pormann, 2007).

According to Ibn Abi Usaibiah (1245/46), contrary to reports in the literature, this tome was actually two books. One, "Provisions for the Traveler," made up of two volumes, and a large, twenty-volume book titled "Nourishment of the Settled/Sedentary (Ibn Abi Usaibiah, 1245/46).

Copies of the Hebrew edition are in Oxford's library and the library in Taurine, Italy. The Latin edition was printed in Basel, Switzerland, in 1516 AD. The Arabic language manuscript is in the Paris Public Library, the Vatican Library, Florence library, and Oxford's library (Al-Samerra'i, 1989).

Tibb al-Fuqara wal-Masakeen (Medicine for the Poor and Destitute):

This is a fifty-eight-chapter book, a collection of cheap compound remedies for the poor, traditional folklore practices, and magical procedures. In the introduction to the book, Ibn Al-Jazzar stated that he collected the recipes and procedures from the works of Galen, Ibn Masaweh, Hunayn Ibn Ishaq, and other excellent physicians. The book was translated into Hebrew. Copies of the book are in the Iraqi National Library (Samerra'I, 1989; http://www.nlm.nih.gov/hmd/arabic/biol.html).

Medical Handbook of Special Pathology

The text of the book includes two aspects:

The first is a classification of apoplexy, which became popular in the late Middle Ages. Apoplexy is divided into "major" and "minor" varieties, based on Hippocratic teachings. In apoplexy major, loss of movement and sensory functions are complete and are associated with loss of consciousness and respiratory compromise. Apoplexy minor is differentiated into two types, a "hard" (dura) type and a "smooth" (lenis) type. In the hard type, caused by repletion of one side of the head with "sticky humor," there is loss of the voluntary motion of the side of the body, as well as the ability to speak. The "smooth, lenis" type, caused by repletion of spinal nerves or a single nerve involved only motion and sensations in the part of the body without impairment of speech (Karenberg, 1998). Modern neurologists recognize this as one of the first descriptions of spastic and flaccid paralysis due to a lesion in the brain or the peripheral nerves, respectively.

The second important aspect of the book is the observation that loss of speech occurs mostly if motion on the right side of the body is affected. Other than a very unclear reference in the Hippocratic writings, this association of aphasia with right-sided paralysis seems to have no known precedent (Karenberg, 1998).

The book was translated into Latin by Constantine the African under the title "Viaticum" (Karenberg, 1998).

Risala fil Nisian wa "Ilagihi (Treatise on Forgetfullness and its Treatment)

This book was translated into English by Gerrit Bos in 1995. The original Arabic manuscript is lost (Al-Samerra'i, 1989; http://www.nlm.nih.gov/hmd/arabic/biol.html).

Kitab Tibb al-Mashayikh wa Hifz Sihhatihim (Book on Medical Care of the Elderly)

Copies of the book are in the Egyptian Book Repository and the private library of Ahmad Khairi in Egypt (Al-Samerra'i, 1989; http://www.en.wikipedia.org/wiki/Ibn_Al_Jazzar).

Risala fi Asbab al-Wafat (Treatise on Causes of death) (Al-Samerra'i, 1989; http://en.wikipedia.org/wiki/Ibn_Al_Jazzar)

Book on Disorders of Sleep: (Al-Samerra'i, 1989; http://en.wikipedia.org/wiki/Ibn_Al_Jazzar).

Siyasat al-Subyan wa Tadbirihim (Book on Pediatrics):

This book is in twenty-two chapters, dealing with care of the newborn in health and disease. It includes sections on breastfeeding and the nature of food taken by the mother. It also addresses common ailments of the infant, such as diarrhea, vomiting, intestinal worms, earache, umbilical infections, childhood epilepsy, bulging fontannelle, teeth pain, and bladder stones (Al-Samerra'i, 1989).

In this book, Ibn Al-Jazzar wrote that one should use the ashes of the Achilles tendon of a calf, instead of ashes of bones of pigs, to sprinkle the umbilical hernia of the infant in line with Islamic law that prohibits use of pigs (Ullmann, 1964).

Kitab al-I'timad fil Adwiyah al-Mufrada (Book on simple Drugs)

This book was criticized by Abdel Rahman Ibn Ishaq Ibn Haytham

Al-Qurtubi in a book titled "Al-Ikhtisar wal Ijad fi Khat'a Ibn Al-Jazzar fil I'timad"(The Brevity and Errors in Ibn Al-Jazzar's Book Al-I'timad). The book was translated into Latin in 1333 AD by the monk Estiphan al-Surcosti, who claimed authorship of the book, and by Costantine the African, who also claimed authorship, and to Hebrew by Moshe Ibn Tibbon. Some parts of the original Arabic manuscript are in the British Museum and in the Algerian Library (Ibn Abi Usaibiah, 1245/46; Al-Samerra'i, 1989).

The following books are also attributed to Ibn Al-Jazzar:

Kitab al-Baghiyah (On Complex Drugs)

This book is on compound drugs. The manuscript is in the private Jarrah Library in Aleppo, Syria (Al-Samerra'i, 1989).

Kitab Sahih al Tarikh (Book of Correct History)—a book about the luminaries of his time and a brief about each (Ibn Abi Usaibiah, 1245/46)

Kitab fil Ma'idah and Mudawatiha (A Book about the Stomach and Its Treatment)

This book was referred to in the author's book "Al-Mashayekh." It is in four sections. Copies are in the Iraqi National Museum. It was published by Salman Qutaba in Baghdad in 1981 (Ibn Abi Usaibiah, 1245/46; Al-Samerra'i, 1989).

Kitab fil 'Ilal Allati Tashtabeh Asbabiha wa Takhtalif 'Aradiha (Book on Diseases with Similar Etiology and Different Signs)

This book was published by the Center for Arabic Scientific Heritage in Baghdad in 1984 (Ibn Abi Usaibiah, 1945/46; Al-Samerra'i, 1989).

Kitab al-Mukhtabarat (Laboratory Book) (Ibn Abi Usaibiah, 1245/46)

Risala fil Juzam (On Leprosy) (Ibn Abi Usaibiah, 1245.46)

Kitab fil Kila wal -Mathana (Book on Kidneys and Bladder)

The original manuscript of this book is lost (Al-Samerra'i, 1989).

Osoul al-Tibb (Fundamentals of Medicine)

The original manuscript of this book is lost (Al-Samerra'i, 1989).

Kitab al-Malinkholia (Book on Melancholy)

Parts of this book are in the Bodlein Library, Oxford (Al-Samerra'i, 1989).

Kitab Qout al-Muqeem fil Tibb (Book for the Trainee in Medicine)

This book, reported to be in twenty volumes, is lost (Al-Samerra'i, 1989).

Kitab al-Sumoum (Book on Poisons)

This book was referred to in Ibn Al-Baytar's book "Al-Jami'" (Al-Samerra'i, 1989).

Kitab al-Khawas (Book on Special Medicine)

This book deals with medicines for the royalty (Al-Samerrai, 1989).

Kitab fil Zukam, Asbabuhu Wa 'Ilajohu (Coryza, Causes and Treatment) (Al-Samerra,i, 1989).

Ibn Al-Jazzar died in Qayrawan at age eighty-two, before taking a trip to the Andalus, which he had planned.

AL-MAJUSI (AL-MAJUS, AI-MAGUSI), ALI IBN ABBASI (HALY ABBAS) (925–994/995 AD)

Al-Majusi was born near Shiraz (in today's Iran) (Freely, 2011), although others (Ibn Abi Usaibiah, 1245/46; Browne, 1962; Al-Samerra'i, 1989; Campbell, 2011) cite Ahwaz, a city in south west Persia (today's Iran) near the famous medical school of Ghondi-Shapour. His name (Al-Majusi) suggested that he belonged to an ancient Persian religion (Zoroaster), although he was Muslim (Freely, 2011).

He is considered the most outstanding Islamic physician in the latter half of the tenth century (Freely, 2011).

He received his medical training in Ahwaz under the physician Abu Mahir Musa Ibn Yousef Ibn Sayyar (Ibn Abi Usaibiah, 1245/46; Al-Samerra'i, 1990; Freely, 2011), after which he went to Baghdad where he directed the Adud Al Dawla Hospital (Freely, 2011).

Al-Majusi was not a prolific writer. His major work was "Kitab Al-Malaki," (Maliki) (The Royal Book, Liber Reguis), which he dedicated to Caliph Adud Al-Dawla (Browne, 1962; Haddad, 2003; Campbell, 2011; Freely, 2011).

Kitab al-Kamil fil-Sina'a al-Tibbiyah (Complete Book of the Medical Art) (Liber Reguis); Kitab al-Malaki (Maliki) (The Royal Book).

The book known also by the name "Al-Qanoun Al-Udadi fil Tibb," embraced everything that the student of medicine needed to know to become master of the art. The book is characterized by brevity and clarity of presentation. It includes a section on anatomy summarizing all known anatomy before him (Haddad, 2003). The book is considered better than Al-Razi's "Al- Mansuris," which was, at the time, the popular book for study. It was of clearer style and up-to-date compared to Ibn Ribn Al-Tabari's "Firdaws Al-Hikma" (Al-Samerra'i, 1989).

The book was written with the intention of applying a theoretical framework that would provide structure and organization (Dallal, 2010).

This book is an encyclopedic work on surgery and medicine, which was translated widely and widely used as a textbook in schools of Europe (Wakim, 1944) until the publication of Ibn Sina's "Al-Qanoun fil Tibb " (Canon of Medicine), which replaced Al-Majusi's Kitab Al-Kamil (Dallal, 2010; Campbell, 201).

The book is made up of twenty discourses (tracts), each of which is divided into numerous chapters. The first three chapters (introduction to the book) include criticism of previous works in medicine, including that of Al-Razi (Brown, 1962; Al-Samerra'i, 1989; Haddad, 2003; Campbell, 2011; Freely, 2011). He considered the writings of Hippocrates too concise and those of Galen too diffuse (Browne, 1962: Al-Samerra'i, 1989). The first ten discourses deal with the theory of medicine and the last ten with the practice of medicine. The nineteenth discourse (110 chapters) is devoted to surgery (Browne, 1962; Campbell, 2011). He is credited of being the first Arab physician to write comprehensively about surgery. His surgical descriptions were described as very clear and definite, as shown in his description of catheterization of male patients (Khairallah, 1942; Keys, 1953), how to excise cysts of tubercular lesions, and of superficial cancer. In the latter, he recommended complete excision with a large border of clear skin (khairallah, 1942). The book also includes one of the greatest contributions Haly Abbas made to medical science, the closest description (prior to Harvey) of capillary circulation (Khairallah, 1942; Wakim, 1944; Keys, 1953). His description of the expulsion of the fetus, during parturition, due to uterine contraction, not spontaneously, is considered to be a first (Khairallah, 1942; Keys, 1953).

The description of pleurisy and its symptoms is accurate and reflects the state of medicine at the time: "Pleurisy is an inflammation of the pleura, with exudation which pours materials over the pleura from the head or chest...." The symptoms of pleurisy are described thus: "There are four symptoms that always accompany pleurisy: fever, cough, pricking in the side, and difficult breathing" (Freely, 2011). He is considered the first to note difficulty in healing of pulmonary tuberculosis attributing that to the movements of the lung during respiration (Al-Samerra'i, 1989).

In the section of the nervous system (Al-Kurdi, 2004), Al-Majusi described the brain as a center of sensation and movement. He discussed headache, stroke, epilepsy, dementia, coma, and schizophrenia. He described the spinal cord and its thirty-one pairs of nerves (eight cervical, twelve thoracic, five lumbar, three sacral, three coccygeal, and a single nerve below the coccyx). He also differentiated between spastic and flaccid paralysis in spinal cord disease.

Al-Majusi stressed the importance of proper diet, hygiene, and exercise for a healthy body and mind. He was one of the leading authorities on dietetics in his time (Wakim, 1944). He stressed the relationship between psychology and medicine and the importance of psychother-apy in the treatment of psychosomatic disorders (Al-Samerra'i, 1989; Freely, 2011).

His description of poisons, their symptoms, and treatment may have been the beginning of medical toxicology (Freely, 2011).

The book includes a discussion on drug addiction and use of opiates (Freely, 2011).

Al-Majusi opposed contraception and induction of abortion by drugs except when the mother's mental or physical health were endangered (Freely, 2011). He stressed the importance of ethical practice in line with the Hippocratic Oath (Al-Samerra'i, 1989; Freely, 2011).

Al-Majusi emphasized the importance of regular attendance of students at the hospital "and of those things which are incumbent on the student of this art and that he should constantly attend the hospital and sick houses; pay unremitting attention to the conditions and circumstances of their inmates, in company with the most astute   professors of medicine; and enquire frequently as to the state of the patients bearing in mind what he has read about the variations, and what they indicate for good or evil. If he does this, he will reach a high degree in this art..." (Browne, 1962).

The Al-Malaki was translated into Latin by Constantine Africanus, who attributed authorship to himself (Keys, 1953; Al-Samarra'l, 1989; Haddad, 2003; Campbell, 2011), and by Stephen of Pisa. The book continued to be studied in Salerno and other European medical schools under the authorship of Africanus until 1127 AD when another translation by Elias Istphan Al-Antaki gave the credit to Al-Majusi, the original author

(Al-Samerra'i, 1989). The book was used in European universities until the eighteenth century, when it was replaced by Avicenna's "Canon" (Haddad, 1975; Campbell, 2011).

A hundred Arabic manuscripts of the book are preserved in such libraries as Berlin, Leyden, Paris, Munich, Florence, Madrid, Al-Khalidiyya in Jerusalem, Welcome in London, Harvard, and the Iraqi museum (Keys, 1953; Al-Samerra'i, 1989; Haddad, 2003).

AL-MAWSILI, AMMAR IBN ALI (CANAMUSALI)

Al-Mawsili was born in Mosul, Iraq (hence his name al-Mawsili) and studied medicine there. He traveled to different places, including Khorasan, Diyar Bakr, Syria, Palestine, Mecca, and Medina in Saudi Arabia, and practiced ophthalmology in all of them. He finally settled in Egypt during the rule of the Fatimid ruler Al-Hakim bi Amr Allah. When he became known for his expertise in medicine, the ruler invited him to join his court and be his personal physician (Al-Samerra'i, 1990).

His scholarship consists of only one treatise on eye diseases, written in 1010 AD, dedicated to Fatimid ruler Al-Hakim, who ruled from 966–1020 AD. The treatise includes a discussion of forty-eight diseases of the eye, with clinical cases and adaptations of surgical instruments in twenty-one chapters. One of the surgical instruments was a hollow needle used to extract cataracts by suction. The book is considered the most original book on the subject of eye disorders. The book was translated into Latin by David Hermanus and was the text on the subject in medical schools of Europe until the mid-eighteenth century. The book was translated into German from its original Arabic copy. Copies of the original Arabic texts are kept in libraries in Rabat (Morocco) and Leningrad (Khairallah, 1942; al-Samerrai, 1990; http://nlm.nih.gov/exhibition/islamic_medical/islamic 09html). The hollow tube for cataract extraction was accredited by some to this oculist Ibn Abi Usaibiah in about 1230 AD in the Nuri Hospital of Damascus (http://nlm.nih.gov/exhibition/islamic_medical/islamic 09.html).

IBN SIWAR IBN AL-KHAMMAR, ABU AL-KHAYR AI-HASAN IBN PAPA IBN BIHNAM (942–1017 AD)

Ibn Al-Khammar (also known by Ibn Siwar) was a Christian Syriac physician and philosopher of Persian origin. Bihnam in Persian means "Khair," or "good luck," and hence he was known by "Abu Al-Khair." Ibn Siwar was born in Baghdad when it was under the religious reign of the Abbasid Caliphate and the secular rule of the Buyids, who were the ruling authority. His father traded in alcoholic drinks (khamr in Arabic), and hence the father was called "Al-Khammar" and his son "Ibn al-Khammar" (son of Al-Khammar) (Al-Samerra'i, 1989; http://en.wikipedia.org/wiki/User: Onciaoncia).

Ibn Al-Khammar became a student of the theological and philosophical school of Yahia bin 'Adi, a monophysite Jacobite. He studied medicine and became a successful physician and philosopher (Al-Samerra'i, 1989; http://en.wikipedia.org/wiki/User:Onciaoncia). In 1001, he moved to Khwarism at the invitation of its Amir Abi Al-Abbas Mamoun Ibn Mamoun Ibn Mohammad. In 1017, he moved to Gizna at the invitation of its Amir Mohammad Ibn Sabkatkeen, where he converted to Islam at an advanced age (Al-Samerra'i, 1989).

He succeeded so much in Gizna that he was called "The Second Hippocrates" (Al-Samerra'i, 1989).

Among his students was Abu Al-Faraj Ibn Hindu, who mentioned him in his book "Miftah Al-Tibb" (Key to Medicine). He was also complimented for his work by Ibn Radwan Al-Masri in his book "Hall Shukuk Al-Razi Ala Jalinus" (Solution of Doubts of Al-Razi about Galen" (Al-Samerra'i, 1989).

Ibn Siwar reportedly suffered regular bouts of epilepsy (http://en.wikipedia.org/wiki/User:Onciaoncia).

Ibn Siwar worked in translating works in Syriac into Arabic, but he is an author in his own right. Most of his books are in philosophy, but he also wrote in medicine and social behavior. His writing style has been described as having definite influences from the Alexandrian school of Neoplatonism. He has been identified as a humanist, and his works are accepted as being superior to his teacher (http://en.wikipedia.org/wiki/User:Onciaoncia; http://syriacstudies.com/AFSS/Syriac_Scholars_and_Writers).

His scholarly works in medicine include:

Kitab fi Khalq al-Insan wa Tarkib A'da'ihi (Book on Creation of Man and His Anatomocal Makeup)

This book is in four sections (Al-Samerra'i, 1989; http://en.wikipedia.org/wiki/User:Onciaoncia).

Kitab Tadbir al-Mashayekh (Book on Dealing with Old People)

This book contains twenty-six chapters in the form of questions and answers (Al-Samerra'i, 1989).

Maqala fi Imtihan al-Atibba' (On Examination of Physicians)

This book was dedicated to Amir Khwarism Shah Mamoun Ibn Mamoun (Al-Samerra'i, 1989; http://en.wikipedia.org/wiki/User:Onciaoncia).

Maqala fil Marad al-Ma'rouf bil-Kahini ay al-Sara' (Work on the Sacred Disease, also known as Epilepsy) (Al-Samerra'i, 1989; http://en.wikipedia.org/wiki/User:Onciaoncia)

AL-BIRUNI, ABU AL-RIHAN MOHAMMAD IBN AHMAD (973–1048 AD):

Al-Biruni was a tenth-century physician, traveler, historiographer, philosopher, mathematician, geographer, astronomer, and teacher of the Greek learning (Afnan, 1958; Landau, 1959; Haddad, 1975; Myers, 1964; Al-Khalili, 2011). Little is known about his early life since he did not leave an autobiography (Al-Khalili, 2011). He was born in Birun, near the city of Kath in Khwarism, hence the name BIRUNI. Others suggest that "Biruni" is a Persian word for "outsider" and could refer either to his family's Tajik origin or to the fact that he came to Kath as a boy from an outlying suburb, or it may be a name given to him later in life (Al-Khalili, 2011). He was a contemporary of Ibn Sina (Avicenna) and corresponded with him and with his associates (see under Ibn Sina) on matters of medicine and philosophy (Ibn Abi Usaibia, 1245/46; Afnan, 1958, Al-Khalili, 2011). With Ibn Sina, he shared total lack of racial prejudice, a broad humanity, devotion to truth, and intellectual curiosity (Afnan, 1958).

As a young man, he worked in the courts of the Banu Iraq princes of Kath, who ruled over that region of Khwarism on behalf of the Samanid dynasty (Al-Khalili, 2011). He had to leave Kath when it was taken over, in 995, by a rival dynasty. He traveled first to Samanid capital Bukhara, where he came under the protection of the Samanid ruler Prince Nuh Ibn Mansur. From Bukhara, he moved to Rayy, where he spent a miserable few years in poverty unable to gain royal patronage. In 999, he was invited by Prince Qabus of Gorganj to join his court, which he did, and to whom he dedicated his great historical text "The Chronology of Ancient Nations," one of the greatest sources of medical history ever written (Al-Khalili, 2011).

In the early years of the eleventh century, he was lured back to Khwarism, and its capital Gorganj. The Mamunid sultans were welcoming of scholarship and were keen at inviting top scholars to work in their court. In Gorganj, Al-Biruni was in a highly intellectual environment where he spent many highly productive years (Al-Khalili, 2011).

Like many luminaries of his time, he fell in trouble with his patron, Sultan Mahmoud (Afnan, 1958). According to anecdote, Sultan Mahmoud commanded him to prophesize. In both cases his predictions turned out correct, contrary to the Sultan wishes, and he was sent to prison (Afnan, 1958).

SCHOLARSHIP:

Al-Biruni was a true scholar bent on reason, understanding, and criticism, refusing to accept belief blindly (Afnan, 1958). His intellectual background and acumen had "no equal except in Ibn Sina" (Afnan, 1958). Along with Al-Razi and Ibn Al-Haytham, he was one of the earliest and leading exponents of the scientific method (Al-Khalili, 201). He was fluent in Greek, Sanskrit, Syriac, and Hebrew (Afnan, 1958). His mother tongue was Chorasmian, an Iranian dialect with a Turkish admixture (Afnan, 1858). He developed an interest in comparative religious beliefs. His interest and writings in comparative religions was described as follows: "It is rare before modern times to find so fair and unprejudiced statement of the views of other religions" (Afnan, 1958).

Al-Biruni, like earlier Muslim astronomers, envisaged the universe as a dynamic "becoming" and thus as a proof of God's eternal manifestations (Landau, 1959).

Al-Athar al-Baqiya 'an al Qurun al-Khaliya (Chronology of Ancient Nations)

This book was written about 1,000 AD. It is a discourse of the calendar and eras of ancient people (Myers, 1964; Haddad, 1975). It contains a picture about Caesarian operation and describes how the mother of Caesar Augustus died in labor and how her abdomen was cut open, and the child was thus delivered through the incision in the abdomen (Haddad, 1975).

Kitab al-Saidala fil Tibb (Book of Pharnacy in Medicine)

A book about medicines used at the time arranged in alphabetical order, with comments made about each medicine by his contemporaries and his predecessors (Ibn Abi Usaibia, 1245/46)

Kitab Tastih Al Kura (Book about the Flat Globe) (Ibn Abi Usaibia, 1245/46)

Kitab al-Tafhim fi Sina'at al-Tanjim (Book of Understanding of Stars) (Ibn Abi Usaibia, 1245/46)

Kitab Al-Qanoun Al-Masoudi

Written for Masoud Ibn Siktakeen (Ibn Abi Usaibia, 1245/46)

Al-Biruni is also credited with being the first to provide careful description of obstetrical monstrosities (Khairallah, 1942).

Al-Biruni wrote an astronomical encyclopedia and a summary of mathematics (Myers, 1964).

His book on astrology and astronomy was translated into Latin by Hugh of Santalla (Myers, 1964). He entertained the question of whether or not the Earth rotates on its axis five hundred years before Galileo but did not reach a definite answer (Myers, 1964).

He estimated the speed of light and concluded that it must be greater than the speed of sound (Myers, 1964).

Al-Biruni's best known, if not most important, achievement in science was his determination of the circumference of the Earth from an ingenious measurement of the height of a mountain done between 1020 and 1025 AD while traveling with Sultan Mahmoud in northwest India in a place called Nanda in modern Pakistan (Al-Khalili, 2011).

In his definitive "Introduction to the History of Science," the historian George Sarton defined the first half of the eleventh century as the "age of Al-Biruni" (Al-Khalili, 2011).

AL-TABARI, ABU HASAN AHMAD IBN MUHAMMAD (932–976 AD)

Not very much has been written about Al-Tabari. He was a private physician to Prince Rukn Al-Dawlah (Haddad, 2003).

Al-Tabari was born in Tabaristan (hence the name Tabari). He moved among the towns of Al-Rayy, Hamadan, and Asfahan. He served Caliph Al-Radi's representative in Al-Ahwaz, then Al-Radi's Vezier, before becoming the personal physician of Rukn Al-Dawla Al-Buweihi (Al-Samerra'i, 1989).

He classified physicians into two categories: philosopher physicians and non-philosopher physicians. According to his classification, philosopher physicians' interest extends into the understanding of pathophysiology and causation of disease. The non-philosopher physicians' interest, in contrast, is in diagnosis and treatment of disease (Al-Mahi, 1959).

SCHOLARSHIP

Mu'alajat Abuqratiyya (Hippocratic Treatments)

As the title of the book suggests, this is a book on diseases and the remedies used by Hippocrates to treat them (Haddad, 2003), which non-philosopher physicians need to know (Al-Mahi, 1959). The book is in ten sections (Al-Samerra'i, 1989; Haddad, 2003):

The first section, of fifty chapters, deals with general topics necessary for the non-philosopher physician to know.

The second section, of thirty-five chapters, deals with skin diseases of the face.

The third section, of forty-three chapters, deals with diseases of internal organs.

The fourth section, of fifty-four chapters, deals with structure and diseases of the eye.

The fifth section, of thirty-three chapters, deals with diseases of the nose and ears.

The sixth section, of fifty-eight chapters, deals with diseases of the mouth, teeth, tongue, throat, and neck.

The seventh section, of sixty chapters, deals with skin disorders.

The eighth section, of thirty-three sections, deals with diseases of the chest, lung, heart, and respiratory pathways.

The ninth section, of fifty-two chapters, deals with diseases of the stomach.

The tenth and last section, of forty-nine sections, deals with diseases of the liver, spleen, and intestines.

A special section of the book is devoted to diseases of children. It is considered one of the first books, if not the first book, in Arabic devoted to childhood diseases, although Ibn Rubn Al-Tabari and Al-Razi before him wrote in detail on the subject (Al-Samerra'i, 1989). The section on pediatrics includes chapters on skin diseases, including scabies, epilepsy, crying in children, and intestinal worms, among many others (Al-Samerra'i, 1989).

The book is considered equivalent in value to that of Ali ibn Sahl Rabbani al-Tabari (Firdous Al Hikma).

AL-KINDI (AL- KINDES), YAQUB IBN ISHAQ (ABU YOUSEF) (801–866 or 873 AD)

Al-Kindi was a descendent of the rich Al-Kindi royal family from Kufa in present-day Iraq (Myers, 1964; Al-Samerra'i, 1989; Haddad, 2003; Freely, 2011). His father, Ishaq Ibn Al-Sabbah, was ruler (Amir) of Kufa (Ibn Abi Usaibiah, 1245/46; Al-Samerra'i, 1989).

Yaqub was born in either Basra or Wasit. He moved to Baghdad, where he studied philosophy, astrology, engineering, and medicine, as well as played music (Al-Samerrai, 1989). Of all his specialties, he excelled in philosophy and is referred to as "Philosopher of Islam" (Al-Samerra'i, 1989). In Baghdad, he founded his own intellectual circle of translators, writers, and teachers (Freely, 2011). Al-Kindi along with Hunayn Ibn Ishaq and Thabet Ibn Qurra were considered among the best translators to Arabic language (Al-Samerra'i, 1989; Freely, 2011).

He was a philosopher, physician, music theorist, mathematician, astrologist, geographer, and astronomer (Ibn Abi Usiabiah, 1245/46; Myers, 1964; Al-Samerra'i, 1989; Haddad, 2003). He was highly regarded by Caliph Al-Mamoun and his successor, Al-Mu'tasim, to whom Al-Kindi dedicated most of his books (Ibn Abi Saibai, 1245/46; Myers, 1964; Al-Samerra'i, 1989; Haddad, 2003; Freely, 2011; Al-Khalil, 2011). Because of his interest and excellence in astrology and astronomy, he was appointed the chief astrologer for the caliph. Although a qualified physician, he did not actively practice medicine but devoted his knowledge to teaching and writing books in medicine (Al-Samerra'i, 1989).

Caliph Al-Mu'tasim and his son Al-Wathiq reigned for only nine and five years, respectively. They were followed by Al-Wathiq's younger brother Al-Mutawakkil, who showed little interest in science in favor of a literalist interpretation of the Quran and Hadith. Al-Mutawakkil started a backlash against freethinking and liberal theologists like Al-Kindi, who fell victim to a conspiracy led by the powerful Bani Musa brothers, who felt jealous of Al-Kindi's extensive library and persuaded the caliph to expel him. Al-Kindi was expelled, physically beaten, imprisoned, and his library confiscated and its contents granted to the Bani Musa brothers (Al-Khalili, 2011). He was released when the caliph fell sick and needed his skills (Al-Samerra'i, 1989), and although his library was restored to him, Al-Kindi lived his remaining years a lonely man (Al-Khalili, 2011).

According to his contemporary, the satirist Al-Jahiz, Al-Kindi was a miser. In his "Book of Misers," Al-Jahiz said that Al-Kindi, though rich, rented rooms in his house to lodgers, and he told a story about a tenent family of six who asked Al-Kindi if two of their relatives could stay with them for a month. Al-Kindi demanded an extra amount of rent for the additional lodgers (Freely, 2011).

In his will to his children, Al-Kindi is reported to have written, "The father is god, the brother is a trap, the paternal uncle is gloom, the maternal uncle is a curse, the son is grief, relatives are scorpions, saying 'no' deflects problems, saying 'yes' deprives of wealth." The wording of the will was interpreted as confirming that he was a miser (Al-Samerra'i, 1989).

SCHOLARSHIP

According to Ibn Al-Nadim, Al-Kindi contributed over 250 scholarly works on mathematics, physics, astrology, mineralogy, zoology, metallurgy, cryptology, politics, theology, alchemy, meteorology, optics, cosmology, geography, music, philosophy, logic, pharmacology, and medicine. Only about 10 percent of his works have survived (Al-Samerra'i, 1989; Freely, 2011). Twenty-two of his publications are in medicine, twenty-six in astrology, and four books were on the use of Hindu numbers (Al-Mahi, 1959; Myers, 1964; Al-Samerra'i, 1989; Goodman, 2003).

Al-Kindi integrated the Greek word "philosophy" with the Arabic word "Falsafa" and defined it as "the knowledge of things as they are in reality." He considered that truth is universal and supreme, thus religion and truth are two versions of truth and are in harmony (Tarabay, 2011). Al-Kindi's most astonishing work was the explanation of Aristotle's six volume book on logic, the "Organon" (Tarabay, 2011).

Al-Kindi was the first Muslim to write on music. He based his musical system on Greek musical theories, including the use of letters of the alphabet to designate the notes of the scale, a system that was adopted a century later in Europe (Myers, 1964; Freely, 2011).

Al-Kindi's theory of light transmission is based on that of Euclid, which suggests that visual images are created by rays transmitted from the eye to the external object (Freely, 2011). This theory was later proved erroneous by the work of Ibn Al-Haytham. His work on visual perception and light reflection was the basis for the laws of perspective developed during the European Renaissance (Freely, 2011).

Al-Kindi tried to explain the reason why the sky is blue. He explained it as the mixture of the darkness of the sky with the reflection of light on particles of dust and vapor in the air, which created the blue color (Tarabay, 2011).

He was considered by Geronimo Cardone (Stalin's physician and mathematician) as one of the twelve great minds of history (Myers, 1964).

On First Philosophy

This is the largest of Al-Kindi's extant work. It is an homage to earlier philosophers, such as Aristotle. The work was dedicated to Caliph Al-Mu'tasim (Freely, 2011).

De Apecticus

This is a manual on ancient Greek optics. This book and "On Burning Mirrors" were translated into Latin in the twelfth century (Freely, 2011).

On Burning Mirrors

The Efficient Cause of the Flow and Ebb

In this book, Al-Kindi discussed the movement of the tides, assuming that it depends on the changes in the bodies due to the rise and fall of the temperature (Tarabay, 2011).

He wrote short treatises on ethics such as (Myers, 1964):

"On Morals"

"On Facilitating the Path to the Virtues"

"On the Government of the Common People"

His medical contributions include:

Risala fi Ashfiyat al-Sumum (On Treatment from Poisons) (Ibn Abi Usaibiah, 1245/46; Al-Samerra'i, 1989)

Risala fi Illat al-Baharrin min al Amrad al- Hadda (On Acute Illnesses of Sea Farers) (Ibn Abi Usaibiah, 1245/46). This Risala may have been attributed to Al-Kindi in error (Al-Samerra'i, 1990).

Risala fi Kayfiyat Al Dimagh (On Structure of the Brain) (Ibn Abi Usaibiah, 1245/46; Al-Samerra'i, 1989)

Risala Fi Illat al- Juzam Wa Ashfiyatuhu (On Leprosy and Its Treatment) (Ibn Abi Usaibiah, 1245/46; Al-Samerrai, 1989)

Risala fi Addat al-Kalb wal-Kalab (On Dog Bites and Rabies) (Ibn Abi Usaibiah, 1245/46; Al-Samerrai, 1989)

Risala fi Waja' al-Mi'da wal-Nokros (On Diseases of the Stomach and Gout) (Ibn Abi Usaibiah, 1245/46; Al-Samerrai, 1989)

Risala fi Aqsam al- Himiyyat (On Classifications of Fevers) (Ibn Abi Usaibiah, 1245/46; Al-Samerra'i, 1989)

Risala fi Ilaj al-Tuhal (On Treatment of the Spleen) (Ibn Abi Usaibiah, 1245/46; Al-Samerrai, 1989)

Ikhtibarat Abi Yusif Al-Kindi fil Adwiyah Al Mumtahana (Experience of Al-Kindi in Tested Medicines)

The material in this book was used by Al-Razi in his book "Al-Hawi." The book was translated into Latin by Gerard of Cremona and printed in Strasburg in 1531 AD. It was also translated into English by Martin Levy in 1966 and published in Arabic with an introduction on simple and compound drugs used by Arab physicians (Ibn Abi Usaibiah, 1245/46; Al-Samerrai, 1989).

Risala fi Ma'rifat Quwa al Adwiya al Murakkaba (On Knowledge of Strength of Compound Drugs) (Al-Samerra'i, 1989)

Risala fil At'ima (On Food) (Al-Samerra'i, 1989)

Risala fil Hammam (On Bathing) (Al-Samerra'i, 1989)

Risala fil Hayat (On Living) (Al-Samerra'i, 1989)

Risala fil Lathga (On Snake Bites) (Al-Samerra'i, 1989)

Risala fi Tibyan Al-A'da' Al-Ra'isiyya fi Gism al-Insan (On the Major Organs in the Human) (Al-Samerra'i, 1989)

Risala fil Ghitha' wa al-Dawa' al-Muhlik (On Food and Fatal Drugs) (Al-Samerra'i, 1989)

Kitab fil Tibb al-Ruhani (Book on Spiritual Treatments) (Al-Samerra'i, 1989)

The book discussed nonmedical treatments used at the time (Al-Samerra'i, 1989)

Risala fil Adwiyah al-Mushila (On Laxative Drugs)

The material in the book was the source on the subject in Al-Razi's book "Al-Hawi" (Al-Samerra'i, 1989).

IBN SAHL, ABU SA'D AL-ALA' (1212-1251)

He was far less known than his contemporaries in tenth-century Baghdad, but he would advance the subject of optics in a way that has until recently been almost completely ignored (Al-Khalili, 2011).

The work of Ibn Sahl is regarded as the first serious mathematical study of lenses for focusing light (Al-Khalili, 2011).

Ibn Sahl is credited with writing a treatise between 983 and 985 titled "A Proof of the Fact that the Celestial Sphere Is Not Perfectly Transparent," in which he correctly stated the law of refraction, which was not discovered in Europe until the seventeenth century (Freely, 2011).

Manuscript pages were discovered in the early 1990s in two separate places, Damascus and Tehran. The two components of the book were put together by the historian Roshdi Rashed, who reconstructed the full original text. The insight in this book is what students at schools call Snell's law of refraction, when, actually, Ibn Sahl arrived at the same results 650 years earlier (Al-Khalili, 2011).

IBN HINDU, ALI IBN AL- HUSAYN IBN HASAN (ABU AL-FARAJ) (d. 1019AD)

Ibn Hindu was born in the city of Qum in Hindujan, Persia; hence he was referred to as "Ibn Hindu" and "Al-Qummi." From Qum, he moved, in 953 AD, to the city of Rayy near Tehran, where he stayed for thirteen years. From Rayy he moved to Baghdad to study medicine under the famous physician Abu Al-Khayr Al-Khammar (Sheik Abi Al- Khair Al-Hasan Ibn Siwar Ibn Al-Baba) and philosophy under Abu Al-Hasan Al-'Amiri. He flourished during the second half of the tenth century and became a well-known medical scholar, philosopher, skillful calligrapher, and poet (Ibn Abi Usaibiah, 1245/46; Farhadi, 1989; Kaadan, 2003; Nasser, 2007).

In 990 AD, he left Baghdad for the city of Naishapur in Persia, where he served in the court of Shams Al-Maa'li Qabous, and he stayed until 1000 AD. During his service in the court, he met the physician and philosopher Al-Biruni (see below) (Kaadan, 2003). He died in 1019/1020 AD and was buried in his own home in Gorganj (Farhadi, 1989).

Ibn Hindu was especially known for his teaching ability. Students came from different parts of Persia to attend his lectures. He taught them medicine, philosophy, letters, and poetry. His lectures and writings were characterized by a clear style (Farhadi, 1989; Nasser, 2007).

SCHOLARSHIP

Ibn Hindu's scholarship falls in three categories: medicine, philosophy, and literature/letters. In his treatises, he encouraged the study of philosophy and logic (Nasser, 2007). He taught that "knowing logic is most essential to a physician, for it is the art of deduction and proof. A true physician is deductive. Neither theoretical nor applied medicine can be realized except by the use of the art of logic, for it is by this art that true and false in words and deeds can be recognized" (Farhadi, 1989).

Miftah al-Tibb Wa Minhaj al-Tullab (The Science of Medicine and Student Guide)

Of all of Ibn Hindu's books, this one enjoyed the most reputation. Ibn Hindu introduced the book by saying that he wrote the book at the request of his students, who wanted him to write an "easy" reference book about medicine. He explained that the task of the physician is to help his patients gain and maintain health but not until they have learned proper methods for doing this. The book is divided into ten chapters (Farhadi, 1989; Kaadan, 2003; Nasser, 2007).

Chapter 1: On prompting learning in general and of the science of medicine in particular

Chapter 2: On proving the validity of the science of medicine; in the chapter, he argued against those who discredit the science of medicine on the basis of mistakes committed by physicians or the difficulty in becoming a physician

Chapter 3: On the definition of the science of medicine

Chapter 4: On the nobility of the science of medicine

Chapter 5: On the various categories of the science of medicine

Chapter 6: On the various schools of the science of medicine

Chapter 7: On ways and methods by which the science of medicine is understood

Chapter 8: On other sciences that a medical student must know in order to fully develop in his profession; in it, he stated that the student of medicine does not need to master all the branches of philosophy, only those related to medical science

Chapter 9: On the stages the student has to go through in his study of medicine, and the significance of the books written on the subject; in it, he also emphasized the importance of the student of medicine to learn about ethical principles in the practice of medicine

Chapter 10: On the definitions, interpretations, and terminology used in medical sciences; it is made of twelve sections, including on weights, measures, and simple and compound drugs; and it is an important part of the book

Ibn Hindu described medicine as consisting of theoretical and practical components. He divided the theoretical component into three branches:

1. The science of natural phenomena as found in the human body

2. The science of causes

3. The science of symptoms and indications

Causes are then divided into two categories. The first affects the body and includes the surrounding atmosphere, movement and stillness, food and drinks, sleep and wakefulness, diarrhea and constipation, and emotions.

The second category affects the body but can be avoided, such as the sword, lion, fire, and the like (Nasser, 2007).

He made clear that the knowledge of theory must be supported by empirical observation (Nasser, 2007).

In chapter seven, Ibn Hindu suggested that the science of medicine is learned in four main ways (Nasser, 2007):

1. Mere accidental occurrence of events, such as while walking in the fields, a group of boys picked laurel seeds, and one of them tasted some. He was later bitten by a snake and did not suffer symptoms. This was proof of the seeds usefulness as an antidote for poison.

2. Knowledge gained by purposeful experimenting, such as trying several medicines one by one on bodies with different natures, time after time, then assigning to each of the medicines the action that kept recurring by its use. Of the four methods of deriving the science of medicine, this is the one that comes close to the empirical observations that guide treatment decisions nowadays. It is believed that it was by this experimental approach that Ibn Hindu came to the conclusion that music could play a useful role in treatment. Quoting from his book: "There is a certain way of singing a tune or performing on the drum and flute which arouses sadness, another which brings joy, one relaxing and captivating, another disturbing, one which keeps one awake, another which induces sleep...."

3. Knowledge arrived at through dreams, the effect of mind over body, such as when patients are told in a dream to take a certain drug, and after waking up, they take the drug and are cured.

4. Knowledge gained by observing animals. This method, as suggested by Ibn Hindu, is different from the current science of animal research. He illustrated this concept by the use of saltwater to treat colics based on observations of a long-beaked bird that used saltwater to treat its colic.

Ibn Hindu stated that the above four methods of deriving medical knowledge can be strengthened through reason and the application of analogy and logic (Farhadi, 1989; Nasser, 2007).

Thus, over one thousand years ago, Ibn Hindu suggested that physicians must utilize designed experiments to support logic and theory in their pursuit of medical knowledge (Nasser, 2007).

As for the quality of gradual learning of medical sciences and the order of studying medical books, Ibn Hindu suggested the following (Farhadi, 1989):

Subjects that are inherently antecedent are to be studied first, such as elements followed by humors, mucus, and limbs.

Subjects that are more basic are to be studied first, such as starting with anatomy, followed by the sciences of humors and elements in this order.

Subjects that are learned more readily should be taught first.

At the end of the book, Ibn Hindu emphasized that a student should learn some ethics so that he may cleanse his own soul from impurities and prepare it for admission and acceptance of excellence.

Towards the very end of the book, Ibn Hindu said, "Anyone who wants to learn a trade or industry needs to learn the terminology developed for it. Since medicine has much in common with philosophy, and as logic is the instrument for philosophy and for any other science, it is proper that we first mention in our books logical and philosophical terms and expressions and then relate the terms that are strictly the business of medical sciences" (Farhadi, 1989).

The book was published in Tehran, Iran, in 1989 (kaadan, 2003).

Kitab al-Shafi (The Book of Healing)

This is a detailed book on medicine (Kaadan, 2003).

Maqala fil Farq

In this article, Ibn Hindu compared the pros and cons of the three schools of learning medicine (Kaadan, 2003).

Kitab al-Kilam al-Ruhaniyyah min al-Hikmah al-Yunaniyyah (Book of Quotes from Greek Wisdom)

This is a book on philosophy in which he contradicted the views of Ibn Sina on the soul (Kaadan, 2003)

IBN HINDU THE POET

Ibn Hindu wrote poems on love, praise, and satire. He was described by some as the prince of poetry (Kaadan, 2003).

IBN AL-HAYTHAM (ALHAZEN), ABU 'ALI MOHAMMAD IBN AL-HASAN (965–1039/1041 AD)

Ibn Al-Haytham was a distinguished physician, mathematician, astronomer, philosopher, and physicist (Masoud, 2006). To some (Al-Khalili, 2011), he was the greatest physicist since Archimedes and the like of which would not be seen until Isaac Newton seven hundred years later. Although well versed in medicine, he did not practice the profession (Ibn Abi Usaibiah, 1245/46; Al-Samerra'i, 1990).

LIFE AND CAREER:

The best and most exhaustive records of Ibn Al-Haytham's life and career are to be found in two biographies, written by Jamal Al-Din Ibn Al-Qufti and Ibn Abi Usaibiah some two centuries after his death (Freely, 2011). Ibn Al-Haytham was born in Basra (hence sometime called "Al-Basri") in southern Iraq in 965 AD, and there he had his early education. The name "Al-Haytham" was his grandfather's name, so in fact, he was ibn Al-Haytham (Gorini, 2003; Al-Khalili, 2011; Tarabay, 2011). His Latinized name, "Al-Hazen," came from his first name, "Al-Hasan," or "Al-Hacen" (Gorini, 2003; Al-Khalili, 2011). In Medieval Latin texts, he was referred to as "Avenatan" and "Avennathan" (Gorini, 2003). He was also known by the name "Al-Misri" in relation to "Misr" (Egypt) (Gorini, 2003).

In Basra, Ibn Al-Haytham received an excellent education, which suggests that his family was financially secure and moved in the right political and social circuits (Al-Khalili, 2011). His father was a civil servant (Gorini, 2003).

He was given a government post in Basra before taking up science and philosophy (Ibn Abi Usaibiah, 1245/46; Al-Samerra'i, 1990; Whitaker, 2004; Freely, 2011). He was offered highly prestigious positions in government by the Abbasid caliph Al-Ta'ih but preferred to devote his time to intellectual pursuits and scientific research (Al-Khalili, 2011). He faked mental illness to get out of the government jobs (Al-Samerra'i, 1990).

The munifecence of Fatimid Caliph Al-Hakim bi Amr Allah to scholars and scientists attracted him to Cairo (Gorini, 2003). He went to Cairo around 1010 AD during the reign of Fatimid Caliph Al-Hakim bi Amr Allah. In Cairo, he lived at the Al-Azhar mosque and supported himself from sales of his translations of Greek books. He wrote an interesting treatise on an ambitious civil engineering project in which he claimed that he could build a dam across the Nile that would control its flow and alleviate the problems of floods and droughts. News of his work reached the young ruler of Fatimid Egypt, Caliph Al-Hakim bi Amr Allah, who charged him with the project. After visiting the site of the project (present-day Aswan Dam), Ibn Al-Haytham discovered that it was an impossible task (Al-Samerra'i, 1990; Al-Khalili, 2011; Freely, 2011; Tarabay, 2011). Out of fear of the caliph's revenge (Caliph Al-Hakim was notorious for being bloodthirsty and known to have executed many of his adversaries), Ibn Al-Haytham again faked mental illness and was confined to a mental asylum under the custody of Al-Hakim's sister Sitt Al-Mulk, who was accused of killing her brother few years later (Tarabay, 2011). After the caliph's death in 1021, the new caliph, Al-Zaher, released him from confinement (Al-Samerra'i, 1990; Whitaker, 2009; Freely, 2011). He then spent the rest of his life in Cairo in an apartment near al-Azhar mosque as a recluse in search of the truth, to gain God's favor. It was at this period of his life that he produced the bulk of his scholarship (Ibn Abi Usaibiah, 1245/46; Al-Samerra'i, 1990; Al-Khalili, 2011; Freely, 2011).

SCHOLARSHIP

According to Ibn Abi Usaibiah, Ibn Al-Haytham's scholarly contributions consist of ninety-two titles, twenty-five of which deal with mathematics, twenty-four with natural science, several articles with astronomy, and only three in medicine (Al-Samerra'i, 1990). Fifty-five of his works are extant, including those on mathematics, optics, and astronomy (Freely, 2011). Other contributions of Ibn Al-Haytham include work on logic, ethics, politics, poetry, music, and theology (Freely, 2011).

Ibn Al-Haytham's most lasting contributions were on light and vision (Al-Samerra'i, 1990; Freely, 2011). Credit goes to Ibn Al-Haytham for having the greatest knowledge of optics in his time (Wakim, 1944; Gorini, 2003). For that, he earned the title of "Father of Modern Optics" (Masoudi, 2006; Tarabay, 2011).

The field of optics was advanced significantly from what the Muslims acquired from Hellenistic scholars with introduction of new methodologies and approaches (Dallal, 2010; Tarabay, 2011). Muslim scholars who contributed to the topic of optics include Yuhanna Ibn Masaweh, Hunayn Ibn Ishaq, Qusta Ibn Luqa, Thabet Ibn Qurra, and Al-Kindi (Dallal, 2010). The creative expansion of optical research reached a peak under Ibn Al-Haytham (Dallal, 2010).

Kitab al-Manazir (Book of Optics)

This book is considered the masterpiece of Ibn Al-Haytham's scholarly work and the most important work ever produced in Islamic science. The book, which established the early scientific method of setting a theory based on observation of recurrent phenomenon, is composed in seven books written between 1028 and 1038 AD (Myers, 1964; Al-Samerra'i, 1990; Gorini, 2003; Masoud, 2006; Al-Khalili, 2011; Freely, 2011; Tarabay, 2011).

In the first book, "On the Matter of Vision in General," Ibn Al-Haytham presented his general theory about light and vision, including his own experiments and observations (chapter 3), and (chapter 5) and described eye structure in detail (Masoud, 2006; Freely, 2011).

Ibn Al-Haytham's "intromission theory" of vision introduced the idea that objects are seen by rays of light emanating from objects and not from the eye, as was believed at the time (Landau, 1959; Skinner, 1961; Masoud, 2006; Freely, 2011; Tarabay, 2011). He began the book of optics thus: "We find that when the eye looks into exceedingly bright lights, it suffers greatly because of them and is injured, for when an observer looks at the body of the sun, he cannot see it well, since his eye suffers pain because of the light..." (Al-Khalili, 2011). "Sight perceives light and color existing on the surface of the contemplated object...vision perceives necessarily all objects through supposed straight lines that spread themselves between the object and the central point of the sight" (Masoud, 2006).

The second book deals with Ibn Al-Haytham's theory of psychology of perception.

The third book, "Errors of Direct Vision and Their Causes," deals with binocular vision.

The fourth and fifth books deal with phenomena involving reflections based on experiments with concave and convex mirrors.

The sixth book deals with perception errors emanating from vision by reflected rays.

The final and seventh book is devoted to dioptics.

In the optics book, Ibn Al-Haytham referred to an earlier work on optics by Abi Said Al-Ala' Ibn Sahl, who wrote a treatise (dated 983–985) on optics titled "A Proof of the Fact the Celestial Sphere Is Not Perfectly Transparent," in which he correctly stated the law of refraction not hitherto known in Europe until the seventeenth century (Freely, 2011).

Ibn Al-Haytham's book "Kitab Al-Manazir" was partly translated into English as "The Optics" (Masoud, 2006) and into Latin in the late twelfth, early thirteenth centuries under the title "De Aspectibus," or "Perspectiva" (Gorini, 2003; Al-Khalili, 2011). The only Latin printed edition of the "Book of Optics" was published by Friedrich Risner in 1572 under the name of "Opticae Thesaurus," which contained, along with Ibn Al-Haytham's "Optics," Witelo's "Perspectiva" and the work of a lesser-known scholar by the name of Ibn Mu'adh, which had been translated into Latin even before any of Ibn Al-Haytham works as "Liber de crepuscules." This short treatise on the nature of dawn and twilight for years was wrongly attributed to Ibn Al-Haytham (Al-Khalili, 2011).

Ibn Al-Haytham's work on optics is believed to have influenced a number of later Western scholars such as John Reckham, whose late-thirteenth-century book on optics is basically taken from Ibn Al-Haytham "Al Manazir"; the Polish contemporary of Roger Bacon, Witelo's "Optics" (Myers 1964 Gorini, 2003; Al-Khalili, 2011); Roger Bacon and Johannes Kepler, whose works on optics represent the beginning of the modern science of optics (Gorini, 2003; Al-Khalili, 2011; Freely, 2011; Tarabay, 2011); as well as the great Italian Leonardo Da Vinci (Tarabay, 2011).

In spite of his work on optics, Ibn Al-Haytham did not appreciate the importance of the lens (Whitaker, 2004).

Until Ibn Al-Haytham, scholars' understanding of how vision works was a confused mess (Al-Khalili, 2011).

The Greeks had several theories of vision. Euclid and Ptolemy believed in what is called the emission theory, in which we saw optics because rays of light are emitted from our eyes to illuminate them; the rays of light leave the eye in straight lines emanating like a cone (Al-Khalili, 2011; Tarabay, 2011).

An opposing view was held by Aristotle, who argued for an "intromission theory" of vision whereby light enters our eyes from the object we are looking at (Al-Khalili, 2011).

Plato and Galen had a combined intromission/emission theory, whereby the eye sends out rays of light to the object being looked at, and this then reflects the light back into the eye (Al-Khalili, 2011).

The Plato/Galen theory was favored by Islamic scholars like Al-Kindi and Hunayn Ibn Ishaq (Al-Khalili, 2011).

Ibn Al-Haytham also helped clarify a famous optical effect known today as "moon illusion." It is the phenomenon in which the moon appears larger near the horizon than it does when higher up in the sky. Before Ibn Al-Haytham's clarification, no one had realized it was an illusion (Al-Khalili, 2011).

The first three volumes of the Book of Optics contain ideas on the psychology of perception, and it was here that Ibn Al-Haytham dismissed the Greeks' idea that the moon appears larger when it is low in the sky because of the refraction of its light through the atmosphere, and presented his theory of optical illusion (Al-Khalili, 2011).

Kitab Taqweem al-Sina'a al-Tibbiya (Book on evaluation of the medical profession)

In this book, Ibn al-Haytham included what he learned from reading Galen's books (Al-Samerra'i, 1990).

Maqala fi Sharh Qanoun Ibn Sina (Article on Explanation of the Canon of Avicenna)

Kitab al-Adwiya al-Mufrada (Book on Simple Drugs)

In addition to optics and medicine, Ibn Al-Haytham contributed the following scholarly works (Ibn Abi Usaibiah, 1245/46; Myers, 1964; Freely, 2011):

Treatise on the Light of the Moon

Treatise on the Rainbow and Halo

Treatise on the Appearance of the Stars "Kitab al-Bari fi Ahkam al-Nujum," translated into Latin by Judah Ben Moses

Treatise on Spherical Burning Mirrors

Treatise on the Quality of Shadows

Treatise on the Light of the Stars

Treatise on the Marks on the Surface of the Moon

Discourse on Light

Discourse on the Burning Sphere

Treatise on the Form of Eclipse

Treatise on Paraboloidal Burning Mirrors

Besides his works on optics, Ibn Al-Haytham wrote twenty-five works on astronomy, which is twice the number he wrote on optics (Al-Khalili, 2011; Freely, 2011), including his most popular:

"Fi Hayat al-'Alam" (On the Configuration of the World), which was translated into Spanish (Castilian) by Abraham of Toledo, and later into Latin, and by Jacob Ibn Maher and Solomon Ibn Pahar into Hebrew (Myesr, 1964; Freely, 2011).

The Model of Motions of Each of the Seven Planets

This work came in three books and outlined a new theory of planetary motion far in advance of anything Ptolemy had written. Modern historians of science now regard it as monumental and cutting-edge science for the time (Al-Khalili, 2011).

Al-Shukuk Ala Batlamyus (Dubitationes in Ptolemaeum) in which he critiqued three of the writings of Ptolemy: Almagest, planetary hypotheses, and optics (Myers, 1964; Al-Khalili, 2011; Freely, 2011)

Among the mathematical problems he explored was the squaring of the circle (Whitaker, 2004).

Ibn Al-Haytham valued meticulous experimentation and careful recording of results. For this reason, a number of historians have referred to him as the first scientist (Al-Khalili, 2011).

Ibn Al-Haytham's approach to learning and investigations is reflected in the following narrative attributed to him (Al-Khalili, 2011): "The seeker after truth is not one who studies the writings of the ancients and, following the natural disposition, puts his trust in them, but rather the one who suspects his faith in them and questions what he gathers from them ,the one who submits to argument and demonstration and not the sayings of human beings whose nature is fraught with all kinds of imperfection and deficiency. Thus the duty of the the man who investigates the writings of scientists, if learning the truth is his goal, is to make himself an enemy of all that he reads and, applying his mind to the core and margins of the content, attack it from every side. He should also suspect himself as he performs his critical examination of it, so that he may avoid falling into either prejudice or leniency."

As a proof of the relevance of his scholarship, there is on the moon, near the east margin of the Mare Crisium, a crater called "Alhazen" (Gorini, 2003).

AL-QAMARI, ABU MANSUR AL-HASAN IBN NOUH

Al-Qamari was a contemporary and mentor of Avicenna. He was in his later years when Avicenna matriculated with him and learned from him. Al-Qamari was highly respected for his knowledge, particularly so with royals of his time (Ibn Abi Usaibiah, 1245/46; Haddad, 2003).

SCHOLARSHIP

He was the author of an unpublished manuscript "Ghina and Muna" (Wealth and Wishes), which is a collection of sayings by Hippocrates,

Galen, and especially Al-Razi, among others, about diseases and their treatments (Ibn Abi Usaibiah, 1245/46); Haddad, 2003).

AL-MASIHI AL-JURJANI, ABU SAHL ISA IBN YAHYA

Al-Masihi was a Christian physician and a contemporary and mentor of Avicenna. He practiced in Khorasan and was respected by its rulers for his acumen and knowledge in the science and practice of medicine. It is said that Avicenna classified some of Al-Masihi's books and claimed authorship. Al-Masihi died at an early age of forty (Ibn Abi Usaibiah, 1245/46).

SCHOLARSHIP

Kitab Izhar Hikmat Allah fi Khalq al-Insan (Book on the Wisdom of God in His Creation of Man)

This book is considered one of the best books of Al-Masihi. It contains information from Galen's books about the body and organs with additions from his (Al-Masihi) experience. In the introduction to the book, Al-Masihi stated, "To appreciate this work one ought to be fully familiar with both Galen's and our work. Otherwise, one is not qualified to make judgment. What we did in this work is to correct what they said, organize it, complete it, and update it" (Ibn Abi Usaibiah, 1245/46).

Kitab al-Miah fil Tibb (Book on Hundred Items in Medicine)

This book was described by Amin Al-Dawlah Ibn Al-Tilmidh (see under Ibn Al-Tilmidh) as very clear in presentation, containing plenty of facts and little repetition (Ibn Abi Usaibiah, 1245/46).

Kitab al-Tibb al-Kulli (Comprehensive Book of Medicine) (Ibn Abi Usaibiah, 1245/46)

Kitab fil Waba' (Book on Infections)

This book was written for King Al-Adel Khwarizm Shah Abi Al-Abbas Mamoun Ibn Mamoun (Ibn Abi Usaibiah, 1245/46).

IBN SINA (AVICENNA), ABU 'ALI AL-HUSAYN IBN ABDAL-LAH IBN HASAN IBN ALI (980–1037 AD; 937–1037 AD)

SYNONYMS: (Krueger, 1963; Al-Samerra'i, 1989; Athar, 1993; Khan, 2006):

Ash-Shaykhu Rais (Chief Master, Chief of the Wise)

Al-Muallimu El-Thani (Second Teacher), the first teacher being Aristotle, or Galen, and some say Prophet Muhammad, but most agree that it refers to Aristotle

Al-Muallimu El-Thalith (Third Teacher), after Aristotle and Al-Farabi

Faylasouf Al-Islam (Philosopher of Islam)

Other synonyms for Ibn Sina include Prince of Physicians, Chief of Chiefs, the Chief of Lords, Prince of Scholars, Prince of Science, and the teacher par excellence (Kreuger, 1963; Campbell, 2011).

The elder of two sons, Ibn Sina was born in august 980 AD (month of Safar of AH 370), date being uncertain , between 979 and 985 AD (Krueger, 1963) and 937 (Campbell, 2011) into a Persian family in the village of Kharmaithan (land of the sun), near Bukhara in present-day Uzbekistan in Central Asia. Through the Europeanized Hebrew (Aven Sina) transliteration, he acquired the name "Avicenna" (Afnan, 1958; Krueger, 1963; Al-Samerra'i, 1989; Tarabay, 2011; Abu-Asab, 2013).

Ibn Sina enjoyed a privileged upbringing, being the son of politically influential parents who were part of the ruling Samanid elite (Al-Khalili, 2011; Tarabay, 2011).

His father, Abdullah, a tax collector, was from Balkh (Bactra in Greek, home of the Bactrian camel, in today's northern Afghanistan) and of

Persian Ismaili origin (Abu-Asab, 2013), and his mother, Sittara ("star," in Persian), from the village of Afshenah, was also of Persian origin. By the time of Ibn Sina's birth, Central Asia had been under Muslim rule for nearly one hundred years. His father (Abdullah) was the governor of Kharmaithan, near Bukhara (Afnan, 1958; Krueger, 1963; Al-Samerra'i, 1989; Athar, 1993; Khan, 2006; Tarabay, 2011). Ibn Sina moved to Bukhara, the permanent residence of his father, when he was five years, and that was where his formative years began (Afnan, 1958; Krueger, 1963; Abu-Asab, 2013). Upon reaching adult age, Ibn Sina converted to Twelve Shiite sect of Islam (Tarabay, 2011).

His early education included learning Arabic to be able to read the Quran, which he was able to recite from memory by the age of ten (Ibn Abi Usaibiah, 1245/46; Wakim, 1944; Afnan, 1958; Landau, 1959; Krueger, 1963; Al-Samerra'i, 1989; Athar, 1993; Tschanz, 2003; Khan, 2006; Campbell, 2011; Abu-Asab, 2013), followed by learning Islamic law (Sharia) and jurisprudence (Fiqh) under Ismail Al-Zahid (Ibn Abi Usaibiah, 1245/46) in addition to Arabic grammer, poetry, and literature (Khan, 2006). The next step in his education was learning the Hadith, the sayings of the prophet (Khan, 2006).

According to his memoirs, "Life of Ibn Sina" (Ibn Abi Usaibiah, 1245/46; Al-Samerra'i, 1989; Khan, 2006; Freely, 2011; Al-Khalili, 2011; Abu-Asab, 2013), which he dictated to his student Abd Al-Wahid Al-Juzjani, he said, "I was out under teachers of the Quran and letters. By the time I was ten, I had mastered the Quran and a great deal of literature, so that I was marveled for my aptitudes." He then learned mathematical methods, including the decimal system and the concept of zero from an Indian grocer recruited by his father for this purpose (Ibn Abi Usaibiah, 1245/46; Krueger, 1963; Khan, 2006; Freely, 2011). Under the tutelage of a resident tutor, Abu Abdallah Al-Natili (Nateli; Al-Natheli), a leading philosopher of his time, he learned Greek philosophical work, including Aristotle's "Organon," Euclid's "Elements," and Ptolemy's "Almagest" (Ibn Abi Usaibiah, 1245/46; Afnan, 1958; Krueger, 1963; Al-Samerra'i, 1989; Khan, 2006; Freely, 2011; Abu-Asab, 2013). Referring to this period of his training, Ibn Sina said in his memoirs, "Al-Natili was extremely amazed at me; whatever problem he posed, I conceptualized better than he, so he advised my father against my taking up any occupation other than learning" (Ibn Abi Usaibiah, 1245/46; Al-Samerra'i, 1989; Khan, 2006; Al-Khalili, 2011). Al-Natili's approach to teaching was to walk Ibn Sina through the first few theorems and leave him to read the rest himself. In his memoirs, Ibn Sina commented on this approach of learning "such autonomy is the mark of truth. Teaching provides only a hint of the problem, which the real intelligence solves for itself" (Khan, 2006). When Al-Natili left Bukhara, Ibn Sina, on his own, immersed himself in the study of philosophy and theology, he read Aristotle's "Enneads" forty times and memorized it but was unable to understand it until he read Al-Farabi's "On the Purpose of the Metaphysics," which he bought reluctantly from a persistent bookseller in the souk who sold him the book at a great discount (Ibn Abi Usaibiah, 1245/46; Afnan, 1958; Krueger, 1963; Al-Samerra'i, 1989; Khan, 2006; Abu-Asab, 2013). He solved philosophical problems through hard work and prayers, strengthened by wine (Afnan, 1958; Krueger, 1963).

He then embarked on the study of medicine when he was sixteen. He matriculated under a famous physician, Abu Mansour Al-Hasan Ibn Nouh Al-Qamari. Al-Qamari was a master of the specialty in his time and author of "Ghina Wa Muna" (Wealth and Desire), which was not published. Several handwritten copies of the book are, however, available. The book is a collection of the sayings of the ancients such as Hippocrates, Galen, and Al-Razi, among others (Haddad, 2003; Tschanz, 2003). Writing about his medical education in his memoirs, Ibn Sina said, "Next I desired to study medicine and proceeded to read all the books that had been written on the subject. Medicine is not a difficult science, and naturally I excelled in it at a very short time, so that qualified physicians began to read medicine with me" (Ibn Abi Usaibiah, 1245/46; Al-Samerra'i, 1989; Dunn, 1997; Khan, 2006; Al-Khalili, 2011; Abu-Asab, 2013). At the age of eighteen or nineteen, his reputation as a physician was such that he was called upon to attend to illnesses of rulers (Athar, 1993; Khan, 2006; Freely, 2011). Such a ruler was Nuh Ibn Mansur (978–1002), the Samanid Sultan of Bukhara, who summoned him in 998 AD to treat an illness that court physicians had failed to cure (Ibn Abi Usaibiah, 1245/46; Wakim, 1944; Afnan, 1958; Krueger, 1963; Al-Samerra'i, 1989; Khan, 2006; Al-Khalili, 2011; Freely, 2011; Tarabay, 2011; Abu-Asab, 2013). Upon his recovery and in gratitude, the sultan appointed Ibn Sina court physician and allowed him free access to the library of the Samanid ruler (a mansion with many chambers, each devoted to a special subject, with chest upon chest of a huge collection of books of the ancients that Ibn Sina had not yet seen) (Ibn Abi Usaibiah, 1245/46; Wakim, 1944; Afnan, 1958; Krueger, 1963; Al-Samerrai, 1989; Khan, 2006; Al-Khalili, 2011; Freely, 2011; Tarabay, 2011; Abu-Asab, 2013). In a short time, Ibn Sina had made his way through the library's storehouse of knowledge. Shortly after that (in 999 AD), the library was destroyed in a fire. Ibn Sina's detractors accused him of setting the blaze so that he could attribute the contents to himself (Afnan, 1958; Krueger, 1963; Al-Samerra'i, 1989; Khan, 2006).

While in Bukara, Ibn Sina, twenty-one at the time, started his first attempt at authorship and completed "Al-Majmu'" (Compendium) in response to a request from a certain prosodist (Afnan, 1958). Next, in response to a request from a neighbor who was interested in jurisprudence, he wrote the twenty-volume "Al-Hasil Wa Al-Mahsul" (The Import and the Substance) and a work on ethics, "Al-Birr Wal-Ithm"(Good Work and Evil), of which he never made copies but presented it to his friend in the original (Afnan, 1958; Krueger, 1963).

Upon the death of his father, when Ibn Sina was twenty-one, his life changed: "My father died and my circumstances changed" (Afnan, 1958). He became involved in the service of a succession of princes that necessitated constant travel for the rest of his life (Freely, 2011).

He left Bukhara and went to Gorgan, a large and flourishing city along the banks of the Oxus, to gain income (Afnan, 1958, Krueger, 1963; Abu-Asab, 2013). Soon, however, and for unknown reasons, he left the city (Krueger, 1963).

For the following few years, Ibn Sina's travels took him to Fasa, Baward, Tus, Shaqqan, Samanqan, Jajarm, and then to Gorgan (Afnan, 1958; Kruger, 1963). There is no record that he entered Baghdad or any other Arab capital (Al-Samerra'i, 1989). In spite of that, he spoke Arabic fluently and wrote all his books in the Arabic language, except his book on "pulse," which he wrote in Persian (Al-Samerra'i, 1989).

While in Gorgan, he was in the service of Abu Muhammad Al-Shirazi, for whom he wrote a treatise, "The Provenance and Destination" (Freely, 2011). It was in Gorgan that he met Abd Al-Wahid Juzjani, his future bi-ographer, and when Ibn Sina started working on his famous book Kitab "Al-Qanoun fil Tibb"(The Canon of Medicine), which he finished later when in Asfahan (Krueger, 1963; Abu-Asab, 2013). Ibn Sina was very well received in Gorgan. A man who loved science bought him a house next to his own. Juzjani used to visit him every day to read the Almagest with him. He dictated a book on the subject of logic, "Al-Mukhtasar Al-Awsat" (The Middle Summary). He also wrote others, among them "Al-Mabda' Wal-Ma'ad" (The Beginning and the Return), "Al-Arsad Al-Kulliya" (The General Observations), and "Mukhtasar Al-Majisti" (Summary of al-Magest) (Afnan, 1958).

Avicenna and Juzjani then moved to Rayy (ancient Ragha, about five miles from present-day Tehran) (Afnan, 1958; Tarabay, 2011), where he was welcomed by Princess Al-Sayyida (the Lady) and her son, Buyid Amir (Prince) Majd Al-Dawlah, still a child, and whom he treated for melank-holia (Afnan, 1958; Krueger, 1963; Freely, 2011). Al-Sayyida was a strong and able woman who refused to hand over power to her son when he came of age, so he (the prince) took to the worldly pleasures of the ha-rem and of literature (Afnan, 1958).

In Rayy, Ibn Sina composed "Kitab Al-Maad" (Book of the Return) (Afnan, 1958; Krueger, 1963) and "The State of the Soul" (Freely, 2011). After three years in Rayy, he was asked to leave after dissension between the princess and her son and the siding of Ibn Sina with the legitimate rights of the prince, which infuriated the mother Al-Sayyida (Afnan, 1958;

Krueger, 1963). The city was attacked by Shams Al-Dawlah, brother of Majd Al-Dawlah (Afnan, 1958).

From Rayy, Ibn Sina moved to Qazwin and from there to Hamadan, where he entered the service of Emir Shams Al-Dawlah (brother of his earlier patron, Majd Al-Dawlah), whom he treated successfully for colic. In Hamadan, Ibn Sina began to dabble with politics (Afnan, 1958; Krueger, 1963). He became an emir's intimate and Vezier (minister). When he left the palace, after forty days, he was loaded with gifts (Ibn Abi Usaibiah, 1245/46; Freely, 2011). While in the service of Shams Al-Dawlah, he antagonized the army chiefs, who considered him arrogant. They surrounded his house, imprisoned him, pillaged his belongings, and demanded that he be put to death. The emir refused their demand but compromised by agreeing to send him out of the state (Ibn Abi Usaibiah, 1245/46; Afnan, 1958; Al-Samerra'i, 1989). Ibn Sina went into hiding in a friend's (Sheikh Abi Saad Ibn Dahdouk) house for forty days, after which the emir sent for him to the palace to treat a recurrence of his colic, and reinstated him as a vezier (Ibn Abi Usaibiah, 1245/46; Grueger, 1963; Al-Samerra'i, 1989; Athar, 1993; Tschanz, 2003). The experience that Ibn Sina gained from treating the emir's colic led him to write a book on "Colic" (Athar, 1993; Freely, 2011).

Ibn Sina left Hamadan for Isfahan in disguise, accompanied by his biographer Al-Juzjani, his brother, and two slaves, all dressed as Sufis (Afnan, 1958). In Isfahan, Ibn Sina was welcomed by his friends and courtiers of the ruler Al'a Al-Dawlah (Afnan, 1958). Al'a Al Dawlah arranged for a meeting to be held every Friday evening for learned men of all classes to discuss, with Ibn Sina, scientific and philosophical topics (Afnan, 1958). In Isfahan, Ibn Sina did not involve himself in politics but devoted his time to writing (Afnan, 1958). Under Al'a Al Dawlah's patronage, Ibn Sina composed "Danish-Nameh Ye Ala'i" (Ala'i Book of Knowledge), dedicated to his patron, and finished "Kitab Al-Shifa" (Book of Healing), which he started while in Hamadan, "Kitab Al-Najat"(Book of Deliverance), "Lisan Al-Arab" (Language of the Arabs), and "Kitab Al-Insaf" (Book of Equitable Judgment) (Afnan, 1958; Krueger, 1963).

Following the fall of Rayy to the army of Sultan Mahmud, Al'a Al Dawlah fled Isfahan in the company of Ibn Sina. During the journey, Ibn Sina developed an intractable colic and died while accompanying Al'a Al Dawlah advance to Hamadan, as detailed under (Last Days) below (Krueger, 1963; Al-Samerra'i, 1989).

Ibn Sina also served Ali Bin Maimun, ruler of Khwarizma in the capacity of vezier (minister) (Athar, 1993).

Ibn Sina was fluent in Greek, Latin, Moorish, as well as Arabic, and mastered a wide range of disciplines, including mathematics, physics, metaphysics, astrology, geology, chemistry, anatomy, physiology, pharmacology, toxicology, philosophy, philology, logic, ethics, poetry, and medicine (Wakim, 1944; Dunn, 1997).

In his writings, Ibn Sina was most influenced by Galen's logical writings. Following Galen's tradition, Ibn Sina elaborated a logic of hypotheticals that absorb the stoic theory of signs. This synthesis enabled Ibn Sina to schematize a conditional with multiple antecedents and a common consequent. "If this man has chronic fever, hard cough, labored breathing, shooting pain, and rasping pulse, he has pleurisy." In this, Ibn Sina thus pioneered the diagnosis of specific diseases (Goodman, 2003).

Ibn Sina was a man of great energy. Some authorities state that Ibn Sina demonstrated a mind like Goethe's and possessed a genius similar to Leonardo da Vinci and a dynamic personality with an insatiable desire to acquire knowledge (Krueger, 1963).

His daily schedule began with rising before dawn for prayers, followed by writing for several hours. He then met with his students for a period of study before attending to his duties in the royal court. At noon, he returned home for lunch, usually accompanied by guests. After lunch, he took a brief rest before attending to the ruler in the court. He returned home by sunset for dinner followed by a study session with students, giving lectures, or working on his books. The evenings were reserved for pleasure with friends, wine, women, and music (Ibn Abi Usaibiah, 1245/46;

Grueger, 1963; Al-Samerra'i, 1989; Khan, 2006). He did not hesitate to display publicly his love of music and wine and to share them with those who shared his intellectual pleasures (Afnan, 1958). He never married but was not celibate and is said to have been a man with striking good looks who enjoyed the company of women and more than the odd glass of wine (Al-Khalili, 2011). He was also arrogant and disrespectful of the "lesser mortals" around him and demanded quick wit and perfection from people associated with him (Khan, 2006; Al-Khalili, 2011; Abu-Asab, 2013).

Ibn Sina was at the same time a devout Muslim who sought to reconcile Greek rational science with Muslim beliefs. His love of wine, coffee, music, an active love life, and social schedules provoked consternation in others. Many of his works were against the mainstream of Muslim religious thinking, which led people to accuse him of Kufr (unbelief) (Khan, 2006).

In the course of time, legends and anecdotes gathered around Ibn Sina representing him as a boon companion ready to drown all worries in a cup of wine; a resourceful spirit to invoke in desperate situations; a man of hidden powers able to inflict harm; a physician able to cure illnesses by auto-suggestion; an atheist able to undermine men's faith in a subtle manner; and an abiding mystic who ridiculed life and all its offerings (Afnan, 1958).

SCHOLARSHIP

Like Aristotle in the Hellinistic world, Leonardo da Vinci for the Renaissance, and Goethe for the Germans, Ibn Sina was the flower of medieval Arabic culture and learning (Tschanz, 2003).

Ibn Sina is the best-known scholar of Islam. He made enormous contributions in several fields, including medicine (sixteen works), philosophy, astronomy and physics (eleven works), theology and metaphysics (sixty-eight works), poetry (four works), as well as law, music, geography, and art (Myers, 1964; Athar, 1993; Tschanz, 2003; Khan.2006; Al-Khalili, 2011; Abu Asab, 2013).

Ibn Sina enjoyed popularity among Western philosophers and theologians well into the thirteenth century and beyond (Lyons, 2009). Four references to Ibn Sina are made in Leonardo's notebook (Myers, 1964). Dante placed him in the company of Hippocrates and Galen (Myers, 1964). The sixteenth-century Italian physician Scalinger considered him superior in philosophy to Galen (Myers, 1964). Roger Bacon considered him the chief authority in philosophy after Aristotle (Myers, 1964). Ibn Sina influenced the work of later Christian philosophers such as Thomas Aquinas, who spoke about him with as much respect as that of Plato (Myers, 1964), as well as Rene Descartes and Immanuel Kant (Khan, 2006). There is little in St. Thomas Aquinas's notions of human knowledge that we do not find already in the theories of Ibn Sina (Landau, 1959). Sir William Osler described him as "the author of the most famous medical text-book ever written" (Krueger, 1963), and the "Qanoun fil Tibb" remained the bible of medicine for the longest time (Al-Samerra'i, 1989). He was counted by Dante in "Inferno" among the greatest minds of the non-Christian world (Krueger, 1963).

Although Ibn Sina had the benefit of drawing on Hellenistic, Byzantine, Persian, and Arabic sources for his scholarly output, his medical experience was transcendentally greater than that of Galen (Krueger, 1963).

A lunar crater on the far side of the moon is named after Ibn Sina, the Avicenna Crater (http://en.wikiperdia.org/wiki/Avicenna_crater).

Ibn Sina is credited with writing two hundred books. One hundred of them are well documented as his (Afnan, 1958). Of these, forty-three are on medicine, the best known of which is "Kitab Al-Qanoun fil Tibb" (The Canon), a summary of Greek and Arab medicine, which he wrote in 1020 AD (Menocal, 2002; Al-Kurdi, 2004; Khan, 2006; Al-Khalili, 2011). Ibn Sina is known in the West as the "Prince of Physicians." The system of medicine he created is what we nowadays call "holistic," in which physical and psychological factors, drugs, and diet were combined in treatment of patient (Majeed, 2005). His medical writings aimed to rid medicine of superstition and base it on empirical observations, objectivity, and rationalism (Abu Asab, 2013).

Ibn Sina was a pioneer in the introduction of the concept of evidence-based medicine (EBM). Testing of efficacy of drugs was first promoted by Ibn Sina in his book "The Canon." He laid down a set of rules for the experimental testing and use of drugs that constitute the basis of clinical investigations today (Shoja, 2011).

They were (Shoja, 2011):

1. The drug must be free from any extraneous accidental quality.

2. It must be used on a simple, not a complicated, disease.

3. It should be tested on two contrary types of diseases.

4. The quality of the drug must correspond to the strength of the disease.

5. The time of action must be observed so that essence and accident are not confused.

6. The effect of the drug must be seen to occur constantly.

7. Experimentation must be done on humans.

Although Al-Razi commented on the utility of clinical trials, it was Ibn Sina's detailed definition of evidence-based medicine that was to exert lasting influence (Shoja, 2011).

Kitab Al-Qanoun fil Tibb (The Canon of Medicine)

This book is by far the major contribution of Ibn Sina to medicine. It served as the medical bible for a longer period of time than any other work (Afnan, 1958; Krueger, 1963). It is a comprehensive and organized presentation of medical knowledge of the time up to the tenth century in five volumes, containing more than a million words, dealing with (1) theoretical medicine, (2) simple medicaments, (3) localized diseases and their treatments, (4) generalized diseases, and (5) composition and preparation of drugs (Wakim, 1944; Haddad, 1993). The book contains constant emphasis on prevention of diseases and preservation of health (Tschanz, 2003; Abu-Asab, 2013).

The book's discussions include the use of oral anesthetics, rabies, hydrocele, breast cancer, tumors, labor, and poisons and their treatment. In the book, Ibn Sina differentiated meningitis from meningismus and described chronic nephritis, facial paralysis, ulcer of the stomach, and various causes of hepatitis. He also exposited the dilation and constriction of the pupils and iris and their diagnostic value. He described the six motor muscles of the eye and discussed the function of the tear ducts (Haddad, 1993; Tschanz, 2003).

The book included a description of some 760 medicinal plants and the drugs that could be derived from them. He laid down the basic rules of clinical drug trials that are still followed today. The drug being tested must be pure, must work on all cases of the disease, and its efficacy must correspond to the dose and the strength of the disease. Testing in humans, with careful notation of the drug's effectiveness under different conditions, was the necessary final step (Tschanz, 2003).

The book was described as perhaps the most studied medical work ever written (Ullmann, 2006; Taylor, 2008). Ibn Sina intended to add his own experience to those of his predecessors, but the record of these experiences was lost (Ullmann, 2006).

"The Canon" was such an influential treasure in the history of medicine that Sir William Osler credited it as a "medical bible" and "the most famous medical textbook ever written" (Shoja, 2009).

The Italian sculptor Michelangelo, who studied anatomy, is quoted as saying, "It is better to be mistaken following Avicenna than to be true following others" (Shoja, 2009).

Ibn Sina began the book with the following words: "It is my heart's desire to start with speaking about the general and common principles of both parts of medicine, that is the theory and practice" (Abokrysha, 2009). As the opening definition of "The Canon," Ibn Sina said "Medicine is the science by which the dispositions of the human body are known so that whatever is necessary is removed or healed by it, in order that health should be preserved or, if absent recovered" (Siraisi, 1990). Ibn Sina started writing the book in his thirties, while he was in Gorgan, and some of it in Rayy, and continued working on it as he traveled in different places. It took him a decade to complete. It was completed when he was in Hamadan (Krueger, 1963; Al-Samerra'i, 1989; Freely, 2011). One of the distinctive features of the book is the system of classification used (Afnan, 1958).

Ibn Sina's great concern throughout the book was to provide a system of medicine that can organize the abundance of available facts and explains all encountered phenomena. The masterly organization of the book and Ibn Sina's ability to integrate general principles and single observations gave the work an appeal that made it the authoritative text on medicine for centuries and overshadowed the works of Galen and the Greek physicians (Mujais, 1987).

When the book was published, there were three other comprehensive books in medicine: the oldest was "Firdaws Al-Hikma" by Ibn Ribn Al-Tabari; the second was "Al-Mansuri" by Al-Razi; and the thid was "Kitab Al-Malaki" by Al-Majusi. Al-Qanoun surpassed all three in popularity (Al-Samerra'i, 1989; Al-Khalili, 2011).

Kitab Al-Qanoun may have been the first book after the Bible to be printed using a mechanical printer (Al-Samerra'i, 1989).

The book was first printed in 1473 AD. A translation of book one of "The Canon" appeared in 1930 (Morton, 1997).

The book was translated from Arabic into Latin by Gerard of Cremona in the second-half of the twelfth century, or possibly by Gerard de Sablonita.

This was the first encounter of the West with "The Canon" (Shoja, 2009; Abu-Asab, 2013). It was translated from Arabic into Hebrew two hundred years later, by Joseph Bin Joshua, and from Latin into Hebrew towards the close of the thirteenth century, by Abraham Abigdor (Afnan, 1958; Myers, 1964). In the last three decades of the fifteenth century, it was published in fifteen printed Latin editions along with one in Hebrew. Twenty editions were published in the sixteenth century and several more in the seventeenth century, along with one in Arabic, issued in Rome in 1593 (Afnan, 1958; Al-Mahi, 1959; Freely, 2011). A recent (Abu Asab, 2013) translation from the original Arabic language text into English has been published. Previous translations into English were from Latin, Urdu, and Farsi (Abu-Asab, 2013). An Uzbek translation of five volumes was published in Tashkent. The ophthalmology section was published in German in 1902. Later in the twentieth century, Dr. Oskar Cameron Gruner translated into English the first book of "The Canon" with the help of the Latin editions of 1595 and 1608 and published in London under the title "Treatise on the Canon" (Abu-Asab, 2013). An Arabic edition, a copy of the standard Boulak's edition, was published in Beirut, Lebanon (Mujais, 1987).

The book was used in Europe one hundred years after Ibn Sina's death and continued to be used for the next six centuries (Ullmann, 2006). It was the textbook of medicine in Europe up to the seventeenth century, being used at the University of Montpellier, Leipzig, Tubingen, and the University of Louvain, where it was still being used as late as 1650 AD (Afnan, 1958; Al-Samerra'i, 1989; Haddad, 2003; Freely, 2011; Campbell, 2011; Abu-Asab, 2013). The lectures of Ibn Sina were in the University of Brussels until 1909 (Haddad, 1993). The medical curriculum in Vienna and Frankfurt in the sixteenth century was largely based on The Canon (Al-Qanoun) of Ibn Sina (Afnan, 1958). It was not until human dissection was allowed in Europe that anatomists detected the anatomical errors of Galen that were transmitted to Europe through the works of Avicenna (Afnan, 1958). It remained the medical bible for a longer period of time than any other work. Kitab Al-Qanoun fil Tibb was far ahead of its time, being concerned with diseases such as cancer and its treatment, environmental influence, psychotherapy, and the benefits of exercise (Freely, 2011).

The style of writing in the book was authoritative, and its statements remained unquestioned by most of the medical men of his time and for several centuries thereafter (Wakim, 1944).

It is interesting to note that Ibn Sina described the contagiousness of phthisis, diagnosed ankylostomatisis, and treatment of various forms of poisoning (Wakim, 1944). He attributed the effects of microorganisms (which he called "malicious bodies," "germs") to body weakness and receptivity to infection, or what we call "host factors" (Abu-Asab, 2013).

At the celebration of Ibn Sina's millenary in Tehran, it became apparent that some of Ibn Sina's contributions to pharmacology were original and important. He introduced many herbs into medical practice that had not been tried before. He was aware of the antiseptic effects of alcohol, as he recommended that wounds should first be washed with wine, a practice known before him, as it was used by Zoroastrians in their rituals. Ibn Sina may have been the first to recognize its antiseptic properties. He also recommended drinking mineral water, still popular today (Afnan, 1958).

Volume 1 of the book is devoted to the general description of the human body, its constitution, members, temperaments and faculties, along with a section on common ailments, their causes, and complications, then one on general hygiene and the "necessity of death," and finally one about the treatment of disease (Afnan, 1958; Al-Samerra'i, 1989; Freely, 2011). In the opening to this volume, Ibn Sina wrote, "Medicine is a science from which one learns the status of the human body with respect to what is healthy and what is not, in order to preserve good health when it exists and restore it when it is lacking" (Khan, 2006). The section on anatomy is devoted to a discussion of general anatomy (skeleton, muscles, nerves, etc.). The anatomy of organs was discussed in volume III of the book (Oataya, http://www.islamset.com/isc/nafis/oataya.html).

Volume II (Materia Medica), devoted to simple drugs, properties and uses, lists about 760 drugs arranged in alphabetical order (Afnan, 1958; Khan, 2006; Freely, 2011).

Volume III (Head to Toe Diseases) is devoted to diseases of organs and systems (twenty-one in all), including the brain, nerves, ears, joints, and even the nails of the fingers and toes (Afnan, 1958; Al-Samerra'i, 1989; Freely, 2011). In this volume, Ibn Sina addressed issues related to over- and underweight and the need to take care of one's hair, nails, and body odor (Khan, 2006). Addressing pollution, he wrote, "As long as the air is good and clean and not mixed with anything that is incompatible with the patient's temperament, health will materialize" (Khan, 2006). This volume contains five chapters on neurology. Chapter one is an introduction to brain disorders. The rest of the section discusses headaches (chapter two), brain tumors (chapter three), sleep (chapter four), and epilepsy (chapter five) (Al-Kurdi, 2004). In the chapter on epilepsy, Ibn Sina differentiated two types of epilepsy, grand mal and petit mal; identified three stages of grand mal (aura phase, clonic phase, and relaxation phase); and recommended swimming in a water tank with an electric eel for treatment of epilepsy (Al-Kurdi, 2004).

This volume contains also a section on anatomy devoted to each individual organ of the body and followed by the pathology of the organ (Oataya http://www.islamset.com/isc/nafis/oataya.html).

Volume IV (Diseases not specific to organs, generalized diseases) addresses symptoms and diseases that affect the body as a whole, such as fevers (types and symptoms) , poisoning, insect bites, snake and animal bites, rashes, wounds, dislocations and fractures (Afnan, 1958; Al-Samerra'i, 1989; Khan, 2006; Freely, 2011).

Volume V is devoted to compound medicines and discusses how to mix substances to produce compound medicines (Khan, 2006). It is a manual of pharmacology (known to the Islamic world as "aqrabadhin," from the Greek origin "graphidion"), saying it is an integral part of medicine (Afnan, 1958; Freely, 2011; Campbell, 2011).

THE KIDNEY

The kidney and its diseases are discussed in three distinct segments in each of three volumes and referred to in conjunction with diseases of other organs or general conditions (Mujais, 1987).

The anatomy of the kidney is treated very briefly in volume two. Ibn Sina perpetuated the classic Galenic mistake of ascribing a higher position to the right kidney: "The right kidney was created higher than the left because of the need to be close to the liver in order to attract the aqueous humor." The vascular supply of the kidney was accurately described (Mujais, 1987).

The function of the kidneys according to Ibn Sina is "to attract blood to itself and to clear the blood from the aqueous humor, failure of the kidney in this function leads to dysfunction of the liver, edema and ascites" (Mujais, 1987).

On urine analysis, Ibn Sina recommended "a fresh early morning specimen is to be examined as soon after micturition as possible. The urine should be collected in a container without contamination. Special attention should be paid to diets that may induce changes in the color of the urine, as well as conditions of the patient such as exercise, intercourse, fasting etc. A foamy urine is a sign of kidney disease" (Mujais, 1987).

Ibn Sina described signs and causes (stones, clot, pus) of ureteral and bladder outlet obstruction (Mujais, 1987).

Stones were described in detail and so were renal colic and its therapy. He invoked many factors in the causation of stones, including crystallization, imbalance of humors, and dietary factors. He suggested a connection between stone formation and drinking of milk in the young.

He differentiated renal from bladder stones on the basis of size, color, association with infection, and constitution (bladder stones being larger and harder and associated with more infection). He prescribed a detailed dietary regimen for the dissolution of stones, with the induction of diuresis as a notable mode of therapy (Mujais, 1987).

PSYCHOLOGY AND MUSIC THERAPY

In the book, Ibn Sina alluded to the importance of psychological and emotional factors in health and disease, as well as the positive effects of music on persons whose health is compromised (Khan, 2006).

The book contains Greek and Persian terms that Avicenna could not find names for in Arabic, such as "Mania, Diabetes, Qoulange, Melankholia, among others" (Al-Samerra'i, 1989).

KITAB AL-QANOUN AND NEONATAL MEDICINE:

Regimen at Birth:

In Kitab Al-Qanoun, Ibn Sina addressed issues related to neonatology: "The umbilical cord should be severed four fingers' breadth from the umbilicus after it has been well but gently tied with a clean woolen ligature....then one should hasten to harden the surface of the skin by the use of slightly salted water until the cord has desiccated....After this, the body should be bathed in tepid water, the nostril thoroughly cleaned with the fingers, nails are cut short, and a little oil should be instilled into the eyes. After the cord has separated....which should be in three or four days....the stump should be treated with a measure of bone ash or powdered lead oxide in wine..."(Dunn, 1997).

On Bathing the Infant:

"In summer time it should be bathed with suave tepid water. In winter, the water should be on the warm side. It is desirable to wash it twice or three times in the day" (Dunn, 1997).

On Sleeping Quarters:

"The infant must be placed in an airy room, with not too cool air. The room should also be shady" (Dunn, 1997).

On Binding the Infant:

"In doing this the limbs must be handled very gently, every part should be molded according to its appropriate form" (Dunn, 1997).

On Feeding the Infant:

"Whenever possible, the mother's milk should be given by suckling. It should suffice for the infant to suck the breast twice or three times in the day at first, and it should not be allowed to take too much" (Dunn, 1997).

On Rocking and Humming:

"…Besides this, there are two other things to be done to help strength-en the constitution: gentle rocking movements, humming music or some old song….The movement is for the benefit of the body, and the music is for the benefit of the mind" (Dunn, 1997).

On Inability to Nurse the Child:

"If there is anything to prevent the mother from giving milk to the baby…a wet nurse should be selected…the child is laid to sleep after feeding, but its cradle must not be rocked vigorously as otherwise one would churn the milk in its stomach. Duration of lactation is normally two years…weaning must not be abrupt" (Dunn, 1997).

KITAB Al-QANOUN and ANESTHESIA

"If it is desirable to get a person unconscious quickly, without his being harmed, add sweet smelling moss to the wine, or lignum aloes. If it is desirable to produce a deeply unconscious state…place darnel-water into the wine; or administer fumitory, opium, hyoscyamus, nutmeg, crude aloes-wood. Add this to the wine, and take as much as necessary for the purpose. Or boil black hyocyamus in water, with mandragore bark, until it becomes red. Add this to the wine" (Dunn, 1997).

KITAB Al-QANOUN and CAUSES of DEFORMITY

"Some of these agents come into play from the beginning because of a defect in the formative power of the sperm. Others come into force later in life, namely in parturition, during the act of traversing the maternal passage. Others operate after birth and still others operate in infancy, before the limbs are hard enough to enable the infant to walk" (Dunn, 1997).

KITAB Al-QANOUN and the MANAGEMENT of the TERMINALLY ILL

"Up to the last moment we should endeavor to soothe, but we must not gamble with a life by powerful remedies or big operations where there is no well-founded hope" (Dunn, 1997).

KITAB Al-QANOUN and LOVE ILLNESS

Love sickness was one of the psychological disorders described by Ibn Sina in Kitab Al-Qanoun. Ibn Sina diagnosed the condition in a prince whose pulse fluttered when the address and name of his beloved were mentioned. He cured the disorder by uniting the prince with his beloved (Keys, 1953).

A chapter in the Al-Qanoun was devoted to the so-called disorder of love. Ibn Sina described the love disorder as an obsessive disorder in which the patient is overloaded with obsessive thoughts. Physically, the disorder is characterized by poor grooming, sunken and dry eyes, repetitive blinking, cardiopulmonary changes such as rapid breathing and pulse, and perspiration. Sleep impairment is common (Shoja, 2007).

Ibn Sina stated that the identification of the beloved one was the corner stone in the management of such patients. As a diagnostic tool, numerous names should be spoken while monitoring the patient's pulse. A change in the pulse rate and its quality upon mentioning the appropriate name might indicate the name of the beloved one. The test should also be repeated for different titles, vocations, places, and cities together with the liable name to further locate the suspected person. Ibn Sina recommended that physicians make the effort to verify a legitimate marriage of the patient and his or her beloved one if the diagnosis was uncertain. If this was not possible, other options must be undertaken. The patient may be provoked to love someone else so that he or she may forget the initial person. Discussion with the patient on the obsessive and manic nature of his or her disease was also useful. The patient may also benefit from outdoor activities such as hunting and gaming (Shoja, 2007).

Summaries, comments, and interpretations of the book are plenty. Ibn Al-Nafis (see below) wrote summaries of the book "Kitab Mujaz Al-Qanoun" (Summary of the Canon): "Kitab Sharhul Al-Qanoun" (A Commentary on the Canon) and "Sharhul Tashreeh fil Qanoun"(A Commentary on the Anatomical Information in the Canon) (Al-Samerra'i, 1989; http://www.islamset.com/isc/nafis/oataya.html).

KITAB Al-QANOUN and VASOVAGAL SYNCOPE

In volume III of the Qanoun, Ibn Sina described patients with symptoms of carotid hypersensitivity syndrome. These patients were subjected to pressure on the carotid artery by Hammam (public baths) staff or masseurs, resulting in unconsciousness and falling. He called the condition "al-Lawa" in Arabic ("torsion," in English). He noted that such patients were generally fatigued and had excessive yawning and flushing. Based on their symptoms, Ibn Sina appears to be the first to describe carotid sinus hypersensitivity (Shoja, 2009).

KITAB Al-QANOUN and FRACTURES

One of the volumes of "The Canon" contains a section on bone fractures. It describes causes, types, and forms of all kinds of fractures, along with all methods of treatments. Ibn Sina was the first to advocate the theory of

delayed splinting by suggesting that fractures should not be splinted immediately but only after several days (Al-Khalili, 2011). He also discussed how
to deal with fractures of the first metacarpal bone of the thumb, which
is now known as "Bennett's fracture," after Bennett, who described it in
1882, nine centuries after Ibn Sina's description (Al-Khalili, 2011).

The book, however, was not spared criticism. Although considered the
"wisdom cabinet" by some, others, like the Andalusian luminary Ibn Zuhr,
considered it an "empty bunch of papers" and described it as vague in
its discussion of disease (Campbell, 2011). Another luminary, Al-Baghdadi,
considered it "a nonsense one could get rid of," and Ibn Al-Nafis criticized
the anatomical information in the book (http://www.islamset.com/isc/
nafis/oataya.html). Arnold of Villanova (1235–1312) described Avicenna
as a professional scribbler whose misinterpretations of Galen stupefied
European physicians (Campbell, 2011).

The book is still in print and is used at the Unani medical schools in India
and Pakistan (Abu-Asab, 2013).

Although Al-Qanoun is Ibn Sina's most famous work, it is not his greatest
contribution to science. That contribution is in the next book, "Kitab Al-
Shifa (Book of Healing) (Al-Khalili, 2011).

Kitab al-Shifa (Book of Healing)

This is Ibn Sina's greatest contribution to science. Although the word "Al-
Shifa" (Cure) in the title suggests that it deals with medicine, it is actually
a general compendium of knowledge in the hope of curing the world of
the disease of ignorance (Al-Khalili, 2011).

The book is an eighteen-volume philosophical encyclopedia based on
Aristotelian philosophy and Islamic theology and is the most celebrated
nonmedical book of Ibn Sina (Myers, 1964; Al-Samerra'i, 1989; Freely,
2011; Abu-Asab, 2013). It was translated into Latin by John Al-Ishbili in the
twelfth century under the title "Sanatio." The book is known in English as
"Book of Healing," "The Cure," and "Cure of Ignorance" (Freely, 2011).

Ibn Sina started the book when he was in Hamadan (Krueger, 1963) in response to pleading from Ibn Sina's biographer, Al-Juzjani, to write a commentary on Aristotle (Khan, 2006; Freely, 2011). Ibn Sina agreed on one condition: "If you will be satisfied for me to compose a book setting forth the parts of those sciences which I believe to be sound, not disputing therein with any opponents, no troubling to reply to their arguments, I will gladly do so" (Khan, 2006). The book is the longest of his extant work (Freely, 2011). The writing of the book was completed when Ibn Sina was in Isfahan under the patronage of Al'a Al-Dawlah (Krueger, 1963).

Like Kitab Al-Qanoun, this book is an encyclopedic work that deals wiht metaphysics, astronomy, and the natural sciences (Khan, 2006). Of particular interest is his discussion of metaphysics and the notion of the soul (Lyons, 2009).

The book contains nine volumes on logic and eight on natural sciences. Other volumes covered mathematics, geometry, astronomy, music, and metaphysics (Al-Khalili, 2011).

In the book, Ibn Sina divided practical knowledge into ethics, economics, and politics, while theoretical knowledge is divided into physics, mathematics, and metaphysics (Myers, 1964).

The opening of the book states: "There is no doubt that there is existence". Ibn Sina, then, went on to argue that there is something that caused the world to exist. He called this something "God, the Necessary Being." He argued that this concept of God is based on intuition and went on to provide a rational argument for the existence of "God" (Khan, 2006).

In proving God's existence, ibn Sina presented a distinction between essence and existence. He defined "Essence" as the defining character of a thing. Humanness makes a mammal human. "Existence," he argued, was the addition of matter to the "Essence." Thus, according to Ibn Sina, "Essence" can exist without "Existence." In God, according to Ibn Sina's argument, Essence and Existence are the same. Ibn Sina viewed

"God" as a remote creator who started the universe but who does not intervene in its functioning. In this, Ibn Sina contradicted Muslim scholars who believe that the course of human life is predetermined (Khan, 2006). Ibn Sina also contradicted Muslim scholars in denying that humans could define God. He argued that the different attributes of God (Most Merciful, All Knowing, All Powerful, etc.) could not be taken literally (Khan, 2006).

Kitab al-Isharat wal-Tanbihat (Book of Directions and Remarks)

The book describes the spiritual journey of mystics, beginning with development of faith all the way to the advanced stage of the vision of God (Khan, 2006). It is the last and best of his philosophical treatises (Ibn Abi Usaibiah, 1245/46).

Kitab al-Hidayah (Book of Guidance)

Ibn Sina composed this book while he was in prison in a Fardakhan fortress, and it contains a philosophical summary (Ibn Abi Usaibiah, 1245/46; Afnan, 1958; Khan, 2006).

Kitab al-Qoulange (Book on Colitis)

This book was also written while Ibn Sina was in prison at the Fardakhan fortress. It is a summary of his experience in treating colic. Only fragments of the book are available (Ibn Abi Usaibiah, 1245/46; Afnan, 1958).

Hay Ibn Yaqzan (The Living Son of the Vigilant)

This is a story of a child who grows alone on an isolated island. Through his intellect and reasoning, he was able, independently through nature, to discover the truth about being and God (Ibn Abi Usaibiah, 1245/46; Khan, 2006). This book was written when Ibn Sina was a prisoner in Hamadan (Afnan, 1958).

Kitab al-Insaf (Book of Equitable Judgment)

This is a twenty-volume book addressing all the books of Aristotle. It is the last detailed work written by Ibn Sina. It was supposed to contain the results of his mature thoughts written in the intention of arbitrating between the conflicting views of contemporary philosophers. It was written when Ibn Sina was in Isfahan under the patronage of Al'a Al-Dawlah. The book was lost when Ibn Sina's home was looted during the sack of Isfahan; only fragments of the book survived (Ibn Abi Usaibiah, 1245/46; Afnan, 1958; Khan, 2006).

Danesh-Nama el Ala'i (Book of Wisdom for Ala'i)

This book, written in Persian, in honor of Sultan Al'a Al-Din Ibn Kakawah (Al'a Al-Dawlah), in Isfahan is a concise premier on philosophy written for the layperson. It was complimented for its conversational style, wit, and humor. In the introduction to the book, Ibn Sina acknowledged the sultan's favors. "In this prince's shadow I have achieved all ambitions for security, dignity, and respect for science" (Ibn Abi Usaibiah, 1245/46; Krueger, 1963).

Al-Urjusa fil Tibb (Cantica on Medicine, The Poem on Medicine)

This is an undated compendium, which is an abridgement of Al-Qanoun (Krueger, 1963). In it, Ibn Sina made use of Arabic poetry as mnemonics to facilitate the learning of medical facts (Haddad, 1975). The Urjusa contains 1326 verses of poetry (Haddad, 1993; Haddad, 2003) and is considered by some to be the most widely read, compared to Al-Qanoun, and almost of equal value (Krueger, 1963). Ibn Zuhr (Avenzoar) considered the principles of science contained in the "Urjusa" made it more valuable than a whole library of books (Krueger, 1963).

The first translation of Al-Urjusa into Latin was by Gerardo of Cremona (1114–1187) in the middle of the twelfth century (Krueger, 1963). A century later, probably about 1281, Armenguad de Blaise of Montpellier made a Latin translation of the poem (Avicenna Cantica), which, when printed later in Venice, included a glossary by Averros (Afnan, 1958;

Krueger, 1963, Myers, 1964). Subsequent translations appeared in 1520, 1522, and 1527 (Krueger, 1963). The "Urjusa" translation into verse was completed in the sixteenth century by Jean Faucher and printed in 1650 (Krueger, 1963). A Latin prose edition of the "Urjusa," which included an approximation of the Arabic text in its preface, was done by Antonius Deusingius in 1649 (Krueger, 1963).

The "Urjusa"was translated into Hebrew by Solomon Ibn Ayyoub and Moses Ibn Tibbon (Myers, 1964).

In the preface to the text of the "Urjusa," Ibn Sina stated, "The Urjusa is a poem which deals with every part of medicine which, when our Majesty looks at it with all his acuteness of mind,…then he will know how to discern the true practitioner from the despicable mob, the apprentice from the perfect savant, and the erudite from the blockhead" (Krueger, 1963).

The Urjusa has been the subject for various commentaries, the most famous written by the Spanish physician Abu Al-Walid Muhammad Ibn Ahmad Ibn Muhammad Ibn Rushd (Averroes). This commentary, most often known as "Sharh Urjusat Ibn Sina fil Tibb" (Commentary on Ibn Sina's Poem on Medicine) or "Sharh manzumah fil Tibb" (Commentary on the Poem on Medicine), is prose interposed with Ibn Sina's poem (Gorini, 2005).

The Urjusa fil Tibb is organized along the following headings (Krueger, 1963):

Preface in Prose

Preface in Verse

On the Definition of Medicine

On Things That Deviate from Normal State

Practice and Its Divisions

Medical Practice

Surgical Practice

Some of the statements in the text include (Kreuger, 1963; Gorini, 2005):

The opening statement: "Medicine is the art of health preservation and, in case, of the body diseases curing," in essence summarizing Ibn Sina's medical theory.

"Wine, wine from dates, and milk nourish the body."

"Among physical exercise, there are some moderate ones; it is to them that one ought to devote himself."

"There is no illusion about prolonged rest: no advantages in its excess; it fills up the body with noxious humors and it does not place it in a state from which to benefit from its nourishment."

"Gargle and cleanse your teeth in order to have your dentition and palate clean."

"Make use of baths in order to carry away impurities."

"Allow sexual relations for young people: through them they will avoid masturbation. On the other hand, forbid them for the weak, old and debilitated people. The abuse of intercourse weakens the body and gives as a reward all kinds of illnesses."

"A great joy makes the body prosperous."

"The healthy mind possesses an accurate imagination, reasoning, and memory; normal movement and feeling indicate the integrity of the brain; their alteration signifies its illness."

"Habit becomes a force. Satisfy your desire. Suppress a detrimental habit only gradually."

"Wine taken in small quantities is useful; in large amounts it is dangerous."

"After the meal, sleep with the head elevated so that your food will take its proper place of digestion."

"Convalescents are men who have enjoyed good health but have become weak. They are like monuments, having suffered insults of weather."

"Try to lift their (the convalescents) spirit through welcome words and pleasant company: obtain happiness and music for them."

"If you discover a prodromal symptom, treat it without waiting for the illness."

At the close of the Urjusa, Ibn Sina wrote, "Behold the entire account of practical medicine! Here I conclude my purpose...I have finished."

Copies of the Urjusa are in the Egyptian Book Depository and the Iraqi Museum, among many others (Al-Samerra'i, 1989).

The Latin translation with a French translation of the Urjusa was printed by the University of Algeria in 1956 (Al-Samerra'i, 1989).

Kitab al-Majmu' (The Compendium)

This book, also known by the name "Al-Hikma Al Urudiyya" (Wisdom of the Urodi), was written when Ibn Sina was twenty-one years of age in response to a request from Abi Hasan Al-Urudi. It is a comprehensive treatise that covers all branches of knowledge except mathematics (Ibn Abi Usaibiah, 1245/46; Khan, 2006).

Kitab al-Hasil Wal Mahsul (Book of Imports and Substance)

This twenty-volume book was written for the Jurist Abi Bakr Al-Burqi. Only the original manuscript is present (Ibn Abi Usaibiah, 1245/46; Khan, 2006).

Kitab al-Birr wal Ithm (Book of Good Work and Evil)

This is a two-volume book written for the jurist Abi Bakr Al- Burqi, who had the only copy of the book (Ibn Abi Usaibiah, 1245/46).

Kitab al-Najat (Book of Deliverance)

This book is an abridgement of Kitab Al-Shifa (Book of Healing), written while Ibn Sina was in Isfahan under the patronage of Al'a Al-Dawlah (Krueger, 1963), in response to a request from an acquaintance who asked him to write a book that contained the absolute minimum of philosophical and scientific knowledge that an educated person should have to attain salvation from drowning in a sea of errors (Freely, 2011).

Kitab al Adwiyah al Qalbiyyah (Book of Remedies for the Heart)

This book was the first ever written on psychopharmacology (Abu-Asab, 2013). Ibn Sina completed writing of this book when he first came to Hamadan (Afnan, 1958; Krueger, 1963) and dedicated it to Sharif Al-Said Abi Al-Hasan Ibn Hussein Al-Husseini (Ibn Abi Usaibiah, 1245/46). The book was translated from Arabic to Latin by Avendeath (Afnan, 1958).

The book was printed by the Institute of Scientific Heritage of Aleppo in 1884 (Al-Samerra'i, 1989).

Kitab al-Aqrabadhin (Book on Pharmacology)

A copy of this book is in Istanbul Harbiyya Library (Al-Samerra'i, 1989).

Kitab Lisan al Arab fil Lugha (Language of the Arabs)

This book was written in Isfahan but never published (Ibn Abi Usaibiah,

1245/46). The manuscript was in the form of a rough draft at the time of his death (Afnan, 1958).

Kitab al-Mabda' wal Ma'ad (Book of the Beginning and the Return)

Ibn Sina wrote this book while he was in Gorgan (Afnan, 1958; Krueger, 1963).

Al-Mukhtasar al-Awsat (The Middle Summary)

This was dictated to his student while in Gorgan (Afnan, 1958).

Al Arsad al-Kulliyyah (The General Observations)

This book was composed while in Gorgan, in honor of his benefactor (Afnan, 1958).

Mukhtasar al-Majesti (Summary of al-Majest)

This book was also written in Gorgan (Afnan, 1958).

Appendices: Notes and Discussions.

These are two collections of writings in logic, physics, and metaphysics in the form of questions and answers completed in 1037 AD, the year Ibn Sina died (Freely, 2011).

In a number of his works, Ibn Sina wrote on light and the theory of vision. He defended the intromission theory of vision, put forth by Aristotle, in which visual rays emanate from a luminous object within the eye (Freely, 2011). This theory was disproved by the work of Ibn Al-Haytham (see under Ibn Al-Haytham).

IBN SINA AND NEUROLOGY

On Headaches

Ibn Sina divided headaches into three types, ordinary, secondary (due to brain damage), and shaqiqa (migraine). "Shaqiqa" is the Arabic word for "hemicranias." He formulated a hypothesis about the pathophysiology of migraine, suggesting that it was caused by hyper-excitability of brain tissue which causes the brain to react unusually to noises and light stimuli. He described coitus headache and described the beneficial effects of cold compressors on headache (Al-Mahi, 1959; Al-Kurdi, 2004). Recent articles on the history of pathogenesis of migraine have ignored Ibn Sina (Abokrysha, 2009). Ibn Sina's speculations about the pathogenesis of migraine almost resembled the neurovascular theory, suggesting that he was the first scholar to address the neurovascular theory of migraine (Abokrysha, 2009).

On Facial Palsy

Ibn Sina differentiated central from peripheral facial palsy and recommended massage of the face as treatment and surgery on the facial nerve when completely paralyzed (Al-Kurdi, 2004). He described three types of facial palsy, spastic, atonic, and convulsive, much earlier than Charles Bell's description of "Bell's palsy" (Koehler, 2000).

IBN SINA'S FIRSTS

Ibn Sina is credited with being the first to describe (Al-Mahi, 1959; Haddad 1993; Al-Kurdi, 2004; Khan, 2006) the following:

The different parts of the eye (conjunctiva, sclera, cornea, choroid, iris, retina, lens, aqueous humor, optic nerve, and chiasma) in minutest details

The ocular muscles—four of them, he stated, are on four sides of the globe, above, below, inside, and outside. Each moves the globe in its special direction. The other two muscles are oblique and rotate the eyeball. He was the first to teach that the first four muscles are inserted by a common band (Khairallah, 1942).

Treatment of lachrymal fistula (Haddad, 1993)

Anthrax—he called it "Persian fire" (Haddad, 1993)

Obstructive as different from nonobstructive jaundice

Meningitis and associated neck stiffness (meningismus). Prior to Ibn Sina, meningitis was confused with acute infection accompanied by delirium. Ibn Sina described symptoms of meningitis with such clarity and brevity that little has been added to it since (Al-Samerra'i, 1989; Athar, 1993; Haddad, 1993; Tschanz, 2003).

Primary (cerebral) as differentiated from secondary (extra-cerebral) paralysis

Germs as being transmitted through air, water, or soil noting in Al-Qanoun "at certain times the air becomes infected and anyone breathing the infected air falls sick." He even said that the cause was tiny organisms that travel through the air or water, a fact verified centuries later through the microscope and the germ theory of disease.

Tuberculosis as a contagious disease, proven to be correct centuries later

Ankylostomatitis (hookworm) as caused by intestinal worms (Tschanz, 2003)

The term "sesamoid"

Carotid sinus hypersensitivity (vasovagal syncope) (Shoja, 2009)

Caressing a woman's breast as erotic foreplay (Miles, 2008)

IDEAS HELD BY IBN SINA CONSIDERED MODERN TODAY (Keys, 1953):
Close relationship between emotions and bodily function

Beneficial effects of music on the physical and psychological states of patients

Sleep physiology

Influence of climate changes on health and disease

Importance of balanced diet in maintaining health

Importance of purifying drinking water

CONDITIONS ACCURATELY DESCRIBED BY IBN SINA (Keys, 1953; Athar, 1993; Al-Khalili, 2011):

Tic Douloureux

Tetanus

Anthrax

Pleurisy

Contagiousness of tuberculosis

Theory of delayed splinting, now attributed to George Perkins

Bennett's fracture, attributed to Edward H. Bennett, who described it in 1882

IBN SINA, THE POET

Ibn Sina was also a poet who composed in both Arabic and Persian. The Persian verses attributed to him are of greater merit. His Arabic poems are elevating in thought and theme (Afnan, 1958). The last poem he wrote in Arabic (The Poem on The Soul), which describes the descent of the soul into the body from the higher sphere that is its home, is considered classical beauty (Brown, 1962; Athar, 1993). A. J. Asberry ranked some verses in the poem as "among the sublimest composed in any language" (Freely, 2011):

"Out of her lofty home she hath come down

Upon thee, this white dove in all the pride

Of her reluctant beauty, veiled is she

From every eye eager to know her, though

In loveliness unshrouded radiant...

And if the tangled net impeded her,

The narrow cage denied her wings to soar

Freely in heaven's high range, after all

She was a lightning flash that brightly glowed

Momentarily o'er the tents, and then was hid

As though its gleam was never glimpsed below"

The following verses, attributed wrongly to Omar Al-Khayyam, were written by Ibn Sina and were introduced into the collection of Omar Al-Khayyam by anthologists (Afnan, 1958; Campbell, 2011):

"Up from Earth's center through the seventh gate I rose,

And on the throne of Saturn sate,

And many a knot unraveled by the road,

But not the master-knot of human fate"

In his prison in a fortress, he wrote scornfully (Afnan, 1958):

"My going in was sure, as you have seen

My going out is what many will doubt".

Another poem attributed to Ibn Sina is "Urjusa Latifah Fi Qadaya Apocrat al-Khamsah Wal Ishrin" (an elegant poem on the twenty-five premises of Hippocrates) (http://www.nlm.nih,gov/hmd/arabic/hippo-cratic.html).

Ibn Sina also composed poetry on aging, love, and stars (Ibn Abi Usaibiah, 1245/46).

IBN SINA, THE MUSICIAN

Ibn Sina wrote a book on music and musical instruments (Haddad, 1975).

QUOTES ATTRIBUTED TO IBN SINA:

"An ignorant doctor is the aid-de-camp of death" (Taylor, 2008).

"Opium is the most powerful of the stupefacients" (Taylor, 2008).

From his memoirs "Events befell me and such trials and troubles came rushing upon me, that had they befallen the mighty mountains, they would have come crashing to the ground" (Khan, 2006).

"How I wish I could know who I am, what it is in this world that I seek" (Afnan, 1958; Khan, 2006).

"I prefer a short life with width to a narrow one with length" (Khan, 2006).

"When I became great, no country had room for me; when my price went up I lacked a purchaser" (Ibn Abi Usaibiah, 1245/46).

IBN SINA AND AL-BIRUNI

In a famous correspondence around the year 1000 AD, two geniuses argued the nature of reality. The younger of the two was Ibn Sina; the other, seven years older, was Al-Biruni (Al-Khalili, 2011).

The correspondence took place when both were in their twenties and working in the Royal Court of Gorganj, the capital of Khwarism in Central Asia (Al-Khalili, 2011).

Al-Biruni considered himself of superior intellect in matters of mathematics, physics, and astronomy and was interested in knowing what Ibn Sina, the younger and more able philosopher, had to say on abstract metaphysical matters. He posed to him, among a long list, the following philosophical questions: (1) What was the justification for saying that the heavenly bodies had neither levity nor gravity, and their orbits were perfectly circular around the Earth? (2) Why did Ibn Sina support Aristotle's rejection of the theory of atomism? (3) Do the sun's rays have material substance? (4) How does Ibn Sina defend the Aristotelian view that rejected the possibility of the existence of parallel universes (Al-Khalili, 2011)?

Ibn Sina dealt with all Al-Biruni's questions, strongly defending his views and those of Aristotle's. In response, Al-Biruni challenged Ibn Sina's answers. The correspondence grew confrontational. Eventually, Ibn Sina left the correspondence to his most able student, Al-Ma'sumi, in a way that seemed a snub to Al-Biruni (Al-Khalili, 2011).

FINAL DAYS

While accompanying Al'a Al-Dawlah, Amir of Isfahan, on a march to occupy Hamadan in 1037 AD, Ibn Sina suffered severe and repeated attacks of colic that did not respond to treatment with excessive rectal injections. He gave up treating himself, saying, "The manager who used to manage me is incapable of managing me anymore, so it is no use trying to cure my sickness" (Ibn Abi Usaibiah, 1245/46; Afnan, 1958; Freely, 2011; Abu-Asab, 2013). He died soon after in Hamadan on the last Friday night of the month of Ramadan, 428 AH (1037 AD) of complications of ulcerated and perforated intestine at the age of fifty-eight (Tschanz, 2003; Abu-Asab, 2013). One of his servants may have given him an overdose of a medicine that made his illness worse. Some claim that he died from colon carcinoma (Krueger, 1963). He was buried in Hamadan (Ibn Abi Usaibiah, 1245/46; Wakim, 1944; Al-Samerra'i, 1989; Dunn, 1997; Khan, 2006); some say that his body was transferred later to Isfahan (Ibn Abi Usaibiah, 1245/46).

In 1949, Ibn Sina's grave was exhumed during a construction procedure to build a new tomb in Hamadan. His remains, including his skull and a part of the skeleton, were removed, photographed, placed in sealed boxes, and kept until being reburied inside a new tomb. All the photographs were registered and recorded by the National Archeology Center. A two-dimensional approach to skull reconstruction was applied to the photographs to reconstruct the facial features of Ibn Sina. The reconstruction was done in the Center for Anatomy and Human Identification in the University of Dundee, United Kingdom (Erolin, 2013).

On his deathbed, he paid his debts, gave his possessions to the poor, and freed his slaves (Al-Samerra'i, 1989; Dunn, 1997).

Ibn Sina is a national icon in Iran today. Countless schools and hospitals are named after him in countries around the world. In 1980, every member country of UNESCO celebrated the thousand-year anniversary of Ibn Sina's birth. As a philosopher, he is referred to as "The Aristotle of Islam"; as a physician, he is known as "the Galen of Islam" (Al-Khalili, 2011).

A monument to his life and works still stands outside the museum in Bukhara (Iran), his birthplace. A portrait of Ibn Sina hangs in the hall of the faculty of medicine of the University of Paris (Afnan, 1958).

A modern historian described him as a "meteor which flashed across the sky, illuminating the whole world with his brilliance, and whose afterglow we still perceive the world around us" (Tschanz, 2003).

In his will, he wrote, "Will promise God Almighty to undertake a number of tasks including observing the ritual acts of worship,...refraining from drinking for entertainment but doing so only for medicinal and therapeutic purposes," thus reserving wine drinking as therapy (Khalidi, 2005).

Avicenna had a troubled life. He did not have many close friends and was not a popular figure. His detractors succeeded in spreading derogatory stories about him notably as a sorcerer and magician (Afnan, 1958). He was not a modest man and had a violent temper, as his disputes with fellow philosophers show. He referred to Razi as the man who should have stuck "to testing stools and urine" (Afnan, 1958).

He was a man of excessive passion who indulged in sexual relations even when his health was deteriorating (Afnan, 1958).

AL-KAHHAL, ALI IBN ISA (d. 1010 AD)

In some references, he is referred to as Isa Ibn Ali (Ibn Abi Usaibiah, 1245/46, Cumston, 1921; Al-Samerra'il, 1989). However, Isa Ibn Ali is another person who lived a century before al-Kahhal (Al-Samerra'i, 1989). Al-Kahhal also carried the name of Sharaf El-Din and is known in the West by the name Jesu Haly (Al-Samerra'i, 1989).

Al- Kahhal was a Christian who came from Harran in north Mesopotamia. He was a physician and astrologist who came to Baghdad during the zenith of Arabic medicine and was employed by Caliph Al-Mansour in Baghdad (Wakim, 1944; Freely, 2011). The name Al-Kahhal (oculist) was given to those who practice ophthalmology. Al-Kahhal studied medicine under Abi al-Faraj Abdallah Ibn Al-Tayyib. He practiced medicine for some time before focusing on ophthalmology, at which he excelled, and is considered the most prominent Islamic opthalmologist (Al-Samerra'i, 1989). He excelled in making mascara (Al-Mahi, 1959). He practiced in Baghdad and wrote one of the most highly regarded ophthalmological works, covering 130 diseases of the eye (http://www.nlm.nih.gov/exhibition/islamic_medical/islamic_09.html).

Tazkarat (Tadkirat) al-Kahhaleen (Treasury for Ophthalmologists, Memorandum Book for Eye Doctors)

This is a book on the anatomy and diseases of the eye. It was a classic in its time and has been preserved in its original language (Cumston, 1921; Wakim, 1944). It contains translations of Ibn Ishaq on the subject from Greek to Arabic, as well as his own observations on the eye and its diseases (Ibn Abi Usaibiah, 1245/46; Cumston, 1921; Wakim, 1944; Al-Mahi, 1959; Freely, 2011). The author described, in a clear style, such diseases as trachoma, conjunctivitis, and cataract and their treatment (Cumston, 1921; Wakim, 1944; Al-Samerra'i, 1989). In each chapter, the author first gave the definition of the morbid process being considered, followed by objective symptoms, etiology, and, lastly, treatment comprising general therapeutic measures and diet, followed by the local treatment of the lesion (Cumston, 1921). The book was translated into Latin "Tractus de Oculis Jesu Ben Hali", published in Venice in 1497, 1499, and 1500 (Cumston, 1921; Freely, 2011). The inaccurate Latin translation of the book has caused some to discredit the Al-Kahhal, but the original Arabic version proves it and his merit (Wakim, 1944).

The book consists of three parts (Al-Samerra'i, 1989):

Part one deals with the anatomy of the eye, nerves, muscles, fluids, and vision.

Part two is devoted to diseases of the lids.

Part three deals with disorders of near vision, night vision, treatment of cataract, optic nerve disorders, exophthalmos, and drugs used in ophthalmology, and includes suggestions on how to maintain a healthy vision.

In chapter twenty-five of the third part of the book, Al-Kahhal provided the first description of temporal arteritis and a surgical method to treat it. Temporal arteritis was not known to the Greeks and was not introduced in Europe until the nineteenth century.

The celebrity of the book is evident from the number of copies kept in libraries all over the world, including libraries of Florence, Paris, Cairo, Beirut, the Vatican, Dresden, and Gotha (Cumston, 1921).

Al-Kahhal is credited with being the first physician to suggest the use of anesthesia in surgery (Freely, 2011) and to practice hypnotism (Al-Samerra'i, 1989).

In addition to his medical contributions, Al-Kahhal is credited with writing a treatise on "Reflection on the Art of Prediction of Stars," the earliest known Islamic work rejecting the notion of astrological prognostication (Freely, 2011).

IBN AL-THAHABI (AL-DHAHABI), ABU MOHAMMED AB-DALLAH IBN MOHAMMED AL-AZDI (d. 1033 AD)

Ibn Al-Thahabi was born in Oman and moved to Basra, then to Persia, where he studied medicine under Al-Biruni and Ibn Sina. He later migrated to Jerusalem and finally settled in Valencia (Al-Andalus) (http://en.wikipedia.org/wiki/Ibn Al Thahabi).

SCHOLARSHIP

Kitab Al-Ma'a (Book of Water)

This is the first known encyclopedia of diseases, their physiology and treatments, arranged in alphabetical order. In this book, he added numerous original ideas about the functions of human organs and how vision takes place. The book also contains information about causes and treatments of psychological illness, beginning with dietary control and exercise, before moving on to the use of specific medicines (http://en.wikipedia.org/wiki/Ibn al Thahabi).

ABU AL FARAJ, ABDULLAH IBN AL-TAYYIB (d. 1043 AD)

Abu Al-Faraj was a Syriac Christian physician and philosopher from the village of Sumaysat in present-day Iraq. He studied medicine under Ali

Ibn Siwar in Baghdad and practiced at the Udadi hospital in Baghdad (Al-Samerra'i, 1989). He worked for the ruler Saladin in Damascus (Jadon, 1970). He also studied theology and had a prominent role in Churches (Al-Samerra'i, 1989).

SCHOLARSHIP

Abu Al Faraj wrote explanatory commentaries on six books by Aristotle, four by Hippocrates, sixteen by Galen, and two by Hunayn Ibn Ishaq (Ibn Abi Usaibiah, 1245/46; Al-Samerra'i, 1989). Because of the clarity of his commentaries, he became known as "Al-Faraj Al-Mufassir" (Abu Al-Faraj the Explainer) (Al-Samerra'i, 1989).

Other contributions include (Ibn Abi Usaibiah, 1245/46; Al-Samerra'i, 1989):

Maqala fil Illah (Commentary on Illnesses)

Ta'aliq fil Ayn (Commentaries on the Eye)

Maqala fil Ahlam (Commentary on Dreams)

Al-Nukat wal-Ta'liqat fil Tibb (Jokes and Commentaries in Medicine)

Abu Al-Faraj was a contemporary of Avicenna who praised abu Al-Faraj's medical contributions but not his philosophical writings (Ibn Abi Usaibiah, 1245/46; Al-Samerra'i, 1989).

IBN BOTLAN (IBN BUTLAN, IBN BATALAN), ABU AL-HASAN AL- MUKHTAR IBN AL-HASAN IBN ABDOUN IBN SAADOUN (d. 1058 AD)

Ibn Botlan was a Christian physician from Baghdad. He was born and grew up in Baghdad. He matriculated in medicine at Al-Udadi Hospital in Baghdad with Abu Al Faraj Ibn Abdullah Ibn Al-Tayyib and Ibn Zahroun Al-Harrani (Ibn Abi Usaibiah, 1245/46; Al-Samerra'i, 1989). He was also well versed in Arabic literature and poetry but is better known as a physician (Al-Samerra'i, 1989).

He was a well-known physician in Baghdad and became famous after he wrote a book on the purchase of slaves (Mernissi, 2006).

Ibn Botlan was also a theologian and wrote a book on monasteries (Al-Samerra'i, 1989).

He left Baghdad in 1048 AD to travel to Aleppo (in Syria), Antioch, Jaffa (in Palestine), Cairo (in Egypt), and Constantinople (in Turkey). While in Aleppo, he was appointed by the ruler of Aleppo to head the Christian community there; however, because of his strict attitude in religious matters, he antagonized the community and had to leave Aleppo. Towards the end of his life, he settled in Antioch as a monk but left it for Constantinople, where he died in a monastery on September 2nd, 1058 (Al-Samerra'i, 1989).

Ibn Botlan was a contemporary of the Egyptian physician Ali Ibn Radwan. The two of them corresponded frequently and commented critically on each other's writings and books (Ibn Abi Usaibiah, 1245/46; Al-Samerra'i, 1989). The two met when Ibn Botlan stayed in Egypt for three years during the rule of Al-Mustansir Bi Allah (Ibn Abi Usaibiah, 1245/46). The main cause of the conflict between the two was the teaching of Ibn Radwan that medicine can be learned from books, while Ibn Botlan promoted exposure to teachers as part of the learning process (Al-Samerra'i, 1989).

He described medicine as "the most useful of crafts and most profitable of enterprises" (Rosenthal, 1978).

Ibn Botlan remained a bachelor and had no known relatives. In his final days, he composed the following: "I have no one to cry my absence except my medical sessions and the books in my library" (Al-Samerra'i, 1989).

SCHOLARSHIP

Taqweem al-Sihhah (Almanach of Health, Tableu of Health, Tacuinum Sanitatis)

This book was written between 1052 and 1063 AD. It describes, in more than 280 articles and 40 synoptic tables, various plants and their beneficial effects on health. The book also contains items and procedures useful in the maintenance of health, including exercise, bathing, fumigation, alteration of air quality, seasonal changes, eating, regulation of sleep, and music. Some historians believe that Al-Zahrawi (see below) consulted this book in his writings (Ramen, 2006; Pormann, 2007).

The book was translated into Latin in the twelfth century and published in Strasbourg in 1531 AD under the title "Tacuinum Sanitatis in Medicine," which had a great influence in Europe (Al-Samerra'i, 1989; Haddad, 1993; (http://www.nlm.nih.gov/hmd/arabic/biol.html).

Kitab al-Madkhal ilal-Tibb (Book of Entry to Medicine) (Ibn Abi Usaibiah, 1245/46; Al-Samerra'i, 1989)

Kitab al-Adyirah/Kitab al Adyirah wal-Ruhban (Book on Monasteries and Monks)

The book includes information about first aid, treatment with food, and simple drugs available in distant places where monks live. Manuscripts of the book are kept at the Vatican, the Goethe Library in Paris, and the National Library of Medicine in Washington, DC (Ibn Abi Usaibiah, 1245/46; Al-Samerra'i, 1989; hmd/arabic/biol.html).

Risala fi Shari al-Raqeeq (On Race and Slaves)

This book addresses the practice of buying and selling slaves and maintaining slave girls (Ibn Abi Usaibiah, 1245/46). The book gives tips for thwarting the tricks of peddlers who changed the features of sick slaves by using makeup and cosmetics to alter hair and skin color according to the prevailing fashion (Mernissi, 2006). He wrote, "Beware of those with wide eyes. They are lazy or voluptuous. Those with deep set eyes are envious. Blue eyes denote stupidity, and the woman who blinks all the time is malice personified. If you have business with a person in whose eyes the black part is larger than the white, you should pick up your feet and run-that person is mad. Too fine hair is a sign of foolishness, and thick, wiry hair denotes courage. Trying to communicate with a person with a large nose is lost effort, because that denotes a fool. A person with high forehead is lazy, but a low forehead is no better. A large mouth denotes courage, and thick lips are the mark of a fool" (Mernissi, 2006).

After the Arabs, it was the Hindu jawari (slave girls) that he recommended, for their faithfulness and tenderness, but he said, "Their problem is that they die very young." He recommended the Turks for their beauty, but they were stocky. The Romans possessed good manual skills. He recommended avoiding the "monster Armenians," who were faithful but thieving, and one had to "use the rod to get something out of them" (Mernissi, 2006).

Risala Da'wat al-Atibba (Call of Physicians)

The book was completed in 1058 AD in Constantinople and dedicated to Amir (Ruler) Ahmad Ibn Marwan Ibn Dustek, the ruler of Diar Bakr. The book covered what went on in gatherings of physicians of medical and nonmedical topics; and what the "Kahhal" (ophthalmologist) should know in anatomy, the pharmacist in drugs, the physician about care of the patient, and the phlebotomist about distribution of vessels. The text was written in a simple, clear, rhythmic style. Copies of the manuscript are kept in the Egyptian Book Repository, Berlin, St. Joseph University Library in Beirut, Lebanon, and Mosul, Iraq (Al-Samerra'i, 1989).

Ibn Botlan remained a bachelor all his life. In a poem he wrote about his life, he said, "No one will cry for my death, except those who shared my books and meetings" (Ibn Abi Usaibiah, 1245/46).

AL-JUZJANI, SAYYID ZAYN AL-DIN (d. 1070 AD)

Al-Juzjani came from the Central Asian region of Khwarizm. He is remembered because of his association with Ibn Sina. He is considered the most influential follower of Ibn Sina (Freely, 2011).

SCHOLARSHIP (Freely, 2011):

Treasury Dedicated to the King of Khawarizm

This is his principal work. It is an encyclopedia of medicine based on the "The Canon" of Ibn Sina.

Medical Memoranda

The Aims of Medicine

AL-GORGANI (AL-JURJANI), ZAYN AL-DIN (SHARAF AL-DIN) SAYYED ISMA'IL IBN HUSAYN (1040/42–1136)

Al-Gorgani (Gorjani) was a prominent Persian eleventh- and twelfth-century physician from Gorgan, in northeast of Iran near the shores of the Caspian Sea. In addition to being a physician, he was adept in theological, philosophic, and ethical sciences (Shoja, 2007; Shoja, 2010; http://en.wikipedia.org/wiki/Zayn_al_Din_Gorjani).

Little is known about his youth, as he did most of his writing after the seventh decade of his life. He studied Ilm al-Hadith (Knowledge of Prophet sayings) and fiqh (jurisprudence) under Abou-al-Qassem Qureishi in Naishapur, a city in northeast present-day Iran, home of the great medieval poet and mathematician Omar Al-Khayyam (Shoja, 2007; Shoja, 2010). He then matriculated in medicine under Ibn Abi Sadegh Al-Naishapuri, a student of Avicenna, who was known in Persia as the second Hippocrates, and Ahmad Ibn Farrokh. He then traveled to Qum, Merv, and other Persian states where he had the chance to interact with physicians, as well as physicians from present-day Iraq, Khozestan as well as other regions. He also had the chance to meet and interact with students of Avicenna (Shoja, 2010). At an advanced age, in 1110, he became court physician to Khwarizm Shah Qutb al-Din Muhammad, a wise and just governer/king of the Persian province of Khwarizm, to whom Al-Gorgani dedicated his most comprehensive work "Zakhira-i-Khwarizm Shahi" (Thesaurus of the Shah of Khwarizm). The governer also appointed him director of the municipal Baha' al-Dawla Hospital (Shoja, 2007; Shoja, 2010). He continued to serve as court physician to Khwarizm Shah's son and successor, Ala' Al-Din Atziz. He ultimately moved to the city of Merv, capital of the rival Seljuk dynasty, where he died in 1136 AD (Shoja, 2007; http://en.wikipedia.org/wiki/Zayn_al_Din_Gorgani).

SCHOLARSHIP

Al-Gorgani wrote a number of important medical and philosophical works in Persian. The exact number of the books that Gorgani wrote is indeterminate. It is known that he wrote five books in Persian in medicine and innumerable number of others in such fields as philosophy and ethics, written for the most part in Arabic (Ardekani, 2005).

Zakira-i-Khwarizm Shahi (Thetharius of the Shah of Khwarizm)

The book is also known as "The Treasure of Khwarizm Shah." It is an encyclopedic work written in Persian in approximately 1112, when he moved to the province of Khwarizm. It is considered to be the oldest medical encyclopedia written in Persian. Much of the work is based on Avicenna's "Canon of Medicine," with Al-Gorgani's own ideas not found in "The Canon." Other preceding writings included in the book were those of Hippocrates, Aristotle, Galen, Dioscorides, Rufus of Ephesus, Aaron of Alexandria, Al-Razi, Rabban Al-Tabari, Haly Abbas, and Jurjus Bukhtishu, among others. Gorgani gave appropriate reference to those sources. The book is in ten volumes and more than 750,000 words, covering ten medical topics: anatomy, physiology, hygiene, diagnosis and prognosis, fevers, diseases of particular parts of the body, surgery, skin diseases, poisons and antidotes, and simple and compound drugs (Shoja, 2007; Hosseini, 2011; http://en.wikipedia.org/wiki/Zayn_al_Din _Gorgani). The book was translated into many languages, was an essential resource for training physicians for centuries, and was revered in distant lands, including Europe (Shoja, 2010; Hosseini, 2011).

In the introduction of the book, Gorgani wrote: "Since it was destined by the Most High that the author of this book should ever pray for Sultan khwarism Shah on account of the bounties that he has received from him, a ruler most erudite and just and stepping stone to success, the succor of the needy, the pillar of faith, the protector of Islam and Muslims... may God continue his rule in prosperity...It was in accordance with this intention that the materials of the book were gathered and the book was named the 'Zakira-i Khwarizm Shahi' that the name and memory of this great and benevolent ruler may live forever in people's minds and his reputation ever increase throughout the world and last therein" (Ardekani, 2005).

In the preface to the book, Gorgani described the purpose for writing the book "for physicians not being in need of any other book for any discourses" (Hosseini, 2011).

Although Gorgani applied Persian terms throughout the book, occasional reference to Arabic and even Greek terms are present (Hosseini, 2011).

The book was translated by Gorgani at an old age into Arabic and by others into Turkish, Urdu, and Hebrew (Shoja, 2007; Hosseini, 2011).

In the book, Gorgani discussed trigeminal neuralgia and two types of facial palsy "Laqwa": a unilateral facial weakness type (Bell's palsy) and a convulsive type (hemi facial spasm) (Shoja, 2010). Gorgani's writings on trigeminal neuralgia included the first suggestion of a relationship between nerve and vessel in its etiology and constituted the basis for the modern surgical approach to treatment of trigeminal neuralgia (Shoja, 2010; Hosseini, 2011).

The book contained extensive discourse on midwifery and neonatal and childhood care, reflecting the medical knowledge of the time (Hosseini, 2011).

Chapter two of book one includes a discussion of cranial nerves, which at the time were believed to be in seven pairs in line with Galen's teachings as follows (Shoja, 2007):

The first pair of Gorgani included the olfactory and optic pairs of cranial nerves.

The second pair is what we currently call the oculomotor cranial nerve (CN III).

The third and fourth nerves of Gorgani probably represent the sensory and motor roots of the trigeminal nerve.

The fifth cranial nerve of Gorgani represents the auditory and facial nerves.

The sixth cranial nerve of Gorgani corresponds to the glossopharyngeal, spinal accessory and vagus nerves.

The seventh cranial nerve of Gorgani corresponds to the twelfth cranial nerve, the hypoglossal.

Gorgani was one of the first to associate exophthalmos with thyroid gland goiter, which was not repeated until Caleb Parry (1755–1822) and, later, Robert James Graves (1796–1853) and Carl von Basedow (1799–1854). Al-Gorgani also established an association between thyroid goiter and palpitations (Shoja, 2007; Hosseini, 2011; http://en.wikipedia.org/wiki/Zayn_al_Din_Gorgani).

Khafi Ala'i

At the request of Qutb al-Din son and successor, Atzos, nicknamed Ala' Al-Dawlah, Gorgani compiled a synopsis of the "Zakira I-Khwarizm Shahi" to accompany a book called "Khafi Ala'i "(Ala'i's Secrets) (Shoja, 2010). In the introduction of the book, Gorgani wrote:"…And after completing the "Zakireh-i-Khwarizm Shahi" acquiring some lesireu and free time, I, Ismail Ibn Ahmad Ibn Alhusayn Gorgani the sincere servant of His Excellency at the request of the Prince Amir al-Asfia al-Ajal Muhammad Al'a Al-Dawlah ...suddenly conceived the passion to read the book wherever chance might place him whether at home or while travelling, but since the original book was composed in lengthy volumes the perusal of which presented many difficulties His Excellency requested me to prepare a shorter version of the original book which task I duly carried out …." (Ardekani, 2005).

Other medical works by Gorgani include:

Al-Iqraz al-Tibbieh wal-Mabahis al-Alaieh

This book was written in Persian, at the request of Majd al-Din Abu Mohammad Salhyin Muhammad AlBukhari, the minister of Atzis. It occupies a middle position between "Zakira-I Khwarizm Shahi" and "Khafi Ala'i", the two books of Gorgani. It is a hotchpotch of the "Zakira- I Khwarism Shah". The author wrote in the introduction: "…And my skill in medicine and earlier I had made a summary of it and now in accordance with His Excellency's order Imam Ajal Majd al-Din Abu Mohammad Bukhari….this task was completed….As for being brief it is yet great in the wealth of knowledge it contains and the detailed explanations it offers touch upon many troubles and diseases to which human flesh is heir. Therefore no scientific matter of importance was omitted. A book so short and brief yet so full of knowledge and information does not exist which claim on my part acquires significance when the book is actually read and perused…" (Ardekani, 2005).

Yadegar Sayyid Ismail (Tibb Yadegar)

This book was also written in Persian and was popular among students and physicians during Gorgani's lifetime. It was written in 1135 AD. It is in one volume of five chapters. Chapter one, with seventeen sections, deals with the scientific benefits that accrue in the science of medicine. The second chapter, thirty sections, deals with curing diseases that may affect the entire human constitution. The third chapter consists of two sections. The fourth chapter consists of eleven sections. The fifth chapter consists of three sections. A few versions of the book are found in different libraries in various parts of the world, and three versions are in Tehran University Central Library, the Tehran University Medical College Library, and Dr. Husayn Miftah Private Library (Ardekani, 2005).

Kitab fi Hifz al Sihha (Book on Preserving Health)

This book was composed with the intention of safeguarding public hygiene and health and has been considered by many scholars as belonging to Gorgani. It was composed in 1101 AD (Ardekani, 2005; http://en.wikipedia.org/wiki/Zayn _al_Din_Gorgani).

Book on Anatomy

This book contains profound insights that the author obtained from his teacher Ibn Abi Sadiq. Medical historians did not take much notice of this book, and some doubt that it was written by Gorgani (Ardekani, 2005).

Zubdat al-Tibb (Basic Medicine)

This book was written in Arabic and addresses all matters pertaining to medicine and pharmacology. In the introduction to the book, Gorgani expressed his avowed aim in composing the book was to present matters pertaining to theoretical medicine in one small volume. In the book, Gorgani divided drugs into three kinds: mineral drugs, herbal drugs, and animal drugs. Many versions of the book are available in Iranian libraries and libraries of other countries (Ardekani, 2005; http://en.wikipedia.org/wiki/Zayn_al_Din_Gorgani).

Al-Zakira al-Ashrafiyyah fi Assina'a al-Tibbiyah (The Profession of Medicine)

This book was written in Arabic and is believed to be the Arabic translation of the book "Khafi Ala'i". A version of the book is in the Paris Public Library (Arkedani, 2005).

Al-Tibb al-Malaki (Royal Medicine)

While medical historians and researchers agree as to Gorgani's author-ship of this book and its Arabic text, no handwritten copies were found in any of the European libraries (Ardekani, 2005).

Kitab al-Manbah (Al-Risala al-Manbah)

This is a book on ethics written in Arabic. It discourses upon resisting de-sires and passions and dwells at length upon worldly pleasures. The book reflects Gorgani's proficiency in the humanities in addition to medicine. A copy of the book is in the Berlin Royal Library. A few versions are in Indian libraries (Ardekani, 2005).

Kitab Tadbeer al-Yawm wa Layla (Book on Managing the Day and Night)

This book, written in Arabic, concerns itself with how human beings ought to conduct themselves ethically and morally day and night (Ardekani, 2005).

Vasiyat Nameh (Kitab Nameh)

This is another book of ethics written in Persian. No handwritten copies were found in European libraries. It is believed that Gorgani wrote the book at an advanced age (Ardekani, 2005).

Fil Qiyas (On Comparisons)

This is another book of Gorgani written in Arabic. It deals with philoso-phy and reflects Gorgani's expertise in the subject. Versions of the book are in Rampour and Pishawar Libraries in Pakistan (Ardekani, 2005).

Fil-Tahleel (On Analysis)

This book, written in Arabic, is concerned with philosophy. It was widely consulted and valued by students and scholars. Copies of the book are found in Indian libraries (Ardekani, 2005).

Al-Kazimieh

This book, written in Arabic, is a philosophical treatise. No handwritten copies of the book have been found (Ardekani, 2005).

In recognition of his contributions, Gorgani's birthday is celebrated each year in Iran as the day of laboratory medicine (Shoja, 2010; Hosseini, 2011).

IBN JAZLA AL-BAGHDADI (BENGESLA, BUHAHYLYHA, BYNGEZLA), ABU ALI YAHYA IBN ISSA IBN ALI (1074/1030–1100 AD)

Ibn Jazla was born in Karkh, a district of Baghdad on the west side of the Tigris River. He was born to Christian parents but converted to Islam under the tutelage of Abi Ali bin Al-Walid Al-Maghribi, the chief of the Mu'tazilite sect. Late in his life, he wrote a treatise in praise of Islam and criticizing Christianity and Judaism for hiding from their books the coming of Prophet Muhammad (Al-Samerra'i, 1989; Tubbs, 2008; http://www.nlm.nih.gov/hmd/arabic/biol.html), which he sent to Pastor Eliya (Ibn Abi Usaibiah, 1245/46).

Ibn Jazla trained in medicine under Said Ibn Hibat Allah, the physician to Abbasid Caliph Al-Muqtadi Bi Amr Allah. Ibn Jazla would later become physician to this caliph (Tubbs, 2008).

He is known as treating the needy, his friends, and acquaintances gratis, providing them with free medicine (Al-Mahi, 1959; Myers, 1964; Al-Samerra'i, 1989). In his last days, he bequeathed his entire book collection to the famous mosque of Imam Abu Hanifeh in Baghdad, where he would be buried (Al-Samerra'i, 1989; Tubbs, 2008). He promoted the value of music in treatment, equating its effects with those of drugs. He stated, "The effect of music on ailing psyches resembles that of medicines on ailing bodies" (Al- Mahi, 1959; Myers, 1964; Tubbs, 2008). He practiced during the rule of Al-Muqtadi Bi Amr Allah (Ibn Abi Usaibiah, 1245/46; Al-Samerra'i, 1989; Tubbs, 2008).

SCHOLARSHIP

Ibn Jazla is credited with writing only three books:

Kitab Taqweem al-Abdan fi Tadbeer al-Insan (Correcting the Body)

This is a book on diseases and therapeutics arranged in tabular form (Al-Mahi, 1959; Haddad, 1975; Al-Samerra'i, 1989; Tubbs, 2008). In forty-four tables, the description and treatment of 350 diseases are presented. Within the tables, diseases were arranged like stars in astronomical tables (Tubbs, 2008).

In the introduction, the author stressed hygienic measures that prevent disease and promote good health. He emphasized the necessity of medical care for a happy life as well as afterlife. He said, "The existence of both worlds (this world and the hereafter) depends on the desire to correct them, as stated in the tradition (khabar). It is best for one not to ignore or abandon either this world for the hereafter, nor the hereafter for this world, but to benefit from both.... If the preservation of health per se is not intended, but rather for the sake of work and knowledge, then man is considered as a tool or means to them (work and knowledge). If he becomes servant to them, then it would be undesirable to devote time to it (health) more than is required" (Tubbs, 2008).

The book was translated from Arabic to Latin in 1280 AD by Faraj Bin Salim (Farragut), a Sicilian Jew (Myers, 1992; Tubbs, 2008; Campbell, 2011). The book was devoted to Al-Muhtadi Bi Amr Allah (Ibn Abi Usaibiah, 1245/46). A German translation was published in Strasburg in 1533 by Hans Schotte (Tubbs, 2008; Campbell, 2011). Copies of the book are kept in the Royal Library of Egypt and Library of St Joseph University in Beirut, Lebanon. The oldest copy, dated 596 AH.was found in Istanbul hundred years after the death of Ibn Jazla (Al-Sammera'i, 1989). The book was not published in Arabic, although the calligraphy of Ibn Jazla was most beautiful (Campbell, 2011)

Minhaj al-Bayan fi ma Yasta'miluho al-Insan (Pathway of Explanation as to that Which Man Uses)

This book, also dedicated to Caliph Al-Muqtadi Bi Amr Allah, dealt with bodily needs. The topics are arranged in alphabetical order. It discusses drugs and nutrition needed by the body in health and disease, with emphasis on treatments with herbs (Ibn Abi Usaibiah, 1245/46; Al-Mahi, 1959; Al-Samerra'i, 1989; Tubbs, 2008). Although the book was intended to be a medical text, some emphasized its culinary contributions (Tubbs, 2008).

The book was translated into Latin in 1532 AD. Copies of the book are in the Egyptian Book Depository, the Vatican, the British Museum, the Welcome Library in London, and the Baghdad University Library (dating back to 1037) (Al-Sammera'i, 1989).

The book was so popular that Ibn Jazla was dubbed "Saheb Al-Minhaj" (Author of Al-Minhaj) (Al-Samerra'i, 1989).

Kitab al Ishara fi Talkhees al-'Ibara (Book on Medical Rules and Regulations for Maintenance of Health)

This book also deals with medical rules used to preserve health (Ibn Abi Usaibiah, 1245/46; Al-Samerra'i, 1989).

IBN JAZLA AND NEUROLOGY

In his Taqweem al Abdan book, Ibn Jazla devoted three of the forty-four sections to the nervous system. He titled them: Headache, Diseases of the Brain, and Nervous Diseases. He stated that brain diseases were attributed to headache, vertigo, and disorders of the humors such as in encephalitis, memory loss, dizziness, lethargy, and nightmares. Headaches were attributed to both local and systemic diseases. He stated that if the headache was over the entire head, then it was due to disease at remote sites. If, however, the headache stemmed from the head itself, then the ache was due to heat, cold, dryness or moisture.

He recommended cephalic vein bloodletting for treatment of vertigo. He attributed epilepsy to obstruction of cerebral veins and the arrest of proper brain circulation. He concurred with Hippocrates that patients with significant stroke would not recover. Diseases affecting the lateral part of the brain were described as affecting the limbs and organs while diseases of the central part of the brain were known to prohibit movement (Tubbs, 2008).

Ibn Jazla recognized that spinal cord diseases often resulted in weakness and numbness. He believed that certain diseases occur in certain seasons. Vertigo was believed to occur more commonly in hot climates during the summer and to be more prevalent in adults. Sciatic pain was differentiated from arthritic joint pain in the spread of sciatic pain to the knee and ankle joints. He identified that injury to the laryngeal nerve results in loss of the voice. He stated that "looseness" following traumatic nerve injury is an indication that such injuries are not curable (Tubbs, 2008).

ILAQI, ABU ABDALLAH MUHAMMAD IBN YUSUF SHARAF AL-DIN (d. 1141)

Ilaqi was from the town of Ilaq, near Naishapur, Persia. He studied medicine under Ibn Sina. There is no general agreement on where he lived (http://www.nlm.nih.gov/hmd/arabic/biol.html).

SCHOLARSHIP

Kitab Al-Fusul Al-Ilaqiya (The Aphorisms of Ilaqi)

This is an epitome of the first books of The Canon of Medicine by Ibn Sina (Avicenna). The book was very popular (http://www.nlm.nih.gov/hmd/arabic/biol.html).

Kitab Al-Asbab wal-Alamat (The Book of Causes and Symptoms) (http://www.nlm.nih.gov/hmd/arabic/biol.html)

IBN MUSA, SULAYMAN

Ibn Musa was a Muslim physician who was very well versed in literature, Arabic poetry, and prose. He studied medicine in Cairo, Egypt, and moved to Damascus to practice medicine. He was considered one of the distinguished physicians, and the only oculist among Saladin court physicians. He accompanied Saladin all the time (Jadon, 1970).

IBN AL-TILMIDH AL-BAGHDADI, ABU AL- HASAN HIBAT ALLAH (d. 1165 AD)

Ibn Al-Tilmidh was also known by the names Amin Al-Dawlah and Muwaffaq Al-Mulk (Al-Samerra'i, 1989; http://www.nlm.nih.gov/hmd/arabic/biol.html).

Al-Tilmidh was his maternal grandfather's name, after whom he was named (Al-Samerra'i, 1989).

Ibn Al-Tilmidh was a Christian from Baghdad, son of an eminent physician. He was well versed in theology, calligraphy, and poetry, as well as medicine. He was fluent in Arabic, Syriac, and Persian. He matriculated in medicine under his father Abi Al-Ala', and Abi Al-Hasan Hibatullah Ibn Said, the famous classifier in medicine. He traveled to Persia in search of more knowledge before settling in Baghdad where he served in the court of Caliph Al-Muqtafi bi Allah and directed the Al-Adudi Hospital, the most famous hospital in Baghdad. Among his students was the luminary physician Ibn Mutran (Ibn Abi Usaibiah, 1245/46; Al-Samerra'i, 1989; http:www.nml.nih.gov/hmd/arabic/biol.html).

Ibn Al-Tilmidh was known to enjoy music and the company of musicians. He composed a poem describing the benefits of drinking wine (Ibn Abi Usaibiah, 1245/46; Al-Samerra'i, 1989).

He was also well-known for not accepting gifts except from caliphs and sultans. He refused a hefty gift from a wealthy merchant treated for and cured of an intractable illness by Ibn Al-Tilmidh (Ibn Abi Usaibiah, 1245/46).

Ibn Al-Tilmidh was known to be a book collector and to love teaching and considered it a duty. He is known to have said, "The scholar who does not teach is a miser." He donated his income from serving in the caliph's court to students, teachers, and the poor (Al-Samerra'i, 1989).

Ibn Al-Tilmidh died in Baghdad in 1165 AD at the age of ninety-four (Ibn Abi Usaibiah, 1245/46; Al-Samerra'i, 1989).

He had a son who studied medicine with his father and excelled in its practice. He converted to Islam and died at the age of eighty years by suffocation in the basement of his house (Al-Samerra'i, 1989).

SCHOLARSHIP

Ibn Al-Tilmidh composed a considerable number of medical texts.

Kitab Aqrabadhin (Book on Pharmacopea)

This twenty-chapter book is the most influential of his books. In it, the author described how to prepare and prescribe a wide variety of medicines. It became the basic reference of practicing pharmacists in their private pharmacies and in hospital pharmacies. Copies of it are in the British Museum, Gothe Museum, and the Egyptian Book Repository (Ibn Abi Usaibiah, 1245/46; Al-Samerra'i, 1989; Tarabay, 2011; http://www.nml.nih.gov/hmd/arabic/biol.html).

Aqrabadhinah Al Mujaz al-Bimarestani (Summary Pharmacopeia of Hospitals) in thirteen chapters

A copy of it is in the Welcome Library in London (Ibn Abi Usaibiah, 1245/46; Al-Samerra'i, 1989).

Kitab Mukhtarat Min Kitab Al-Hawi li Al-Razi (Selections from Al Hawi by Al-Rhazis) (Ibn Abi Usaibiah, 1245/46; Al-Samerra'i, 1989)

Kitab Mukhtasar al-Hawashi ala Kitab Al-Qanoun li al Rais Ibn Sina

(Summary of Notes in Kitab Al-Qanoun by Avicenna) (Ibn Abi Usaibiah, 1245/46; Al-Samerra'i, 1989)

Sharh Ahadith Nabawiyyah Tashtamil ala al-Tibb (Explanation of Prophets Sayings Related to Medicine) (Ibn Abi Usaibiah, 1245/46; Al-Samerra'i, 1989)

Sharh Masa'el Hunayn Ibn Ishaq (Explanation of Questions by Hunayn Ibn Ishaq) (Ibn Abi Usaibiah, 1245/46; Al-Samerra'i, 1989)

Ibn Al Tilmidh left a substantial collection of books to his son. Following Ibn Al Tilmidh's death, the collection of books was moved by twelve camels to the house of Al-Majd Ibn-Saleh (http://www.nml.nih.gov/hmd/arabic/biol.html).

Kitab Khalq al-Insan (Book on Creation of Man) (Al-Samerra'i, 1989)

Kitab Zubda Fi Ilm Al-Tibb (Book of the Cream in Medicine) (Al-Samerrai, 1989)

IBN AL-TILMIDH, MU'TAMAD AL-MALEK ABU AL-FARAJ YAHYA IBN SA'ED IBN YAHYA

Ibn Al-Tilmidh belongs to a family known for their excellence in medicine and literature. He was a practitioner and teacher of medicine, as well as a poet. Several poems were written about him in appreciation of his skills (Ibn Abi Usaibiah, 1245/46).

IBN ALI MALKA AL-BALADI, AWHAD AL-ZAMAN ABU AL-BARAKAT HIBATU ALLAH

Ibn Ali Malka Al-Baladi was born in Balad but lived in Baghdad. He was a Jew and converted to Islam. He matriculated in medicine with Abu Al-Hasan Ibn Hibatu Allah Ibn Al-Hussein. Initially, Ibn Al-Hussein would not admit him to his class because he was a Jew. Al-Baladi started to frequent Ibn Al-Hussein's classes by sitting in the corridor outside the classroom to listen and write the lessons. After a year of sitting in the corridor, he was permitted to enter the class to provide an opinion on a medical problem that puzzled Ibn Al-Hussein students. His participation in the discussion impressed Ibn Al-Hussein, who inquired about the source of his information. When Al-Baladi told him about listening to his lessons in the corridor, Ibn Al-Hussein decided to admit him to his class (Ibn Abi Usaibiah, 1245/46; Al-Samerra'i, 1989).

His conversion to Islam was voluntary and happened in the court of Caliph Al-Mustanjid Bi Allah. It was triggered by the refusal of the qadi (judge) to rise from his chair to greet Al-Baladi when Al-Baladi entered the court. Al-Baladi addressed the khalifeh, saying that if Al-Qadi refused to salute him because of his Jewish faith, he declared in the presence of the khalifeh his conversion to Islam, and he did (Ibn Abi Usaibiah, 1245/46).

Ibn Malka became blind towards the end of his life but continued to dictate his books to his students. He died about 1164 AD at the age of ninety years (Al-Samerra'i, 1989).

SCHOLARSHIP

Ibn Malka is credited with the following books:

Kitab al-Mu'tabir fil Hikma (Book of Reverence)

Ibn Malka completed this book after he became blind by dictating it to his student Yousef Abi Abdel-Latif Al-Baghdadi. The book is in three parts. The second part contains sections on body parts and their functions, advantages of animals over plants, plant growth in different lands, commonalities among animals and plants, and reflections on Aristotle's writings on animals and plants (Ibn Abi Usaibiah, 1245/46; Al-Samerra'i, 1989).

Kitab Ikhtisar al-Tashrih (Book of Dissection Summary)

This book is basically a collection of statements made by Galen on the subject (Ibn Abi Usaibiah, 1245/46; Al-Samerra'i, 1989).

A summary from Galen's books

Kitab al-Aqrabadhin (Book of Pharmacology) (Ibn Abi Usaibiah, 1245/46; Al-Samerra'i, 1989)

Risala fil Aql Wa Mahiyatahu (On the Brain and its Function) (Al-Samerra'i, 1989)

Kitab Hawashi ala Qanoun Ibn Sina (Commentaries on Avicenna's Canon) (Al-Samerra'i, 1989)

AL-SURI, RASHIDUN (1177–1241)

Al-Suri was born and brought up in the town of Sur (Tyre) in southern Lebanon and derived his name (al-Suri) from his town (Sur).

He was a leading physician and botanist of the thirteenth century.

After completing his studies in Sur, he moved to Jerusalem, then under Mamluk's rule, where he served as a physician in one of the hospitals. From Jerusalem, Al-Suri moved to Cairo at the invitation of the Ayyoubid Sultan Al-Adil, where he bacame the sultan's personal physician. He also served Al-Adil's son, Al-Muazzam, and grandson Al-Nasir Dawud, the successive governors of Damascus.

Al-Suri held an interest in plant life and was a botanist. He used to roam about and study herbs and plants in their natural surroundings. He also employed a professional painter to sketch and paint the plants in different stages of their growth using different colors and dyes (http://en.wikipedia.org.wiki/Rashidun_al=Suri).

SCHOLARSHIP

Al-Suri has one book "Al-Adwiya al-Mufradah" (The Simple Medicines) (http://en.wikipedia.org/wiki/Rashidun_al-Suri).

IBN AL-MUTRAN (IBN AL-MATRAN), MUWAFFAQ AL-DIN ABU NASR AS'AD IBN Al-FATH ILYAS IBN JIRJUS (d. 1191 AD)

Ibn Al- Mutran was a Christian physician, the son of a famous traveling physician. Two of his brothers (Hibat Ul Allah and Ibn Elias) were also physicians (Ibn Abi Usaibiah, 1245/46; Jadon, 1970).

Ibn Al- Mutran was born and grew up in Damascus. From Damascus, he went to Baghdad to study medicine and matriculated, in addition to his physician father, with Amin Al-Dawla Ibn Al-Tilmidh and Muhazzab Al-Din Ibn Al-Nakkash, after which he returned to Damascus (Ibn Abi Usaibiah, 1245/1246; Al-Samerra'i, 1990; http://www.nlm.nih/hmd/arabic/biol.ktml).

He studied Arabic literature and grammar with Sheikh Imam Taj Al-Din Abi Al-Yaman Zeid Ibn Al-Hasan Al-Kindi (Ibn Abi Usaibiah, 1245/46; Al-Samerra'i, 1990).

He served in the court of Salah Al-Din Ibn Ayyoub (Saladin) in Egypt and accompanied him on his campaigns (Ibn Abi Usaibiah, 1245/46; Jadon, 1970). He was so close to Saladin that his tent during travel was colored red to differentiate it from the tents of others in the entourage of Saladin (Samerra'i, 1990).

He was very well compensated by Saladin and is reported to have gathered great wealth. Princesses competed for his service and rewarded him with large sums of money. His house was filled with carpets, and the pipes of the fountains were made of gold. When Ibn Al-Mutran converted to Islam, Saladin gave him one of his wife's finest handmaids (Joza) in marriage. She brought along her jewelry and valuable gifts, thus adding to his wealth (Jadon, 1970; Al-Samerra'i, 1990).

Al-Mutran was jealous of others. Upon hearing about a generous gift given by Saladin to Dr. Abu Al-Faraj Al-Nasrani, court physician of Saladin's household, Al-Mutran neglected his duties until the ruler noticed his neglect, understood the reason, and gave him a like sum (Ibn Abi Usaibiah, 1245/46; Jadon, 1970).

Ibn Al-Mutran served also in Bimaristan Al-Nuri, where he is reported to have attended to a patient with paralysis of one arm and the contralateral leg (Ibn Abi Usaibiah, 1245/46), conceivably a case of crossed paralysis from a motor decussation lesion.

He had a reputation of haughtiness even with kings (Ibn Abi Usaibiah, 1245/1246), but he was praised for his humility when seeking knowledge (Jadon, 1970). He always visited the sick and gave them free medicine.

Ibn Al-Mutran converted to Islam when he was in the service of Saladin (Ibn Abi Usaibiah, 1245/46; Al-Samerra'i, 1990). He was described by the historian Al-Qufti as a "good Muslim." A Syriac Christian, however, declared "this man, for the sake of the honor of the transient world, abandoned the faith and became a Muslim." A contemporary poet, Ibn Hunayn, who disliked Ibn Al-Mutran, accused him of converting to Islam because he loved a boy (Ghulam) who was his servant (Jadon, 1970).

SCHOLARSHIP

Ibn Al-Mutran was known for his collections of manuscripts and books. It was estimated that, upon his death, his library contained over ten thousand volumes (Ibn Abi Usaibiah, 1245/46; Al-Samerra'i, 1990).

Ibn Al-Mutran's best-known publications are:

Kitab Bustan al-Atibba Wa Rawdat al Alibba (Garden of Physicians and Medows of the Wise)

This is a medical anthology containing quotations and extracts from a large number of early medical writings (http://www.nlm.nih.gov/hmd/arabic/biol.html). The book was unfinished when Ibn Al Mutran died (Ibn Abi Usaibiah, 1245/46; Al-Samerra'i, 1990). Ibn Abi Usaibiah reported that he saw the handwritten copy of two volumes of the book dedicated to Saladin (Ibn Abi Usaibiah, 1245/46).

Al-Maqala al-Najmiyyah fil Tadbeer al-Sihiyyah (Health Regimen)

This book, basically one of the two volumes of Kitab AL-Bustan, was written for Saladin (Ibn Abi Usaibiah, 1245/46; Al-Samerra'i, 1990; http://www.nih.nlm.gov/hmd/arabic/biol.html).

Al-Maqala al-Nasiriyyah fi Hifz al Omour al-Sihiyyah (The Nasiriyyah article on Preservation of Health)

This book was dedicated to King Saladin (Al-Samerrai, 1990).

Kitab al-Adwiyah al-Mufrada (Book of Simple Drugs)

This is another book that was not completed, in which he intended to list the available medicines and their uses (Ibn Abi Usaibiah, 1245/46; Al-Samerrai, 1990).

Kitab Adab Tibb al-Muluk (Book of Ethics of Royal Medicine) (Ibn Abi Usaibiah, 1245/46)

Ibn Abi Usaibiah reported that one of Ibn Al-Mutran relatives informed him that after Ibn Mutran's death, his family found several drafts of manuscripts that were subsequently lost (Ibn Abi Usaibiah, 1245/46; Al-Samerrai, 1990).

IBN JUMAY' AL-ISRAEII, ABU MAKAREM HIBAT ALLAH IBN ZEID IBN HASAN IBN EFREIM IBN YACOUB (d. 1198)

Ibn Jumay' was an Egyptian Israeli physician and one of the famous physicians in Egypt during the Ayyoubid's rule (Al-Samerra'i, 1990). He was born in Fustat (old Cairo) and matriculated under Ibn Al-Ayn Al-Zurbi (Al-Samerra'i, 1990). He received honorific titles such as "Ustath Zamaneh" (Teacher of his age). He served the Egyptian ruler Saladin and

King Al-Saleh Najm Al-Din Al-Ayyoubi, who ruled from 1240 to 1249 AD. He gained fame from having prevented a person with cataleptic fit from being buried alive (http://www.nlm.nih.gov/hmd/arabic/biol/html). He practiced medicine in a clinic in the market place in Cairo and taught students of medicine in his house (Al-Samerra'i, 1990).

When the practice of medicine deteriorated in Egypt, Saladin consulted with Ibn Jumay' about the cause of the deterioration and ways to ameliorate it. Ibn Jumay' attributed the decline to the absence of anatomical dissection in the teaching of medicine and replacement of the books of Hippocrates and Galen with summaries of these books. He recommended to Saladin that teaching of medicine should depend on reading original sources and not summaries and that practical clinical teaching in hospitals should be emphasized. He also suggested that graduates should be examined for their proficiency in the profession before being allowed to practice and that practicing physicians should be followed up to insure quality of care (Al-Samerra'i, 1990).

SCHOLARSHIP

Ibn Jumay' is credited with several medical writings, including the following:

Al-Irshad li Masalih al Anfus wal-Ajsad (Advice Regarding the Body and Mind)

This book in four chapters was dedicated to Al-Baysori, the Vezier of Saladin (Al-Samerra'i, 1990; http://www.nlm.nih.gov/hmd/arabic/biol/ html).

A Treatise on "What to Do When a Physician Is Not Available" (Al-Samerra'i, 1990; http:www.nlm.nih.gov/hmd/arabic/biol/html)

A Treatise to Salah al-Din on the Revival of the Art of Medicine

In this book, he wrote, "The best and most excellent way to train medical students is in the hospitals, as they are the places where the doctors and the sick gather and where students can perfectly train themselves in the practice of this art under the supervision of teachers skilled in it" (Al-Samerra'i, 1990; Pormann, 2007).

Sam'a Al-Tasrih bil-Maknoun fi Tanqih al-Qanoun (Book on Describing the Being in The Canon (of Avicenna)

In this book, the author attacks some concepts expressed by Avicenna which contradicts Hippocrates and Galen. When the book arrived in Baghdad, a supporter of Avicenna wrote a poem attacking Ibn Jumay' (Al-Samerra'i, 1990).

Risala lial-Qadi Abi Al-Qasim Ali Ibn Al-Hussein fi ma Ya'tamiduhu Heena la Yajid Tabiban (Letter to Judge Abi Al-Qasim Ali Ibn Al-Hussein concerning What to do in the Absence of a Physician) (al-Samerra'i, 1990)

Maqala fil Laymoun wa Sharabihi Wa Manafihi (Article on the Lemon Drink and its Benefits) (Al-Samerra'i, 1990)

Al-Risala al Saifiah fil Adwiyah al Mulukia (The Saifiah Message on Royal Drugs)

The manuscript was dedicated to King Saif Al Din (hence the Saifiah in the title) Abi Bakr Al-Ayyoubi on the treatment of colitis (Al-Samerra'i, 1990).

AL-NASRANI, ABU AL-NAJM IBN ABI GHALIB (d. 1202 AD)

Al-Nasrani, as the name suggests, was a Christian physician. He was born in the village of Shafa in the district of Houran in Syria. His father was a peasant of meager means. He was brought to Damascus as a child by a physician who taught him the profession. He distinguished himself as a physician and served in the court of Saladin in Damascus to treat his household. He was in poor financial state and could not afford to buy clothes for his daughter. When the caliph became aware of it, he asked for the list of clothes his daughter needed and provided them to her (Ibn Abi Usaibiah, 1245/46; Jadon, 1970).

SCHOLARSHIP

Kitab al-Mujaz fil Tibb (Summary of Medicine)

The book addresses both the science and practice of medicine (Ibn Abi Usaibiah, 1245/46).

IBN HUBAL AL-BAGHDADI, MUHADHIB AL-DIN ABU'L HASAN (1122-1213 AD)

Ibn Hubal, an Arab physician and scientist was born in Baghdad (hence the name Baghdadi) but lived most of his life in Mosul in Iraq. He is also known by the name Al-Khilati, with reference to the city of Khilat in Azerbaijian where he stayed with its ruler. From there he went to Mardin before returning to Mosul at an old age and poor vision. He died in Mosul in 1213 AD at an age of over hundred years. (Al-Samerra'i, 1989; http://www.nml.nih.gov/hmd/Arabic/biol.html).

He learned the Quran in the Nazimiyya School in Baghdad, Arabic literature with Ali Ibn Al-Qasim Ismail Al-Samarqandi of the Hanafi sect of Islam, and medicine with Abi Al-Barakat Ali Malka (Al-Samerra'i, 1989).

SCHOLARSHIP

Kitab al-Mukhtarat fil Tibb (Book of Selections in Medicine)

Ibn Hubal was best known for this compendium, which was written in Mosul in 1165 AD before he left for Azerbaijia. The book is in four parts. The first part is devoted to anatomy and physiology of the body from head to toe, with symptoms and signs of diseases that affect each part. The second part is devoted to reproductive organs in males and females, intercourse, and drugs used for it. The third part is devoted to diseases, their presentations, diagnosis, and treatment modalities, with detailed discussions of headaches, neurological and mental disorders; eye, nose, and throat disorders; liver disorders; kidney disorders; and sexual desires. The fourth part is devoted to simple drugs, poisons, cancer, surgical emergencies, and fevers. The book is highly dependent on Ibn Sina's

"Al-Qanoun," with occasional passages quoted verbatim;The Royal Book of Al-Majusi and Kitab Al-Tasrif of Al-Zahrawi (Al-Samerra'i, 1989; http://www.nlm.nih.gov/hmd/Arabic/biol.html).

Manuscripts of the book are in the Egypt Book Repository, Leydin, Iraqi Museum, the Baghdad Institute of Islamic Studies, and Paris Library (Al-Samerra'i, 1989).

The book was published in two volumes in Pakistan in 1943 (Al-Samerrai, 1989).

HOMSI, KAMAL AL-DIN (d. 1215)

Al-Homsi matriculated in medicine with Sheikh Radiy Al-Din Al-Rahbi and in literature with Al-Kindi. He was a good physician; most of his income came not from medical practice but from commerce and from a shop he had in Damascus. He was sought by a lot of people, including the ruler of Damascus,Al-Malik Al Adel Abu Bakr Ibn Ayyoub. He turned down an invitation from Al Malik Al-Adel to join his court as court physician. He limited his medical practice to the hospital built in Damascus by Al-Malik Al Adel Nour Al-Din Zinki where he treated patients free of charge (Ibn Abi Usaibiah, 1245/46).

SCHOLARSHIP

Al-Homsi is credited with the following scholarly works (Ibn Abi Usaibiah, 1245/46):

Sharh Kitab al 'Ilal wal A'rad (Explanations of Galen's book on Dieases and Treatments).

Ikhtisar Kitab Al-Hawi li Al Razi (Summary of Razes Book Al-Hawi)

Ikhtisar Kitab al-Masa'el li Hunayn Ibn Ishaq (Summary of Hunayn Ibn Ishaq Book on Questions)

Maqala fil Istisqaq (Article on Masturbation)

Ta'liq fil Boul (Commentary on Urine)

Maqala fil Bah (Article on the Penis)

Al-Risala al-Kamila fil Adwiyah al Musahilla (A Complete Communication on Laxative Medications)

IBN AL-MASIHI, ABU NASR SAID IBN Abi Al-Khair Ibn ISA

Ibn Al-Masihi came from Al-Hazira, a village between Baghdad and Takrit in Iraq. He lived in Baghdad, where he studied Arabic literature, and medicine. He excelled in the practice of surgery and joined the court of Caliph Al-Nasir (Al-Samerra'i, 1989). His fame is related to treatment of Caliph Al-Nasir Li Din Allah in 1201 AD, who suffered from a bladder stone. The caliph's physicians advised him to undergo surgery, which the caliph did not favor. Ibn Al-Masihi was consulted. He recommended conservative medical treatment, which worked. The caliph, his mother, and the rest of his family were so impressed and grateful that Ibn Al-Masihi was overwhelmed with money and gifts. When the caliph recovered, he sought revenge from physicians who advocated surgery. Ibn Al-Masihi appealed to the caliph to forgo the revenge, arguing that their recommendations were one of the standards of care for his condition (Ibn Abi Usaibiah, 1245/46: Al-Samerra'i, 1989).

SCHOLARSHIP

Ibn Al-Masihi wrote two books:

Kitab Al-Iqtidab fil Tibb (Summaries of Medicine)

This book was based on Avicenna's "Kulliyat Fil Tibb" in the form of questions and answers about medical problems. Copies of the book are in Petersburg Library, the Book Repository of Egypt, Al-Zahirriya Library in Damascus, St. Joseph University Library in Beirut, Lebanon, and the Mosul Library (Ibn Abi Usaibiah, 1245/46; Al-Samerra'i, 1989).

Kitab Intikhab Al-Iqtidab (Selections of Summaries)

This book is a summary of his other book "Kitab Al-Iqtidab fil Tibb". Copies of it are in Munich, Oxford, and Paris (Ibn Abi Usaibiah, 1245/46' Al-Samerra'i, 1989).

Ibn Al-Masihi died in Damascus in 1202 AD. He had a son who also practiced medicine (Ibn Abi Usaibiah, 1245/46).

AL-DAKHWAR, MOHAZAB AL-DIN ABD UL-RAHMAN IBN ALI IBN HAMID AL-DIMASHKI (1170–1230 AD)

Al-Dakhwar was a leading Arab physician in the thirteenth century. He was born and brought up in Damascus, Syria. The son of an oculist and brother (Hamid Ibn Hamid) of an oculist, he initially was an oculist at the Great Al- Nuri Hospital in Damascus and later became its director. He studied medicine with his father and with Ibn Mutran, Radiy Al-Din Al-Rahawi, Al-Baghdadi and Al-Mardini and became a famous teacher of medicine and educated or influenced most of the prominent physicians of Egypt and Syria in the thirteenth century, including Ibn Abi Usaibiah and Ibn Al-Nafis (Al-Samerra'i, 1990; Haddad, 2003; http://en.wikipedia. org/wiki/Al-Dakhwar).

Al-Dakhwar was the first to establish a school (Madrassa) devoted exclusively to teaching medicine (the Dakhwarian School). He bequeathed his house in Damascus as a charitable trust (Waqf) to establish the school, and provided endowment for its maintenance, teachers' salaries, and students' grants. The school opened on January 12, 1231 AD, and was still in existence in 1417 AD (Al-Samerra'i, 1990; Pormann, 2007). Among those who attended the school were Ibn Abi Usaibiah and Ibn Al- Nafis (Al-Samerra'i, 1990; http://en.wikipedia.org/ wiki/Al-Dakhwar).

Al-Dakhwar served various rulers of the Ayyoubid dynasty. He declined an initial invitation from Sultan of Egypt Al-Adil to practice there because the pay was less than that of his contemporaries. When the sultan became ill, he called for Al-Dakhwar to treat him. When the sultan recovered, Al-Dakhwar became the sultan's personal physician and chief medical officer of the Ayyoubid State (Al-Samerra'i, 1990; http://en.wikipedia.org/wiki/Al-Dakhwar).

Al-Dakhwar died in Damascus in 1230 AD from intracranial hemorrhage (Al-Samerra'i, 1990).

SCHOLARSHIP

In medicine: (http://en.wikipedia.org/wiki/Al-Dakhwar)

Kitab Al-Janineh fil Tibb (Book on the Embryo in Medicine)

This is a book devoted to embryology (Al-Samerra'i, 1990).

Sharh Kitab Taqdimat al-Ma'rifah li Apocrat (Commentary on Hippocrates' "the Introduction of Knowledge") (Al-Samerra'i, 1990)

Mukhtasar Kitab Al-Hawi fil Tibb li Al-Razi (Resume of "Al-Hawi" by Al-Razi) (Al-Samerra'i, 1990)

A summary of Al-Razi's book "Al-Hawi" (Al-Samerra'i, 1990)

Kitab Al-Radd ala Sharh Ibn Abi Sadek Li Masa'el Hunayn (Book on the Response to Ibn Abi Sadek Explanation of "Questions" by Hunayn) (Al-Samerrai, 1990)

Maqala fil Istifragh (Article on Vomiting) (Al-Samerra'i, 1990)

Ta'aliq Wa Masa'el fil Tibb (Commentaries and Questions in Medicine) (Al-Samerra'i, 1990)

Shukouk Tibbiyya wa Radd Ajwibatiha (Medical Doubts and Answers) (Al-Samerra'i, 1990)

In poetry: (http://en.wikipedia.org/wiki/Al-Dakhwar)

Kitab al-Aghani (Book of Songs)

This book is a summarized version of Al-Isfahani's book by the same name.

AL-BAGHDADI, MUAFFAQ AL-DIN ABDEL LATIF IBN YUSUF (1160–1231 AD)

Al-Baghdadi, as his name suggests, was born in Baghdad and traveled extensively in Iraq, Syria, and Egypt (Khairallah, 1942; Al-Mahi, 1959; Haddad, 1975). He was also known as Ibn Al-Labbad and Ibn Al-Labban (Al-Samerrai, 1990).

His father was well versed in Quranic and Hadith (sayings of the Prophet) studies and had his son (Muwaffaq) tutored in Hadith, Quranic studies, and calligraphy when he was a child (Ibn Abi Usaibiah, 1245/46; Al-Samerra'i, 1990). He matriculated in medicine with Amin Al-Dawla Ibn Al-Tilmidh (Al-Samerra'i, 1990).

At age twenty-eight, he left Baghdad for the city of Mosul in Iraq, only to leave it after one year for Damascus, and from there to Akka (Acre, in Palestine). After a short stay in Akka, he went to Egypt to meet other scholars there. He had with him a letter of recommendation from the qadi (judge) of Saladin's army to Saladin's representative in Egypt. In Egypt, he developed relations with Maimonides. While in Egypt, he used to teach religious studies in the Azhar mosque in Cairo from morning till midafternoon, after which he would teach medicine to students who came to him until the end of the day, after which he would return to the mosque to teach some more (Dallal, 2010).

From Egypt, he moved to Jerusalem and back to Damascus and Aleppo. While in Jerusalem, he frequented the Al-Aqsa mosque, where students came to learn from him. While in Damascus, he was appointed by Saladin to teach medicine at the Umayyad mosque. He finally returned to Baghdad after an absence of forty-two years and died there in 1231 AD and was buried there (Ibn Abi Usaibiah, 1245/46; Jadon, 1970; Al-Samerra'i 1990).

The frequent movements of Al-Baghdadi are attributed to the instability and uncertainties in the region during which the influence of the Fatimid dynasty was in decline and the Seljuks controlled Syria (Al-Samerra'i, 1990).

SCHOLARSHIP

Al-Baghdadi was a scholar of independent thought. He is known to have made fierce attacks on his colleagues, including Avicenna, accusing them of being uncritical disciples of Galen (Al-Samerra'i, 1990; Ullmann, 1997).

He specialized in the study of skeletons and corrected earlier misconceptions about the skeleton (Al-Mahi, 1959; Haddad, 1975).

He was a proponent of learning from scholars and less from books. He is quoted to have said, "Those who do not sweat at the doors of scholars will not know excellence and will not shine" (Al-Samerra'i, 1990).

PUBLICATIONS:

Al-Baghdadi wrote over 170 books on language, jurisprudence, medicine, biology, mathematics, history, and logic (Al-Samerra'i, 1990).

His medical books include:

Kitab fil Adwiyah al Mufrada (Book on Simple Drugs)

This is a book dealing with simple drugs (Ibn Abi Usaibiah, 1245/46).

Mukhtasar fil Himiyyat (Summary on Fevers)

This is a summary on the subject of fever (Ibn Abi Usaibiah, 1245/46; Al-Samerra'i, 1990).

Ikhtisar Kitab al-Himmiyat li Ishaq al-Isreali (Summary of Ishaq al- Israeli on Fevers)

This is a summary of the book by Ishaq al-Israeli on the subject of fevers (Ibn Abi Usaibiah, 1245/46; Al-Samerra'i, 1990).

Kitab fi Alat al Tannafus wa Af'aliha (Book on Breathing Equipments and Their Uses)

This book deals with respiratory equipment and their uses, as described by Galen (Ibn Abi Usaibiah, 1245/46; Al-Samerra'i, 1990).

Ikhtisar Kitab Manafi' al A'da' li Galinos (Summary of Galen's Book on Benefits of Body Organs)

This book summarizes the book on organs and their functions by Galen (Ibn Abi Usaibiah, 1245/46; Al-Samerra'i, 1990).

Ikhtisar Kitab al Nabd li al-Israeli (Summary of Ishaq Al-Isreali's Book on Pulse)

This is a summary of Ishaq Al-Israeli's book on pulse (Ibn Abi Usaibiah, 1245/46; Al-Samerra'i, 1990).

Sharh Kitab al-Fusul li Apocrat (Explanation of the Book "Al-Fusul" by Hippocrates)

This book explains Hippocrates's book of seasons (Ibn Abi Usaibiah, 1245/46; Al-Samerra'i, 1990).

Ikhtisar Kitab al-Hayawan of Jahiz (Summary of Jahiz's Book on Animals)

This book is a summary of Al-Jahiz's book on animals (Ibn Abi Usaibiah, 1245/46; Al-Samerra'i, 1990).

Kitab al-Ifada wal-I'tibar fil Umor al-Mushahada wal-Hawadith al-Muay-inah bi Ard Misr (Book on Benefits and Lessons Learned from What Was Seen and Examined in the Land of Egypt).

This book, the largest of Al-Baghdadi's works, is a description of the geography of Egypt, including the floods of the river Nile, and its effects on agriculture and economics of Egypt, and the changing seasons and their effects on the psychology of the people. In this book, he described the famine that affected the country in 1200 AD. He described his findings in the skeletons of people who died from starvation and were buried on a hill near Cairo. He counted more than two thousand skulls and established that the lower jaw consists of one piece, not two pieces, as Galen had suggested (Ullmann, 1997). He wrote, "For while we have the greatest respect for Galen, what we see with our own eyes is more trustworthy" (Ibn Abi Usaibiah, 1245/46; Khairallah, 1942; Al-Samerra'i, 1990).

Risala fil Marad al-Mussama Diabetes (Letter on Diabetes)

This is a short letter on diabetes with an introduction on what the ancients knew about the disorder. Absent from this work is any reference to disorders, other than diabetes, that are associated with polyuria. Absent also is a mention of the sweetness of the urine in diabetes (Al-Samerra'i, 1990; Ullmann, 1997).

Kitab al-Nakhba (Book of Acute Illnesses)

This book is a summary about acute illnesses (Al-Samerra'i, 1990).

Kitab al-Rad ala Ibn Al-Khatib's Explanations of Al-Qanoun of Ibn Sina (Book of response to Ibn Al-Khatib's Explanations of Avicenna's "Canon of Medicine") (Al-Samerra'i, 1990)

Kitab Ta'qib of Ibn Jumay' ala Al-Qanoun (Book of comments on Ibn Jumay' Notes on the "Canon of Medicine") (Al-Samerra'i, 1990)

Kitab al-Nasihatayn li al Atibba' wal-Ulama' (Book on Advice to Phyicians and Wise People) (Al-Samerra'i, 1990)

Ikhtisar Kitab al Hayawan li Ibn Al-Ash'ath (Summary of Al-Ash'ath Book on Animals) (Al-Samerra'i, 1990)

Maqala fil Hawas (Essay on the Senses)

This is actually two articles on the senses. In the first, the author described the known five senses, their functions, and how senses are perceived. The second article is in the form of questions and answers dealing with thirst after eating fish, obesity following illness, overeating with age, relation of size of body part to the function for which the part is used, and developmental delay, among many others (Al-Samerra'i, 1990).

Ikhtisar al-Adwiyah al-Mufrada li Ibn Samajoun (Summary of Ibn Samajoun's Simple Drugs) (Al-Samerra'i, 1990).

Ikhtisar Kitab al Boul li Ishaq Al-Israeli (Summary of Ishaq al Israeli's Book on Urine) (Al-Samerra'i, 1990)

Maqal fil Atash (Essay on Thirst) (Al-Samerra'i, 1990)

Maqala fil Badi' fi Sina'at al Tibb (Essay for the beginner in the Medical Profession) (Al-Samerra'i, 1990)

Nonmedical works include (Al-Samerra'i, 1990):

Kitab fil Qiyas (Book of Analogy)

This is a four-volume book on analogy (Ibn Abi Usaibiah, 1245/46).

Kitab Gharib al-Hadith (Book of Strange Sayings of the Prophet)

Kitab al-Wadihah fi I'rab al-Fatiha (Book of Grammar of the al-Fatiha Sura)

AL-RAHBI, RADIY AL-DIN ABU AL-HAJJAJ YUSUF IBN HAIDARA IBN AL-HASAN (1137–1234 AD)

Al-Rahbi was a physician from Al-Rahba in Iraq. He was born in Ibn Umar Island but lived many years in Al-Rahba (Ibn Abi Usaibiah,

1245/46; Al-Samerra'i, 1990). He studied medicine in Baghdad and accompanied his father, the physician and oculist, to Damascus (during the rule of NurAl-Din Ibn Al-Zinki), then to Cairo, Egypt, where he matriculated with Hibat Allah Ibn Jumay' Al-Masri, the famous Jewish physician. After that, he returned with his father to Damascus, where he became the preferred student of the famous physician Muhazzab Al-Din Ibn Al-Naqqash (Ibn Abi Usaibiah, 1245/46; Jadon, 1970; Al-Samerra'i, 1990). His father died and was buried in Damascus (Ibn Abi Usaibiah). Al-Rahbi served in the court of Saladin and was one of his physicians. Because he refused to accompany Saladin on his travels, he did not attain a higher post in the court (Ibn Abi Usaibiah, 1245/46; Jadon, 1970).

Al-Rahbi practiced medicine at the Great Al-Nuri Bimaristan (hospital) in Damascus as well as at the Citadel of Damascus (Jadon, 1970; Al-Samerra'i, 1990).

Besides Saladin Al-Rahbi served three other rulers of Damascus. He treated Nur Al-Din Mahmoud Ibn Zinki for angina, which caused his death. Thereafter, he served Saladin. Upon Saladin's death, he served his brother Al-Malik al-Adel Abi Bakr Ibn Ayyoub, and finally he served Isa Ibn Al-Malik al-Adel (Ibn Abi Usaibiah, 1245/46; Jadon, 1970).

Besides serving rulers and practicing at the Nuri Hospital and the citadel, Al-Rahbi gave private lessons to medical students. He refused, however, to teach non-Muslim students or those he thought were not fit to become physicians. There were two exceptions, Omran al-Israeli and Ibrahim ibn Khalaf al-Samiri, a Jew and a Christian, because he could not resist pressure put on him to teach them (Ibn Abi Usaibiah, 1245/46' Jadon, 1970).

TheArab historian Ibn al-Jawsi accusedAl-Rahbi of causing Caliph Saladin's death. Ibn al-Jawsi claimed that al-Rahbi bled Saladin against the advice of other physicians. This narrative was challenged by Saladin's biographer, who stated that bleeding Saladin was the consensus of all physicians who attended to the Caliph (Jadon, 1970).

Al-Rahbi was careful to follow strict dietary rules. He is reported to have hired the best cooks to serve at his home and used to invite his friends to share meals with him. He ate only when he was hungry and instructed his cooks not to serve food before he called for it (Ibn Abi Usaibiah, 1245/46).

Al-Rahbi also used to devote Sundays for rest in his orchard. He was known to refuse attending to patients when he had to climb stairs to reach them. He is quoted to have said, "Stairs are the saws of life" (Ibn Abi Usaibiah, 1245/46).

Al-Rahbi died in 1234 AD at the age of ninety-seven years. He was buried in Damascus next to his father (Ibn Abi Usaibiah, 1245/46; Al-Samerra'i, 1990). He maintained good vision and hearing, but his memory for recent events failed shortly before his death. His distant memory remained intact, suggesting the possibility of Alzheimer's disease (Ibn Abi Usaibiah, 1245/46).

SCHOLARSHIP

Tahzib Sharh Ibn al-Tayyib li Kitab al-Fusul by Apocrat (Polishing of Ibn al-Tayyib's Book on Explanation of al-Fusul by Hippocrates) (Ibn Abi Usaibiah, 1245/46; Al-Samerra'i, 1990).

Ikhtisar Kitab al-Masael li Hunayn (Summary of Hunayn's Book of Questions) (Ibn Abi Usaibiah, 1245/46; Al-Samerra'i, 1990)

Maqala fil Istifragh (Essay on Vomiting) (Al-Samerra'i, 1990)

Mukhtasar Al Hawi li Al-Razi (Summary of Al Razi's Book al-Hawi) (Al-Samerrai, 1990)

AL-HALABI, KHALIFEH IBN AL-MAHASIN

Al-Halabi was a very skillful and confident ophthalmologist who never hesitated to operate on cataracts in a one-eyed person (Khairallah, 1942).

AL-HALABI, SUKARRA

Al-Halabi was a Jewish physician from Aleppo, Syria. He gained a reputation when he succeeded in treating a favorite slave of Al Malik Al Adel Nour al Din Mahmoud Ibn Zinki. She was losing weight and refusing to eat in spite of treatments by court physicians. She confided to Al-Halabi that she was Christian and missed the foods that Christians eat. Upon this information, Al-Halabi provided her, from his home, beef and wine for two days. She got much better and told the ruler that Al-Halabi was able to cure her when all the other physicians failed. The ruler was impressed and gave him property and money that made him and his progeny rich (Ibn Abi Usaibiah, 1245/46).

SUKARRA, AFIF IBN ABDEL QAHIR

Afif Sukarra was a Jewish physician from the Sukarra family in Aleppo, Syria. He came from a family known for a number of prominent physicians.

SCHOLARSHIP

Kitab fil Qoulange (Book on Colitis)

This book was written in honor of Al-Malik Al-Nasir Salah al-Din Al-Ayyoubi in 1188 AD.

IBN AL-SALAH, NAJM EL DIN ABU AL- FUTUH IBN MO-HAMMED IBN AL SARRY (d. 1188 AD)

Ibn Al-Salah was originally from Hamadan in Persia but lived in Baghdad where he practiced medicine for a while before moving to Damascus, where he died. He was very well versed in the science and practice of medicine. While in Baghdad, he served Husam Al-Din Tamartash Ibn Al-Ghazi Ibn Arnaq, who treated him very generously (Ibn Abi Usaibiah, 1245/46).

IBN ELYAS, MANSUR

Ibn Elyas is known for his anatomy book in Persian, Al- Mansuri, dedicated to the Persian provincial ruler. The book consists of an introduction followed by five chapters on the systems of the body (bones, nerves, muscles, veins, and arteries). Each of the chapters included full-page labeled illustrations. Interestingly, the anatomy presented is that of Galen and does not include the refinements introduced by Ibn Al-Nafis or Al-Baghdadi (Pormann, 2007).

The concluding chapter is devoted to compound organs and the formation of the fetus, with a diagram showing a pregnant woman (Pormann, 2007).

AL-KAHHAL, AL-SHARIF BURHAN AL-DIN ABU AL-FADL SULEIMAN

Al-Kahhal was originally from Egypt and moved to Damascus to serve in the court of Saladin. He was a respected ophthalmologist and poet, well versed in philosophy, literature, and Arabic language. He was close to Saladin and continued to serve him until his death (Ibn Abi Usaibiah, 1245/46).

SUHRAWANDI, SHIHAB AL-DIN (born 1155 AD)

Suhrawandi was a Persian physician, a wandering Sufi, who stood out among his colleagues for his peculiarities. He seemed dirty in appearance, never cut his hair or nails, and lice crept over his face and clothes. He was described by Ibn Abi Usaibiah as having more knowledge than wisdom. Some described him as a unique genius. He went from Baghdad to Damascus and finally to Aleppo, Syria, where he served Al-Malik Al-Ghazi, Saladin's son. His mystical disposition appealed to Al-Malik Al-Ghazi but not to his father, Saladin, who ordered his death. Suhrawandi isolated himself and died from hunger at age thirty-six (Jadon, 1970).

ABU MANSUR

He was a Christian physician who practiced in Damascus and was for several years in the service of Saladin (Jadon, 1970).

IBN ABI AL-BAYAN, ABU AL-FADL DAUD AL-ISRAELI (d. 1240 AD)

Ibn Al-Bayan was a Jewish physician working in Cairo. He composed "The Dustur Al-Bimaristan (Dispensary for the Hospital) for use in the Nasiri Hospital in Cairo, and a treatise on his medical experience (http://www.nlm.nih.gov/hmd/arabic/biol.html).

DA'UD AL- ISRAELI, ABU Al-FADL (1161–1242)

Da'ud Al-Israeli was a Karate Jewish physician who lived in Egypt in the twelfth century AD. He was born in Cairo in 1161 and died there about 1242. He studied medicine under the Jewish physician Hibat Allah Ibn Jumay' and became the court physician of the Sultan Al-Malik Al-Adil Abu Bakr Ibn Ayyub, the brother and successor of Saladin. He was also chief physician at the Nasiri Hospital in Cairo where he had many students, among them Ibn Abi Usaibiah, who described Da'ud Al-Israeli as the most skillful physician of the time and his success in curing the sick was miraculous (http://en.wikipedia.org/wiki/Da%27ud_Abu_al-Fadl).

SCHOLARSHIP

Da'ud Al-Israeli is the author of an Arabic pharmacopeia in twelve chapters, entitled "Aqrabadhin". It was chiefly of antidotes (http://en.wikipedia.org/wiki/Da%27ud_Abu_al-Fadl).

AL-QAYSI, FATH AL DIN (d. 1259 AD)

Al-Qaysi was an oculist in Cairo. He was chief physician in Egypt and served the Ayyoubid rulers, including Saladin. He was one of three generations of court physicians in Cairo (http://www.nlm.nih.gov/exhibition/islamic_medical/islamic_09 html).

SCHOLARSHIP

Natijat al-Fikr fi Ilaj Amrad al-Basar (The Results of Thinking about Cure of Diseases of the Eye)

The book consists of seventeen chapters dealing with anatomy and physiology of the eye, etiology, symptoms, and treatment of 124 eye conditions, some of which were not described previously (http://www.nlm.nih.gov/exhibition/islmic_medical/islamic_09 html).

AL-RAHBI, GAMAL AL-DIN UTHMAN IBN RADY Al Din YUSUF IBN HAYDARAH (d. 1259 AD)

Gamal Al-Din Al-Rahbi was born in Damascus. He studied medicine under his father as well as other physicians. He distinguished himself in his practice and served for several years at the hospital built by Al Malik Al Adel Nur Al Din Ibn Zinki in Damascus. He had a particular interest in commerce and used to travel to Egypt for this purpose. He left Damascus to Egypt in 1256 when the Mongols occupied Damascus. He died in Cairo in 1259 AD (Ibn Abi Usaibiah, 1245/46; Al-Samerra'i, 1990).

AL-RAHBI, SHARAF AL-DIN ABU AL-HASAN ALI IBN AL-HASAN (1187–1268 AD)

Sharaf Al-Din Al-Rahbi was born in Damascus, son of Rady El Din Al-Rahbi the physician (see above). He was a physician and poet. He matriculated in medicine under his father as well as under Muwaffaq al-Din Al-Baghdadi (Ibn Abi Usaibiah, 1245/46; Al-Samerra'i, 1990). He preferred staying by himself and reading medical books and literature. He was not interested in affiliating with rulers and courts. He worked for a while at the hospital built by Al-Malik Al Adel Nur Al-Din Ibn Zinki. He then taught in the medical school of Damascus. He died in Damascus in 1268 AD. He correctly predicted the time of his death and told his students to make the prediction public so that people will know the extent of his knowledge in life as well as at his death bed (Ibn Abi Usaibiah, 1245/46).

SCHOLARSHIP

Kitab Khalq al Insan wa Hayat A'daihi wa Manafi'aha (Book on Creation of Man, His Organs and Their Benefits) (Ibn Abi Usaibiah, 1245/46; Al-Samerra'i, 1990)

Hawashi Ala Kitab Al-Qanoun li Ibn Sina (Commentary on Avicenna's Canon on Medicine) (Ibn Abi Usaibiah, 1245/46; Al-Samerra'i, 1990)

Hawashi Ala Sharh Ibn Abi Sadeq Al-Naishapuri li Masa'el Hunayn (Commentary on Ibn Abi Sadeq Al-Naishapuri's Explanation on "Questions" by Hynayn) (Ibn Abi Usaibiah, 1245/46; Al-Samerra'i, 1990)

IBN ABI USAIBIAH, MUWAFAK AL-DIN ABU AL ABBAS AHMAD IBNUL QASIM (1203–1269/1270 AD)

Ibn Abi Usaibiah, physician, ophthalmologist, and medical historian, was born in Damascus, Syria, to a family of physicians associated with the Ayyoubid dynasty. His name means "the son of the six-fingered," which derived from the fact that his father, who was also a physician oculist, had a little supernumary sixth finger. His grandfather served Saladin in Egypt. His father and uncle, otolaryngologist, practiced in Egypt before moving back to Damascus in 1200 AD. He studied medicine in Damascus's famous school of al-Dakhwar, as well as in Cairo, Egypt. His schoolmate in Damascus was Ibn al-Nafis, of pulmonary circulation fame. One of his teachers was Radiy Al-Din Al-Rahbi, the famous physician of Saladin, as well as the famous Ibn Al-Baytar, and Al-Kahhal (Al-Mahi, 1959; Jadon, 1970; Haddad, 1975; Haddad, 1993; Campbell, 2011; http://en.wikipedia.org/wiki/Ibn_Abi_Usaibia).

In 1236, Ibn Abi Usaibiah was appointed physician in the Al-Salahi hospital, a new hospital in Cairo where his classmate in medical school, Ibn Al-Nafis, also worked. He returned the following year to Damascus to take a post given to him by Izzedine, the amir (ruler) in Sarkhad (Sarkhar) (Houran region) near Damascus, where he spent the rest of his life. While in Damascus and Sarkhad, he started and completed the writing of his book "Uyoun Al-Anba' Fi Tabaqat Al- Attiba" (Lives of the Physicians; Glimpses of Medical Strata) (Al-Samerra'i, 1990; Campbell, 2011; http://en.wikipedia.org/wiki/Ibn_Abi_Usaiba).

SCHOLARSHIP

Ibn Abi Usaibiah is the most famous biographer of Arab physicians, and has the distinction of being the first historian of Arabian medicine (Campbell, 2011).

Uyoun al-Anba' fi Tabaqat al-Attiba' (Lives of the Physicians; Glimpses of Medical Strata)

This is the only book authored by Ibn Abi Usaibiah and available. It is unique in being the only book of its kind. No other author had attempted an encyclopedia of physicians as Ibn Abi Usaibiah did. The book is made of fifteen chapters and includes the biographies of four hundred Arab physicians and one hundred Greek, Indian, and Alexandrian physicians. The first five chapters are devoted to the historical development of the medical profession and the early physicians. The remaining ten chapters are devoted to Arab physicians at the early days of Islam, the Syriac physician at the beginnings of the Abbasid caliphate, and the translation activities in Baghdad; physicians of Iraq; those in Persia; those in India; those in North Africa and Spain; those in Egypt; and finally those in Damascus (Al-Mahi, 1959; Haddad, 1975; Haddad, 1993; http://al hakawati.net/Personalities/PersonalityDetails/4/, accessed on April 24, 2017).

The first edition of the book, published in 1245/46 AD, was dedicated to the Vezier of Damascus. Ibn Abi Usaibiah continued to revise the book until he died twenty-four years later. It is uncertain whether the new edition was made public during his life (Haddad, 1993; Campbell, 2011; http://en.wikiperdia.org/wiki/Ibn *Abi* Usaibia).

The book included the best of Arab physicians. He obviously had prejudice against certain of the physicians in the book. He told of the disappointment in the book of Rafi' Al-Din Al-Jili, a philosophy teacher and medic, and the chief judge of Damascus, who upon examining a copy of the work found himself not mentioned (Jadon, 1970).

Manuscripts of the book are in the British Museum and at Leyden (Campbell, 2011).

The book was translated into Latin under the title "Fontes relationum de classibus medicorum" (Campbell, 2011).

Ibn Abi Usaibiah has been quoted as claiming the authorship of three other books, none of which is available (http://al-Hakawati.net/Personalities/PersonalitiesDetails/4/).

They are:

Kitab Hikayat al Attiba' fi Ilagat al Dawa' (Book of Stories about Doctors and Treatments)

Kitab Isabat al- Munajjemin (Book of Illnesses of Astrologers).

Kitab Al Tajarub Wal-Fawa'ed (Book of Trials and Benefits)

This book was never completed.

(Al-Samerra'i, 1990; http://al-Hakawati.net/Personalities/PersonalityDetails/4/)

Ibn Abi Usaibiah died in al-Sarkhad, a town near Damascus, in 1269 AD, at the age of seventy years (Al-Samerra'i, 1990).

IBN AI-NAFIS, ALA' UDDINE ABUL HASAN ALI IBN ABI AL-HAZM-AL- QARSHI AI-DIMASHQI (ANNAFIS) (1210/1213–1288 AD)

Ibn Al Nafis's birth date was variously recorded as 1208 (Freely, 2011), 1210, and 1213 (Al-Samerra'i, 1990; Haddad, 1993; Morton, 1997;

Al-Ghazal, 2002; Loukas, 2008; Al-Khalili, 2011; Campbell, 2011; Tarabay, 2011; http://en.wikipedia.org/wiki/Ibn_al_Nafis).

Ibn Al Nafis was born and brought up in a village near Damascus called "Qarsh, Kersh," which is now the Al-Qarshi Quarter south of Damascus. The Al-Qarshi in his name is thus attributed to the town Al-Qarsh (Khairallah, 1942; Athar, 1993; Nagamia, 2003; Loukas, 2008; http://www.angelfire.com/md/takrouti,Ibn_al_Nafis.htm; http://en.wikipedia.org/wiki/Ibn_al_Nafis).

He grew up in a time (thirteenth century) of political turmoil in Islamic history. It was made especially turbulent by the Mongol's sack of Baghdad in 1258. It was made worse by the continuous strife with the Crusaders (Nagamia, 2003; http://en.wikipedia.org/wiki/Ibn_al_Nafis). In his time, in Al-Andalus (Spain), Islamic culture was declining. Cairo and Damascus were the only centers left for education and medical science. He moved to Cairo in 1236, where he spent most of his professional life (Khairallah, 1942; Al-Samerra'i, 1990; Athar, 1993; Al-Khalili, 2011; Taraby, 2011). He built a house in the El-Hussein district of Cairo and remained single. He willed his house and library to Al-Mansuri Hospital, in which he served close to fifty years (Al-Samerra'i, 1990; Haddad, 1993; Al-Ghazal, 2002; Haddad, 2003; Nagamia, 2003). His house in El-Hussein district of old Cairo was made of marble with a fountain in the center in line with Islamic architecture. In it, he entertained princes, ministers of state, leading physicians, and colleagues (Ather, 1993; Haddad, 1993; Nagamia, 2003).

Ibn Al Nafis began his day with dawn prayers, followed by rounds in the hospital and case discussions with students and colleagues. He then attended to hospital administrative issues. In the evenings, he spent the time reading, writing, and discussing medicine and philosophy with his guests at his home.

Ibn Al Nafis was an orthodox Sunni Muslim, and a scholar of the Shafi'i School of jurisprudence and Shari'a (Islamic Law). He disliked the misuse of wine as self-medication, for medical and religious reasons. He is quoted as saying to his physicians when they advised him to drink wine during his illness, "I will not meet God, the Most High, with any wine in me" (Al-Samerra'i, 1990; Haddad, 1993; http://en.wikipedia.org/wiki/Ibn_al_Nafis).

One of the anecdotes about Ibn Al-Nafis states that while he was in the midst of taking a bath in a Hammam (public bath) in Cairo, he stopped his bath and went to the dressing room, asked for a pen and paper, and sat down to write a commentary on the pulse before returning to complete his bath (Haddad, 2003, Nagamia, 2003).

He was a prolific writer with a beautiful style. When he wanted to write, it is said, he would have several pens sharpened and ready before him before he sat at his desk facing the wall to write from memory, picking one pen after another as soon as they got blunted, without stopping for a second (Al-Samerra'i, 1990; Haddad, 1993; Nagamia, 2003).

Ibn Al-Nafis matriculated in 1232 AD in the famous School of Medicine in Damascus under the able mentorship of Muhazzab Al-Din Al-Dimashqi (popularly called Al-Dakhwar). The famous medical historian Ibn Abi Usaibiah was his schoolmate. He practiced medicine in Al-Nuri Bimaristan (Hospital) in Damascus, and in 1236, at the invitation of the sultan, he departed to Egypt to work as an oculist in Al-Naseri Hospital. He also worked in Qalawoun Hospital and Al-Mansuri Hospital. Later he became Egypt's chief physician. Between 1260 and 1277, he was Sultan Bebar's personal physician (Al-Samerra'i, 1990; Haddad, 1993; Al-Ghazal, 2002; Nagamia, 2003; Loukas, 2008; http://www.angelfire.com.md/Takrouti/Ibn_al Nafis.htm; http://en.wikipedia.org/wiki/Ibn al Nafis).

In 1284, Ibn Al Nafis became the first chief of Cairo's Al-Mansuri Hospital and Dean of its School of Medicine (Khairallah, 1942; Ather, 1993).

SCHOLARSHIP

Ibn Al-Nafis was a notable historian, linguist, astronomer, philosopher, logician, and author of fiction (Al-Khalili, 2011). He was also well versed in jurisprudence and the Arabic language (Haddad, 1993). He is reputed to have had a tremendous memory and to have written most of his books from memory without reference to any books or compendia (Nagamia, 2003). His writing sessions were described in this way: "He used to turn his face to the wall and to write as fluently as a waterfall. And when the quill in his hand got blunt, he discarded it and took a fresh one from the collection made ready and placed before him. In this way he lost no time" (Nagamia, 2003).

Ibn Al-Nafis made many contributions in medicine, philosophy, and jurisprudence. His fame stemmed from his discovery of the minor (pulmonary) circulation three hundred years before William Harvey (Al-Samerra'i, 1990; Haddad, 1993; Majeed, 2005; Freely, 2011; Al-Khalili, 2011). He was the first to develop the concept of body's metabolism and is regarded by many historians of science as the greatest physiologist of the Middle Ages, and one of the greatest anatomists in history (Al-Khalili, 2011).

Ibn al-Nafis's works can be divided into five categories (Nagamia, 2003):

Scholarly contributions on old Greek texts

Commentaries on early Islamic texts

Original contributions to medical texts of his time

Writings on nonmedical subjects, including theology and philosophy

Pioneering discoveries like those about the pulmonary and coronary circulations

Among his books are (Haddad, 2003; http://www.angelfire.com/md/takrouti/Ibn_alNafis.htm):

Kitab al-Shamil fil Tibb (Comprehensive Book of Medicine)

An eighty-volume encyclopedia of medicine that was originally intended to be made up of three hundred volumes but could not be completed due to death (Al-Ghazal, 2002; Haddad, 2003; Nagamia, 2003). The manuscript is available in Damascus (Al-Ghazal, 2002), and some of the volumes are in the Iraqi museum (Al-Samerra'i, 1990). It is the most voluminous of Ibn Al Nafis's books and one of the largest known medical encyclope-dias in history (Al-Samerra'i, 1990; Al-Ghazal, 2002). It is much larger than Avicenna's "The Canon of Medicine," which it eventually replaced as the medical authority in the Medieval Islamic World (Al-Samerra'i, 1990; http://en.wikipedia.org/wiki/Ibn_al_Nafis).

N. Heer made a study of the book and identified its contents. Albert Zaki Iskander analyzed and presented the surgical sections in the book from a manuscript (MS # Z 276) in the Lane Medical Library at Stanford University (Nagamia, 2003).

IL-Muhazzab fil Kuhl (Perfected Book on Ophthalmology)

This is a treatise on eye diseases, which includes treatment of trachoma and eye infections. It is largely an original contribution and is extant. A copy of the manuscript is kept in the Vatican Library (Al-Samerra'i, 1990; Al-Ghazal, 2002; Nagamia, 2003).

The book was composed of two main parts. The first was a more general overview of ophthalmology. The second main part focused the reader's attention on specific diseases of various parts of the eye (Loukas, 2008).

Al-Mukhtasar min al-Aghthia (Choice of Nutritional Items)

This is another of Ibn Al-Nafis's famous books embodying his original contributions. The book is on the effect of diet on health, in which em-phasis is placed on diet, nutrition, and food consumption by a patient, rather than on drug prescriptions. A copy of the manuscript is kept in the Berlin Library (Al-Samerra'i, 1990; Al-Ghazal, 2002; Nagamia, 2003; http://en.wikipedia.org/wiki/Ibn_al_Nafis).

Sharh Fusul Apocrat (Commentary on Aphorisms of Hippocrates)

This book is a commentary on the aphorisms of Hippocrates. Copies of the manuscript are kept in Dar Al-Kutub of Egypt, Aya Sofia, and the Gothe Institute. The book was printed in Tehran in 1876 AD (Al-Samerra'i, 1990; Nagamia, 2003).

Sharh Kitab Taqdimat al Ma'rifah li Apocrat (Commentary on Prognostica of Hipocrates)

This book is a commentary on the "Prognostica" of Hippocrates. The "Prognostica" was translated from Greek by Hunayn Ibn Ishaq. A number of commentaries were written on the "Prognostica," including the one by Ibn Al Nafis, which consists of three chapters. It is considered one of the most influential of the Hippocratic writings in the Islamic World (Al-Samerra'i, 1990; Nagamia, 2003; http://www.nlm.nih.gov/hmd/arabic/hippocratic.html).

Ibidymia li Apocrat wa Tafsiruhu li Amrad al-Wafideh (Commentary on the Epidemiology of Hippocrates) (Nagamia, 2003)

Sharh Masail Hunayn Ibn Ishaq (Commentary on the Questionary of Hunayn Ibn Ishaq)

This is a commentary on the Questionary of Hunayn Ibn Ishaq. A copy of the manuscript is kept in the Library of Leyden (Al-Samerra'i, 1990; Nagamia, 2003).

Sharh al-Hidayah fil Tibb

This book is a commentary on Avicenna's "Canon," in which Ibn Al-Nafis developed his theory of pulmonary circulation in 1268 (Morton, 1997; Nagamia, 2003).

Al-Rajul al-Kamil (The Perfect Man)

In this book, Ibn Al-Nafis expounded on his beliefs and teachings supporting Unitarianism (Haddad, 1975; Ather, 1993).

Al-Mujaz bil Tibb (Summary of Medicine (http://en.wikipedia.org/wiki/
Ibn_al_Nafis)

This is a five-hundred-page book on medicine, organized in four sections,
as follows:

Section I: General Principles

Section II: Medicaments and Diets

Section III: Diseases of Organs and Systems

Section IV: Diseases not Specific for a Particular Organ

Kitab Moujaz Al-Qanoun (Epitome of Kitab al Qanoun of Avicenna)

This is an edited version of Avicenna's original "Canon" intended for
medical students in which Ibn Al Nafis criticized the shortcomings of
Avicenna's work and Galen's views. The book was popular in the Islamic
world and was translated into several languages, including Turkish, English,
and Hebrew. This book gave Ibn Al-Nafis fame.

Ibn al-Nafis deleted from Avicenna's original "Canon" the sections on
anatomy and physiology due to "inaccuracies" in these sections, and he
did not include his own commentary on Avicenna's "Canon" (Haddad,
1975; Al-Samerra'i, 1990; Ather, 1993; http://en.wikipedia.org/wiki/Ibn_
al_Nafis). A number of commentaries were written on this book. A copy
of the manuscript is kept in The National Library in Paris (Al-Samerra'i,
1990; Haddad, 1993; Al-Ghazal, 2002; Nagamia, 2003).

Kitab Sharh Tashrih Al-Qanoun (Commentary on the Anatomy in
Avicenna's Canon)

Published in 1242, this book is a commentary on anatomy found in
Avicenna's "Canon." It contained many medical discoveries, most importantly those about the pulmonary and coronary circulations. Ibn Al-Nafis

was twenty-nine years when he wrote the book (http://en.wikipedia.org/wiki/Ibn_al_Nafis).

The book did not get the recognition it deserves at the time of publication probably because it addressed basic science issues (anatomy) rather than clinical matters and because it contained sharp criticism of Galen's and Avicenna's anatomical views. The book describes Ibn Al Nafis discovery of the "minor circulation." The introduction of the book includes five sections. Section one is on the variation of organs among animals. Section two deals with rules of anatomical dissection. The third section is about proof of the benefits of organs. The fourth section is about the role of anatomical dissection in discovering the benefits of organs. The last (fifth) section is about instruments and techniques used in anatomical dissections (Al-Samerra'i, 1990). Copies of the original manuscript are kept in libraries in Berlin, Istanbul, Paris, Tehran, Mosul, and London (Al-Samerra'i 1990).

Risalat al-'Ada' (Essays on Organs)

Al-Risala al-Kamiliyyah fil Seera al-Nabawiyyah (Treatise of Kamil on the Prophet's Biography)

Written between 1268 and 1277, this book is also known as "Risalat Fadl Ibn Natiq" (Essay of Fadl Ibn Nastiq). An early example of science fiction, it is considered to be the first theological Arabic novel. It was translated in the West as "Theologus Autodidactus" (http://en.wikipedia.org/wiki/Ibn_al_Nafis).

Ibn Al-Nafis described the book as a "defense of the system of Islam and the Muslims'doctrines on the mission of the Prophets, religious laws, the resurrection of the body, and the transitoriness of the world."

In this book, Ibn Al Nafis counteracted the philosophical views of Avicenna as expressed in his book "Hai Ibn Yaqzan" (Al-Samerra'i, 1990; Ather, 1993).

In its plot and content, it is similar to "Hay Ibn Yaqzan," written by the Andalusian physician and philosopher Ibn Tufayl a century before (Nagamia, 2003).

Mukhtasar Ousoul al-Hadith (Brief Account of the Methodology of Hadith)

This book is a synopsis on the foundation of the science of the Prophet's Hadith. In the book, Ibn Al- Nafis classifies Hadith into four categories: decidedly true; probably true; probably false; and decidedly false. This is in contrast to traditional Hadith scholars who classified Hadiths into three categories: sahih (sound); hasan (fair); and dai'f (weak). The book is notable for its use of ijtihad (reason) in the evaluation of a Hadith and of its isnad (chain of transmission) (http://en.wikipedia.org/wiki/Ibn_al_Nafis).

Sharh Kitab Tabi'at al Insan li Apocrat (Nature of Man of Hippocrates)

This book is a commentary on the Hippocratic treatise on the Nature of Man (De Natura Hominis) (Nagamia, 2003; http://www.nlm.nih.gov/hmd/arabic/hippocratic.html).

THE PULMONARY CIRCULATION

The prevailing teachings about the pulmonary circulation during Ibn Al-Nafis's time were those of Galen (second century) and Avicenna (eleventh century) that the right and left heart ventricles communicated by means of invisible pores. According to this theory, blood from the right ventricle reached the left ventricle through pores in the septum that separated the two ventricles. In the left ventricle, the blood mixed with air in order to create spirits and then was distributed to the whole body.

Ibn Al-Nafis rejected the concept of septal pores and suggested, instead, that the blood from the right side of the heart must flow through the pulmonary artery to the lungs, where it mingled with air and then was distributed to the whole body (Wakim, 1944; Haddad, 1993; Al-Ghazal,

2002; Loukas, 2008; Al-Khalili, 2011; http://www.anglefire.com/md/
Takrouti/Ibn_alNafis.htm; http://en.wikipedia.org.wiki/Ibn_al_Nafis).

Describing his findings, Ibn Al-Nafis wrote, "But there is not a vent
between them (heart ventricles). The mass of the heart there (in the
septum) is thick with neither an apparent vent, as some thought, nor an
invisible vent through which blood might pass as Galen believed". Then
he goes on "Their claim to have dissected and seen what they say they
have seen is something that I do not believe or can be certain about. On
many occasions, I have seen what disproves their claims which are based
on what they have allegedly found out by repeated dissection" (Qataya,
http://www.islamset.com/isc/nafis/qataya.htm).

While Ibn Al-Nafis described "pulmonary transit," he did not describe
"pulmonary circulation," for there is no explanation in Ibn Al-Nafis's
work of the circular return of the blood from the left ventricle to the
right (Al-Khalili, 2011).

The accurate description of the heart anatomy by Ibn Al-Nafis raised the
question of whether he did indeed practiced dissection of the heart and
other body organs (Qataya, http://www.islamset.com/isc/nafis/qataya.
htm).

Commenting on Ibn Al-Nafis's anatomical descriptions, Charles
Leschtantiller, professor of medical history at Lousan and Hamburg,
said, "No body could have given such a full description unless he had
actually put his finger in the heart cavities" (Qataya, http://www.islamset.
com/isc/nafis.qataya.htm).

There are three different views about the question of whether Ibn Al-
Nafis did indeed practiced dissection (Qataya, http://www.islamset.com/
isc/nafis.qataya.htm):

1. Whether Ibn Al-Nafis or any other Muslim Arab scholar has ever practiced dissection.

2. Ibn Al-Nafis, like Galen, practiced dissection only on animals.

3. Ibn Al-Nafis did dissect human bodies.

Criticism of Galen's anatomical teachings went beyond the heart. In commenting on Galen's anatomy of the gallbladder, Ibn Al-Nafis wrote, "He (Galen) claims that another canal goes from the gallbladder to the intestinal cavities. This is completely wrong. We have seen the gallbladder several times and failed to see anything from it either to the stomach or to the intestines" (Qataya, http://www.islamset.com/isc/nafis.qataya.htm).

In a similar vein, Ibn Al-Nafis corrected Galen's views about the crossing of the optic nerve in the chiasm. According to Galen, "the optic nerve which comes from the right side of the brain goes to the right eye, and the nerve which comes from the left side goes to the left side." Ibn Al-Nafis wrote, "In fact it is not like that, but each nerve goes to the opposite side" (Qataya, http:// www. Islamset.com/isc/nafis.qataya.htm).

The fact that Ibn Al Nafis made the discovery of the pulmonary (minor) circulation (transit) was not known until 1924 when an Egyptian physician (Dr. Muhyo al-Din al Tawi) discovered a script, No. 62243, titled "Commentary on the Anatomy of Canon of Avicenna" (Sharh Tashrih Al-Qanoun of Ibn Sina) in the Prussian state library in Berlin while studying the history of Arab Medicine at the medical faculty of the Albert Ludwig University in Germany, in which Ibn Al Nafis decribed the minor (pulmonary) circulation (transit) of the blood (Al-Ghazal, 2002; Freely, 2011; Raju, 2012).

Ibn Al-Nafis's description of the pulmonary (lesser) circulation preceded by three centuries those of Spanish anatomist Miquel Servetus, Realdus Colombus, Carlo Ruini, Andrew Cesalpino, Andrea Vesalius, and Francois Rebelais (Al-Mahi, 1959; Ather, 1993; Haddad, 1993; Al-Ghazal, 2002).

The first European to write about the minor circulation was Michael Servetus (ca. 1510–1553), who was burned at the stake in Geneva because of his unorthodox religious views (Freely, 2011). He published his description in 1553 (Haddad, 1993). That of Vesalius was in 1555 and Combo in 1559, all in close proximity and following the Latin translation of Ibn Al-Nafis's work on the pulmonary circulation published in 1547 (Haddad, 1993).

The definitive theory of the pulmonary circulation was finally given in 1628 by the English physician William Harvey (1578–1657) in his "Exercitio Anatomica de Motu Cortis et Sanguinis" (Freely, 2011; Al-Khalili, 2011).

It is postulated that European physicians may have first learned about the pulmonary circulation through a Latin translation of Ibn Al-Nafis's work by Andrea Alpago of Belluno (d. 1520) (Al-Ghazal, 2002; Freely, 2011). Thus, his work may have been known to sixteenth-century European scholars such as Michael Servetus, who described the pulmonary circulation in his theological book "Christianismi Restitutio" in 1553. He wrote, "Air mixed with blood that is sent from the lungs to the heart through the arterial vein, therefore, the mixture is made in the lungs. The bright color is given to the sanguine spirit by the lungs, not by the heart." Andreas Vesalius described in his book "De Fabrica" the pulmonary circulation in a manner similar to Ibn Al-Nafis's description. It is interesting that in the first edition of "De Fabrica" in 1543, Vesalius agreed with Galen that the blood "soaks plentifully through the septum from the right ventricle into the left." Then, in the second edition (1555), he omitted the above statement and wrote instead, "I still do not see how even the smallest quantity of blood can be transfused through the substance of the septum from the right ventricle to the left." Another similar description was given by Realdus Colombo in 1559 in his book "De re Anatomica." All of these would influence Harvey (Al-Ghazal, 2002; Al-Khalili, 2011), who, in 1628, demonstrated by direct anatomic observation in laboratory animals the movement of blood from the right ventricle to the lung and then observed the blood returning to the left side of the heart via the pulmonary vein and stated that he could not find any pores in the interventricular septum. In the "Exercitatio Anatomica de Moto Cordis et Sanguinis in Anamalibus," he stated the following: "I began to think there was a sort of motion as in a circle. I afterwards found true, that the blood is pushed by the beat of the left ventricle and distributed through the arteries to the whole body and back through the veins to the vena cava and then returned to the right auricle, just as it is sent to the lungs through the pulmonary artery from the right ventricle and returned from the lungs through the pulmonary vein to the left ventricle, as previously described." Harvey, however, did not understand the physiology of the pulmonary circulation (dissipation of carbon dioxide and replacement with oxygen), which was fully elucidated by Lavoisier in the eighteenth century (Al-Ghazal, 2002).

Some believe that Servetus described the pulmonary circulation independent of Al-Nafis. They point to the following differences between the reports of Ibn Al-Nafis and Servetus. Ibn Al-Nafis denied the existence of pores in the septum of the heart. Servetus was silent on this point and did not exclude the possibility of blood sweating through. Ibn Al-Nafis reported that the blood filters through the wall of the pulmonary artery, mixes with the air in the lungs, and then filters into the pulmonary vein. Servetus believed that the blood passes from the pulmonary artery into the pulmonary vein by way of intermediate vessels. Thus, Servetus differed in two important anatomical details from Ibn Al-Nafis, thus supporting those who claim that Servetus had no knowledge of Ibn Al-Nafis observations (Bosmia, 2013).

In addition to contradicting Galen's and Avicenna's views about the septal pores, Ibn Al-Nafis also disagreed with both on the number of ventricular cavities in the heart, suggesting that the heart has two, not three, ventricles, as Galen and Avicenna believed (Khairallah, 1942).

CAPILLARY AND CORONARY CIRCULATION:

Ibn Al Nafis had insight into what would become the capillary circulation. He stated, "There must be small communications or pores (manafidh in Arabic) between the pulmonary artery and vein," a prediction that preceded the discovery of pulmonary capillaries by Marcello Malpighi in 1661 by four hundred years (http://en.wikipedia.org/wiki/Ibn_al_Nafis).

Ibn Al-Nafis is also credited with description of the coronary circulation as follows: "Again his (Avicenna's) statement that the blood that is in the right side is to nourish the heart is not true at all, for the nourishment to the heart is from the blood that goes through the vessels that permeate the body of the heart" (Al-Ghazal, 2002; http://www.angelfire.com/md/takrouti/ibn_alNafis).

Ibn Al-Nafis was the first to correctly describe the constitution of the lungs and gave a description of the bronchi. He stated, "The lungs are composed of parts, one of which is the bronchi, the second, the branches of the arteria venosa and the third, the branches of the vena arteriosa, all of them connected by loose porous flesh." Then he added, "The need of the lungs for the vena arteriosa is to transport to it blood that has been thinned and warmed in the heart, so that what seeps through the pores of the branches of this vessel into the alveoli of the lungs may mix with what there is of air therein and combine with it, the resultant composite becoming fit to be spirit when this mixing takes place in the left cavity of the heart. The mixture is carried to the left cavity by the arteria venosa" (Al-Ghazal, 2002).

Because of his contributions to the pulmonary, coronary, and capillary circulations, Ibn Al-Nafis earned the title of "Father of Circulatory Physiology" (http://en.wikipedia.org/wiki/Ibn_al_Nafis).

RELIGIOUS SCHOLARSHIP:

Ibn Al-Nafis was also a religious scholar in the Shafei school of Fiqh (jurisprudence) and taught theology in Al-Massrouriah School for Shafei's doctrine in Islam. He was particularly interested in reconciling reason with revelation (http://en.wikipedia.org/wiki/Ibn_al_Nafis).

Ibn Al Nafis died in Cairo after an unknown short (six days) illness at the age of eighty. His physician friend advised him to take a little wine, but he refused, saying that he would not face God with wine in his stomach (Haddad, 1993; http://www.angelfire.com/md/takrouti/ibn_alNafis.htm).

IBN Al-QUFF AL-KARAKI, ABU Al-FARAJ AMIN AL-DAWLA IBN MUWAFFAQ aL-DIN IBN ISHAQ (1233–1286 AD, also listed as 1210–1288)

Born (1210? 1233?) in Karak (Jordan), son of a learned Melkite Christian court official, he was part of a family that moved to Damascus. He became one of the leading thirteenth-century physicians in Syria and enjoyed the patronage of Syrian rulers (Al-Samerra'i, 1990; http:// www.nml.gov/hmd/ arabic/biol.html).

Ibn Al-Quff matriculated with Ibn Abi Usaibiah with whom he studied "Fusul Apocrat", "Masael Hunayn",and Al-Razi's books. He was a class-mate of Ibn Al-Nafis at the Nuri Hospital in Damascus (Huff, 2003; Al-Samerra'i, 1990; http://www.nlm.nih.gov/hmd/arabic/biol. html).

When he completed his medical studies, he practiced in Ajloun, a town in modern Jordan before moving to Damascus (Al-Samerra'i, 1990).

Like Ibn Al-Nafis, Ibn Al-Quff worked in hospitals in Damascus and Cairo and became the most famous surgeon of his age (Huff, 2003). He was the first Arab physician to call for a standard set of weights and measures in medicine and pharmacy (Huff, 2003).

SCHOLARSHIP

Ibn Al-Quff's best-known treatise pertains to his discovery (though chal-lenged) of the capillaries and their role in blood circulation accurately and with much care four hundred years before the first European sci-entist to make this discovery, Marcello Malpighi (1628–1694), an Italian from Bologne who, in 1661, used a microscope to detect capillaries and explain their role in circulation (Huff, 2003; Freely, 2011).

Ibn Al-Quff also excelled in describing the anatomy of the heart and circulatory system. Describing the structure of the heart, Ibn Al-Quff stated, "The heart has four outlets of which two are on the right side. The one branching from the vena cava carries the blood. In the orifice of this blood vessel-which is thicker than any of the other openings-there are three valves which close from the outside in. The second blood vessel is connected with the arterial vein and through it nourishment from the lung comes. I heretofore, know of no one ever describing these valves" (Huff, 2003).

Kitab al-Shafi fil Tibb (Book on Healing in Medicine)

This is considered the first book written by Ibn Al Quff. In it he discussed body organs, physical and mental disorders, and poisons (Al-Samerra'i, 1990).

Al-Umda fi Sina'at al-Jiraha (The Dependable in the Practice of Surgery)

This book on surgery is in twenty chapters and deals with the theoretical and practical aspects of general surgery. In it he described in detail the anatomy of organs, four techniques for circumcision, the treatment for infants with imperforate anus, and an instrument to rinse the urinary bladder (Khairallah, 1942; Haddad, 2003). In contrast to other surgical treatises of the time, Al-Umda omitted reference to ophthalmologic procedures and internal medical disorders because Ibn Al-Quff considered such issues to fall in the domain of ophthalmologists and internists (Al-Samerra'il, 1990; http://www.nlm.nih.gov/exhibition/islamic_medical/islamic_09.html).

Sharh al-Kuliyyat min Kitab Al-Qanoun li Ibn Sina (Explanation of Kuliyyat Section of Avicenna's "Canon of Medicine")

Kitab al Usul fi Sharh al-Fusul li Apocrat (Book of Basis on Hippocrates "Explanation of Fusul")

This book was reprinted in Alexandria, Egypt, in 1902 (Al-Samerra'i, 1990).

Jami' al Gharad fi Hifz al-Sihha wa Daf' al Marad (Compendium on Maintaining Health and Avoidibg Illness)

This is a book on public health and prevention of illness (Al-Samerra'i, 1990).

Ibn Al-Quff provided the general characteristics of the human fetus for the first six to seven days and for thirteen to sixteen days, following which "the fetus is gradually transformed into a clot, and in 28–30 days into a small 'chunk of meat.' In 38–40 days, the head appears separate from the shoulders and limbs; the brain and heart are formed before other organs and are followed by the liver. The fetus takes its food from the mother in order to grow and to replenish what it discards or loses." He also spoke of "three membranes covering and protecting the fetus, of which the first connects arteries and veins with those in the mother's womb through the umbilical cord. The veins pass food for the nourishment of the fetus, while arteries transmit air… by the end of the seventh month all organs are complete" (Hamarneh, 1971; Huff, 2003).

Ibn Al-Quff also composed a popular commentary on the aphorisms of Hippocrates (http://www.nml.nih.gov/hmd/arabic/biol.html).

AL-SADHILI, SADAQA IBN IBRAHIM

Al-Sadhili was a fourteenth-century physician in Mamluk Cairo. He wrote on ophthalmology, the last work on medical scholarship carried out in Cairo during the Mamluk dynasty (Freely, 2011).

AL-AKFANI, SHAMS al-DIN

Al-Akfani was a fourteenth-century physician who practiced in Cairo during the Mamluk dynasty rule of Egypt.

SCHOLARSHIP

Al-Akfani wrote a pioneering work on first aid (The Refuge of the Intelligent during the Absence of the Doctor) (Freely, 2011).

ANDALUSIAN (UMAYYAD WEST) (711–1492 AD)

The establishment of a Muslim state in Spain was an off-shoot of the overthrow of the Umayyad Caliphate in Damascus by the Abbasids. One of the Umayyads managed to travel to North Africa and led the effort to establish a Muslim Caliphate in Spain (Al-Andalus) to replace the lost caliphate in Damascus. Cordoba became the capital in which the Caliph palace and great mosque were built to re-create what had been lost in Damascus (Landau, 1959; Brown, 2010).

Muslim rulers in the Andalus, like their predecessors in the East, were tolerant towards other faiths. They established a pact "Dhimma," a covenant between the ruler and the subjects, by which Christians and Jews were not forced to convert to Islam and were free to practice their religion. They were not excluded from social or economic life and could occupy the highest political posts, including that of vezier (Landau, 1959; Brown, 2010). When Muslims and Jews were expelled from Spain in 1492, the Muslim emperor of the Turks sent his fleet to save them and settled them in his domain (Shadid, 2012).

IBN SHARPUT, HASDAI (915–970)

Ibn Sharput was born in Cordoba. He was prince of the Jewish community that prospered, both financially and culturally, under Arab rule in Andalus (Menocal, 2002).

He was a gifted physician and a diplomat. He served in the post of vezier for Caliph Abdul Al-Rahman the Third, who ruled from 912 to 961. In 949, Ibn Sharput was head of delegation representing the caliph in delicate foreign negotiations (Menocal, 2002).

SCHOLARSHIP

Ibn Sharput's specialty was antidotes to poisons. He is credited for translation of the important work of Dioscorides " On Medicine" from Greek into Arabic (Menocal, 2002).

AL-ZAHRAWI, KHALAF IBN AL-ABBAS (ABU AL-QASIM, ABULCASIS) (931/936–1013)

Al-Zahrawi was born in Medinat Al-Zahra' (hence his name), a village near Cordoba in Spain, where he grew up and lived all his life. He studied medicine at the University of Cordoba. At the time of his birth, Al-Andalus (Spain) was the center of flourishing culture of Muslim science and philosophy (Haddad, 1976; Al-Samerra'i, 1990; Athar, 1993; Haddad, 1993; Aschoff, 1995; Ramen, 2006; Freely, 2011; Tarabay, 2011).

Al-Zahrawi was probably of Spanish, not Arab, descent and converted to Islam (Ramen, 2006).

He became a luminary physician, and, in 961, when he was only twenty-five years of age, he served as the royal physician to the court of Caliph Al-Hakim the Second (914–976) (Al-Samerra'i, 1990).

It is not known who Al Zahrawi's mentor was, but it is obvious that he read Al-Razi's "Al-Hawi" and "Al-Mansuris," as well as Al-Majusi's "Al-Malaki" and Avicenna's "The Cannon" (Al-Samerra'i, 1990).

He was known to be ascetic and frequently attended to sick people without charging fees (Al-Samerra'i, 1990).

SCHOLARSHIP

Al-Zahrawi was one of the greatest Moorish physicians and the greatest figure in Arabic surgery of that day (Wakim, 1944). Some say that he was not a surgeon himself but compiled the surgical knowledge of his Greek, Roman, Indian, and Byzantine predecessors. Others maintain that his works in surgery described operative technics hitherto unknown in medical science and his comments and personal experience prove that he was an excellent surgeon himself (Wakim, 1944).

Al-Zahrawi's understanding of the human body is believed to have surpassed both Aristotle's and Galen's. He made original contributions to almost all fields of medicine (Wakim, 1944; Ramen, 2006). He resurrected surgery from the hands of barbers and helped integrate it into scientific medicine (Haddad, 1993; Al-Kurdi, 2004; Ramen, 2006).

His work had a great impact on the teaching of medicine in Europe during the Renaissance. His impact can be compared with that of Al-Razi and Ibn Sina (Al-Khalili, 2011).

Like Avicenna before him, Al-Zahrawi believed that the doctor had to closely observe his patient. Reviving the spirit of Hippocratic medicine, he urged doctors to behave ethically towards their patients, and he denounced quacks, or physicians who offered treatments of doubtful use in return for money (Ramen, 2006).

Kitab al-Tasreef Leman 'Ajeza 'an al-Taleef (Practical Guide for Those Unable to be Authors, The Method of Medicine, The Arrangement of Medical Knowledge for One Who is Unable to Compile a Book for Himself)

A literal translation of the title of the book is "An Aid to Him That Lacks the Capacity to be an Author." The book is also known by the title "Kitab Al-Zahrawi" (Al-Samerra'i, 1990; Al-Khalili, 2011).

This, his only known work, completed in the year 1000 AD, was a comprehensive encyclopedia of medicine in thirty volumes that include anatomical descriptions, patient-doctor relationship, mother and child care, classifications of disease, as well as sections on orthopedics, ophthalmology, pharmacology, nutrition, and surgery. Most importantly, it was the first work in the Muslim world to treat surgery as a separate field of study. It represents his experience of nearly half a century as a physician and was written as a practical guide to his students, whom he referred to as "my children" (Al-Samerra'i, 1990; Athar, 1993; Haddad, 1993; Ramen, 2006; Al-Khalili, 2011; Freely, 2011; Tarabay, 2011).

The book distinguished Al-Zahrawi in instructing future physicians in the preparation of drugs. Just as Galen had modified the learning of antiquity, so did Al-Zahrawi codify all that had been learned since Galen by Muslim physicians (Ramen, 2006).

Volume one of the book deals with medical generalities; volume two and three deal with diseases (from head to toe) and their causes. The two volumes were translated into Hebrew in the thirteenth century and printed in Latin in 1915 (Al-Samerra'i, 1990).

Volumes four through twenty-seven deal with compound drugs; volumes twenty-eight and twenty-nine deal with simple drugs (Wakim, 1944; Al-Samerra'i, 1990).

The last volume (volume thirty) deals with general surgery and contains two hundred illustrations of surgical instruments used by the author or invented by him (Wakim, 1944; Al-Samerra'i, 1990; Haddad, 1993; Al-Khalili, 2011; Tarabay, 2011). It is divided into three sections: cauterization, operations, and the treatment of fractures and dislocations (Al-Khalili, 2011). The book includes what is believed to be the earliest accurate account of the syringe in the history of medicine: "When there occurs an ulcer in the bladder, or there is a clot of blood or a deposit of pus in it, and you wish to instill into it lotions and medicaments, this is done with the help of an instrument called a syringe. It is made of silver or ivory, hollow, with a long fine tube, fine as a probe. The hollow part containing the plunger is exactly of a size to be closed by it, so that any liquid is drawn up with it when you pull it up; and when you press it down it is driven in a jet" (Al-Khalili, 2011).

The work as a whole is remarkable, although the last volume, dedicated to surgery, became widely known in the West (Ramen, 2006). It contained all the surgical knowledge of the time (Greek, Indian, Greco-Roman, and Byzantine) (Khairallah, 1942). It was translated into Latin by Gerard of Cremona in the twelfth century and went through no less than six editions, the last being in 1881. A Hebrew translation from the Latin edition was printed in Oxford in 1778 (Al-Samerra'i, 1990; Haddad, 1993).

Although cautery was an ancient technique, it probably became more widespread in the medieval West after the influential surgical manual of Albucasis, which devoted much attention to the subject (Siraisi, 1990).

The book was used in Europe, along with Al-Razi's "Al-Hawi" and Ibn Sina's "The Canon," for five to six centuries. The three books were the basis of European medical knowledge during the Middle Ages (Al-Khalili, 2011). It was translated into Latin in 1778, French in 1861, English in 1908, and Turkish (Al-Samerra'i, 1990). It is considered by some to be the first book on neurosurgery. An incomplete manuscript is found at the National Museum in Damascus, Syria (Al-Kurdi, 2004; Majeed, 2005; Ramen, 2006). Original copies in Arabic are kept in the National Library in Paris and the Iraqi museum in Baghdad (Al-Samerra'i, 1990).

Al-Zahrawi was accused of copying Paul of Aegina had merely copied his predecessors, while Al-Zahrawi added a great deal from his personal experience (Khairallah, 1942).

Other, less known, works include (Al-Samerra'i, 1990):

Risala fi Amrad al-Nisa' (Letter on Diseases of Women)

Maqala fi A'mal al-Yad (Essay on Functions of the Hand)

This report was translated into Latin under the title "Jirahat Abul Qasim" (Surgery of Abul Qasim). It was printed in its original Arabic text with English translation in Oxford in 1778.

AL-ZAHRAWI, THE GENERAL SURGEON

Al-Zahrawi is considered Islam's greatest medieval surgeon, one of the fathers of modern surgery, and one of the most frequently quoted surgeons of the Middle Ages (Khairallah 1942; Haddad, 1993;http://en.wikipedia.org/wiki/Al-Zahrawi).

Al-Zahrawi recommended that surgeons acquaint themselves with the anatomy of the region prior to surgery. He recognized pain as a symptom, not a diagnosis, and considered cleanliness essential to wound healing and promoted alcohol for this purpose. He insisted on having all surgical instruments sterilized at all times for use in emergencies. He used a combination of plants to put people to sleep during surgery (Al-kurdi, 2004). He perfected cauterization to seal blood vessels, as well as the technique of ligation of major blood vessels to prevent bleeding, almost six hundred years before Anbroise Pare (Wakim, 1944; Majeed, 2005; Ramen, 2006; http:// en.wikipedia.org/wiki/Al-zahrawi). His description of varicose vein stripping is almost like that used in modern surgery (Athar, 1993). He was a pioneer in the use of catgut and cotton for stitching, both of which are still practiced in modern surgery (Haddad, 1993; Majeed, 2005; http:// wikipedia.org/wiki/Al-zahrawi). He was the first to use salt solutions to wash wounds (Haddad, 2003).

Al-Zahrawi is also considered to be the first surgeon in history to use cotton (an Arabic word) in surgical dressings to control bleeding, as padding in splinting of fractures, and as vaginal padding in the tearing of the pubes during delivery (Athar, 1993).

AL-ZAHRAWI, THE NEURO-SURGEON

Al-Zahrawi was the first to describe skull fractures and their complications, including intracranial bleeds. He was the first to describe tennis ball (Ping-Pong) skull fractures in children. He introduced instruments to make burr holes in the skull and described currently used methods to expose the brain at surgery by connecting burr holes (Al-Rodhan, 1986; Al-Kurdi, 2004).

He used wax and alcohol to stop bleeding during cranial surgery (Athar, 1993). He devised an instrument to treat vertebral slippage (Al-Kurdi, 2004).

He divided skull fractures into axial, comminuted, hair type, and depressed (Athar, 1993). He identified sword strokes as a common cause of penetrating injuries. He divided crushing injuries into those that lacerated the meninges and those that remained superficial (Al-Rodhan, 1986).

In head injuries, he described vomiting, seizures, mental derangement, loss of speech, fainting, high fever, and protrusion of the eyes as signs of poor prognosis (Al-Rodhan, 1986).

He cleansed abscesses and hemorrhagic sites and soaked the areas in wine and the oil of roses (Al-Rodhan, 1986).

For spinal injuries, he described methods of immobilization and traction and noted involuntary urination and defecation as poor prognostic signs (Al-Rodhan, 1986).

Al-Zahrawi also addressed the etiology of infantile hydrocephalus and its treatment:"The skull of the newborn baby is often full of fluid, either because the newborn has compressed it excessively, or for other unknown reasons.The volume of the skull then increases daily, so that the bones of the skull fail to close. In this case, we must open the middle of the skull in three places, make the liquid flow out, then close the wound and tighten the skull with bandage" (Khairallah, 1942; Aschoff, 1999).

AL-ZAHRAWI, THE NEUROLOGIST

Al-Zahrawi described migraine and other chronic headaches. He treated chronic headaches by removal of the superficial temporal artery (Al-Rodhan, 1986).

He treated facial palsy by making the other side of the face paretic through cauterization at one or more sites—root of the ear, a little below the temple, or at the junction of the lips—to affect branches of the facial nerve so as to reduce tone on the normal side and make the face less distorted (Al-Rodhan, 1986). He differentiated between facial palsy and facial spasm (Al-Kurdi, 2004).

He classified strokes into chronic (ischemic), recoverable (transient ischemic), and fatal (hemorrhagic) (Al-Kurdi, 2004).

He defined coma as absence of brain function with loss of sensation and of voluntary movement (Al-Kurdi, 2004).

He classified anosmia into acquired and inherited (Al-Kurdi, 2004) and described Pott's disease (Al-Kurdi, 2004).

AL-ZAHRAWI, THE DENTIST

Almost alone among physicians of the ancient and medieval world, he was interested in dentistry. He described misaligned teeth and ways to correct them. He demonstrated techniques to re-implant teeth that had been knocked out of the mouth and described how to make artificial dentures from bones of cows, a better alternative to the wooden dentures worn by George Washington, first president of America (Wakim, 1944; Athar, 1993; Ramen, 2006: Tarabay, 2011).

He was the first to write about oral congenital anomalies and the anomalies of the dental arch (Haddad, 1993).

AL-ZAHRAWI, THE PLASTIC SURGEON

Al-Zahrawi was among the first surgeons in Europe to practice plastic and reconstructive surgery. In his book "Al-Tasrif," he described several methods of plastic and reconstructive surgery that are still practiced today. He used ink to mark where to make incisions on the faces of patients. He described methods of breast reduction surgery that resemble contemporary technics (Ramen, 2006).

AL-ZAHRAWI, THE ORTHOPEDIST

Al-Zahrawi wrote about methods to set bones in simple and compound fractures. He described the technique for patellectomy, a technique that was not introduced to the West until 1937. He also described what we know today as the Kocher's technique for repair of a dislocated shoulder that the West discovered in the late nineteenth century (Haddad, 1993; Ramen, 2006; Tarabay, 2011).

AL-ZAHRAWI, THE UROLOGIST

Al-Zahrawi described technics for bladder and kidney surgery. He invented a device to examine the urethra, a version of which is still in use, and introduced a technique using a fine drill inserted through the urinary passages for treating impacted calculi in the urethra (Haddad, 1993; Ramen, 2006; Tarabay, 2011; http://www.nlm.nih.gov/exhibition/islamic_medical/islamic_09.html).

Following ancient authors, Al-Zahrawi called for the surgeon to insert his finger into the patient's rectum in order to work the stone down towards the neck of the bladder and then to make a perineal incision through which the stone could be extracted, an operation that demanded a high level of dexterity and a good working knowledge of complex regional anatomy (Siraisi, 1990).

AL-ZAHRAWI, THE OTOLARYNGOLOGIST

Al-Zahrawi knew how to set fractures of the nasal bones. He performed delicate surgeries on the ear and developed tools to examine and operate on the tiny components of the ear. He gave details on transverse tracheotomies (Wakim, 1944; Haddad, 1993; Ramen, 2006).

AL-ZAHRAWI, THE GASTRIC SURGEON

Al-Zahrawi was the first surgeon to operate successfully on the bowels. He perfected surgical technics for gallstones (Ramen, 2006) and is thought to be the first to use hooks for extracting polyps (Wakim, 1944)

AL-ZAHRAWI, THE OBSTETRICIAN-GYNECOLOGIST

Al-Zahrawi showed special interest in women's illnesses. It is said that the reason was the paucity of female obstetricians (Al-Samerra'i, 1990). He was an accomplished obstetrician and gynecologist. He was the first to describe the lithotomy (Walcher's) position for vaginal surgery. He was also the first to use a mirror to reflect light on a structure to be examined, which he developed to examine the cervices of women. He is credited with being the first to describe surgery to resect breast cancer and to devise a vaginal speculum (Khairallah, 1942; Wakim, 1944; Haddad, 1993; Ramen, 2006).

AL-ZAHRAWI, THE PHARMACOLOGIST

Al-Zahrawi described medicinal plants and the preparation of pharma-ceuticals from chemical substances. He was a pioneer in the use of drugs in psychotherapy and made an opium-based medicine that he described as "the bringer of joy and gladness, because it relaxes the soul, dispels bad thought and worries, moderates temperament, and is useful against melankholia" (Freely, 2011). He pioneered the preparation of medicines by sublimation and distillation (http://en.wikipedia.org/wiki/Al-Zahrawi).

AL-ZAHRAWI, THE EDUCATOR

Al-Zahrawi was also a great educator. He encouraged young people to study medicine after completing their studies in the humanities, philoso-phy, astronomy, and mathematics (i.e. real "Hukama," the name Hakeem, for doctors in Arabic, which means "wise") (Freely, 2011).

He recommended that physicians be specialized in a particular branch of medicine because "too much branching and specializing in many fields before perfecting one of these causes frustrations and medical fatigue" (Freely, 2011).

He emphasized the importance of bedside medicine and the bond be-tween doctor and patient "only by repeated visits to the patient's bedside can the physician follow the progress of his medical treatment" (Freely, 2011).

OTHER CONTRIBUTIONS

Al-Zahrawi distinguished between thyroid goiter and thyroid cancer (Wakim, 1944; Keys, 1953: Haddad, 1993). He was the first to identify hemophilia as a hereditary condition (Haddad, 1993; Ramen, 2006). He worked on the eye and extracted cataracts (Ramen, 2006).

INSTRUMENTATIONS AND TECHNIQUES

Al-Zahrawi invented more than two hundred surgical and dental instruments, some of which are on display in the museum in Cordoba, Spain. Among his inventions are tooth extractors, obstetric devices (including forceps), a hook to extract nasal polyps, syringes to perform enemas, and various surgical knives and saws. He developed the innovative use of silk and catgut (made from sheep intestine) to stitch wounds. He may have invented the tongue depressor (Athar, 1993; Ramen, 2006). Others include a bevel-level cannula, instead of the earlier straight one, for use in draining off liquid when treating abdominal dropsy; he designed a concealed knife for opening abscesses in a manner that would not alarm the nervous patient; and he introduced variations in the design of vaginal speculum. He introduced a technique using a fine drill inserted through the urinary passages for treating an impacted calculus in the urethra (http://nlm.nih.gov/exhibition/islamic_medical/islamic_09.html).

AL-ZAHRAWI'S FIRSTS

Al-Zahrawi is credited with the following firsts (Al-Samerra'i, 1990; Haddad, 1993):

Description of hemophilia as a hereditary condition

Removal of urinary bladder stones through the female urethra

Description and treatment of mouth and palate malformations

Use of silk in suturing blood vessels

Forceps delivery (five centuries before it was used in the West)

Description of missed heart beats

Performance of transverse tracheotomy

Lithotomy technique

Kocher's method of reducing hip dislocation way before Kocher

Extraction of fetal bones from the abdomen

Description of extra-uterine pregnancy

Description of placenta accrete and its extraction

The use of hooks in the extraction of a dead fetus

Description of cancer of the breast and its complete removal, preferably by cautery

AL- ZAHRAWI'S LIFE

Al-Zahrawi lived a life full of scientific contributions and firsts in medicine. During his life, he witnessed the collapse of the Caliphate, weakness of Muslim power, and the beginning of the end of the golden age of Al-Andalus. His hometown, Medinat Al-Zahra, was destroyed by Berber armies from North Africa in 1010, three years before his death from natural causes in 1013 (Ramen, 2006).

The street in Cordoba where he lived is now named Calle Albucasis, in his honor. His house is preserved by the Spanish Tourist Board with a bronze plaque (awarded in January 1977), which reads, "This was the house where lived Abul-Qasim" (http://en.wikipedia.org/wiki/Al-Zahrawi).

IBN JULJUL, ABU DAWUD SULAYMAN IBN HASSAN AI-ANDALUSI (944–994 AD)

Ibn Juljul was born in Cordoba, Spain. He started the study of medicine at the age of fourteen years and studied for ten years with a group of Hellinists who had formed in Cordoba around the monk Nicolas under the mentorship of the vezier and physician Abdul Rahman the Third, Hasdai Ibn Sharput. He later became the personal physician of Caliph Hisham Al-Muayyad Bi Allah (Hishan the Second, 976–1009 AD) during whose rule Ibn Juljul wrote most of his books (http://en.wikipedia.org/wiki/ibn_Juljul; Al-Samerra'i, 1990; Vemet, 2008).

SCHOLARSHIP

Ibn Juljul was an influential Andalusian physician and pharmacologist. His work in pharmacology was frequently quoted by Andalusian physicians during the tenth and eleventh centuries. The famous pharmacologist Ibn al- Baghunish was his disciple (Vemet, 2008).

Ibn Juljul was not a prolific writer. The following are the books attributed to him:

Tabaqat al-Atibba' wal-Hukama (Generations of Physicians and Wise Men)

This is an important work on the history of medicine, covering Western and Eastern sources. It includes fifty-seven biographies on nine genera-tions of Greek and Islamic physicians and philosophers. The book was composed in 987 AD. It is considered the second oldest and most com-plete collection of biographies of physicians written in Arabic. The earliest such book was "Ta'rikh al-Atibba" (History of Physicians) by Ishaq Ibn Hunayn. In his book, Ibn Juljul addressed the causes for the decline of science in the Abbasid empire: "The Abbasid empire was weakened by the power of the daylamites and Turks, who were not concerned with science: scholars appear only in states whose kings seek knowledge." The book is the best known of Ibn Juljul's books

(http://en.wikipedia.org/wiki/ibn_juljul; Al-Samerra'i, 1990; Vemet, 2008).

Tafseer Asma' al-Adwiyah al-Mufrada min Kitab Dioscorides (Explanation of Names of Simple Drugs from the Book of Dioscorides)

This book was completed in 982 AD and deals with Materia Medica of Dioscorides (Vemet, 2008). In the book, Ibn Juljul stated that Dioscordes book was first translated into Arabic in Baghdad by Istiphan Ibn Baseel and edited by Hunayn Ibn Ishaq (Ibn Abi usaibiah, 1245/46). Another copy of the book in the Greek language was given as a gift to Al Nassir Abdel Rahman Ibn Mohammad, ruler of the Andalus, from the king of

Constantinoble, king Armanius. This copy of the book remained without translation until King Armanius sent monk Nicolas to Cordoba. This monk collaborated with the court physician and scholar Hasdai and with Ibn Juljul to translate the Greek nomenclature of drugs into Arabic (Ibn Abi Usaibiah, 1245/46; Al-Samerra'i, 1990).

Maqala fi Dhikr al- Adwiyah al- Mufrada lam Yathkuraha Dioscorides (Essay on Simple Drugs not Mentioned by Dioscorides)

This work focuses on simple drugs not listed in the "Materia Medica" of Dioscorides (Vermet, 2008). Ibn juljul attributed those unlisted drugs to neglect by Dioscorides to mention them, or his unfamiliarity with those drugs, or the possibility that such drugs were not in use at his time (Ibn Abi Usaibiah, 1245/46; Al-Samerra'i, 1990).

Risalat al-Tabyeen fi ma Ghaleta fihi Ba'd al- Mutattabibeen (Letter about Mistakes of Some Practitioners)

This work concerns errors committed by quacks (Al-Samerra'i, 1990; Vemet, 2008).

Other scholarly work by Ibn Juljul include a number of treatises and letters on pharmacology and multiple translations and commentaries on the work of Dioscorides (http://en.wikipedia.org/wiki/Ibn_juljul).

IBN AL-KATTANI, ABU ABD ALLAH MUHAMMAD IBN HUSAIN (951–1029)

Ibn Al-Kattani was born in Cordoba and moved to Zaragosa, where he died. He was mentored in medicine by his uncle Mohammad Ibn Al-Husain. He was an important physician and scholar (Ibn Abi Usaibih, 1245/1246)

Unfortunately, almost all of his medical writings are lost.

"Mu'alajat al-Amrad al-Khatera al-Badiya ela al-Abdan min al- Kharig (Treatment of Dangerous Diseases Appearing Superficially on the Body)

This is the only one of Ibn Al-Kattani's writings extant today and is found in the United States National Library of Medicine (http://www.nlm.nih.gov/hmd/arabic/biol.html).

IBN SAMAJUN, ABU BAKR HAMID

Ibn Samajun lived and worked in Cordoba in the second half of the tenth century. Very few details are known about his life. He was a physician with special interest in medicinal substances (http://www.nlm.nih.gov/hmd/arabic/biol.html).

SCHOLARSHIP

AL-Jami' fi Aqwal al- Qudama' wal-Muhtadeen min al-Atibba wal-Mutafalsifeen fil Adwiyah al-Mufrada (Compendium on Simple Drugs with Statements of the Ancients and Modern Physicians and Philosophers)

In this book on simple drugs from ancient and modern sources, Ibn Samajun quoted a large number of authorities on the subject (http://www.nml.nih.gov/hmd.arabic/biol.html).

Kitab al- Aqrabadhin (Book on Compound Remedies)

This second book addresses the compound drugs and their uses (http://www.nml.nih.gov/arabic/biol.html).

AL- LAKHMI, ABDUL KARIM IBN WALID (d. 1075)

Al-Lakhmi, a native of Toledo, was a physician and vezier.

SCHOLARSHIP

Treatise on fever

This work was lost in its Arabic original but preserved in its Latin, Catalan, and Hebrew translations.

Treatise on Causes and Treatment of Visual Difficulties

This work was cited by later authors, particularly ophthalmological writers of the thirteenth century (http://www.nml.nih.gov/hmd/arabic/biol.html).

ABU AL-SALT, UMAYYA IBN ABDEL-AZIZ IBN ABI AL-SALT (d. 1126)

Abu Al-Salt was born in the city of Dania on the east coast of southern Spain. He left Spain for Tunisia (Tunis) at the age of thirty to join the Mahdi religious movement there and became a member of the Amir Abi Taher Yahya Ibn Tamim Ibn Badis Al-Zabri (Al-Samerra'i, 1989).

Abu Al-Salt was a competent physician, astronomer, poet, and philosopher. He was sent to Egypt during the Fatimid period as an ambassador for the amir. In Egypt, he claimed that he can salvage a ship that sank in the waters off Alexandria. When he failed to salvage the ship after a lot of money spent, he angered the ruler there who put him in prison for over two years during which time, he continued to read and write books. After his discharge from prison, he returned to Tunis to continue his scholarly work and died there in 1126 AD. Of the three places he lived in, Spain, Tunisia, and Egypt, he was most productive scientifically during his Tunisian stay (Al-Samerra'i, 1989).

SCHOLARSHIP

The following works are credited to Abu Al-Salt:

Kitab al-Adwiyah al-Mufrada (Book on Simple Drugs)

Copies of this book are at the Great Mosque in Sana'a (Yemen), and the Bodlian Library, Oxford (Al-Samerra'i, 1989).

Kitab al-Intisar li Hunayn Ibn Ishaq (Book of Support for Hunayn Ibn Ishaq)

This book is in support of Hunayn Ibn Ishaq's views in his book "Masael" and against the views expressed by Ali Ibn Radwan on the book (Al-Samerra'i, 1989).

Al-Risala al-Masriyyah (The Egytian Letter)

This book is the best known of Abu- Al-Salt. It is considered a historical document on Egypt and its people. It includes the history of Egypt from the period of the Pharoes to the Islamic period. It includes sections on medicine in Egypt, the good and bad practitioners in Egypt, and the en-chantment of the Egyptians with astrology (Al-Samerra'i, 1989)

Risala fil Musiqa (Letter on Music) (Al-Samerra'i. 1989)

THE IBN ZUHR FAMILY OF PHYSICIANS

The Bani Zuhr family became famous in the twelfth and thirteenth cen-turies and had six successive generations of physicians including two women physicians. Members of the family reached high ranks in the en-tourages of princes, and were the "ulama" (scholars), "ruasa" (chiefs), "hukama" (wise men), and "veziers" (ministers) (Al-Rubiay, 2005).

The family "Banu Zuhr" belongs to Arabic tribes called "Iyad" and their surname was "Iyadi".They came from the Arabian Desert, then dispersed in Iraq. A group of them went and settled in the East Desert in Andalus (Spain) in the tenth century AD. Ibn Zuhr was the nickname of the family , and Zuhr Al-Iyadi was the greatest grandfather of it (Al-Rubiay, 2005).

IBN ZUHR (AVENZOAR, ABYNZOAR), ABU MARWAN ABDUL MALIK IBN ABI AL-ALA' ZUHR IBN ABI MARWAN (1091/1094/1111/1113- 1160/1162)

Ibn Zuhr's date of birth is variably reported as 1091, 1094, 1111, and 1113. His death is reported as occurring in 1160 and 1162. He was born and lived in Seville (Haddad, 1993; Al-Rubiay, 2005; Pormann, 2007; Al-Khalili, 2011; Freely, 2011). He was one of the great Andalusian physicians.

He is known in Europe as "Abomeroan" (Al-Samerra'i, 1990). The name "Al-Iyadi" refers to his original Arabian tribe "Iyad" descenfdents from Nizar, son of Maad and son of Adnan. Zuhr Al-Iyadi moved from Arabia to Andalusia in the ninth century snd from him issued Abu Bakr Muhammad Ibn Marwan Ibn Zuhr, the famous Muslim scholar in Fiqh (Islamic Jurisprudence) and Hadith (Prophetic traditions), and the great grandfather of six successive generations of physicians (Abdel-Halim, 2005).

Ibn Zuhr's family produced five generations of physicians (including two female physicians) who served the Almoravid dynasty in the Maghreb and al-Andalus (Azar, 2002; Freely, 2011). In Europe, he is the most known among other physicians in his family. Like his father, he was a devout Muslim, and did not like liberal interpretations of the Shari'a of Islam. Also, like his father, he was not fond of Avicenna and did not use Avicenna's "Canon in Medicine." His favorite books were those of Galen (Al-Samerra'i, 1990; Azar, 2002), although he questioned many of the beliefs of Galen (Wakim, 1944). He had nothing but scorn for surgery and left that for barbers (Wakim, 1944). He did not believe it compatible with his dignity to prepare his own medicines, although he is credited with writing a work "Itersir" or "Theisir" which gives information on preparing medicines (Wakim, 1944).

From reading his book "Al-Tayseer" we discover some snippets about his early life. He had smallpox as a child at a time when his physician father was absent. He was attended to by his grandparents who gave him honey to console him. As a youth he had a prolonged fever, perhaps what we now call typhoid fever. He was treated with watermelon splurged in smelling water lily, and camphor sprinkled over apple. He also fell from his mount while in the company of his father and broke a bone in the right forearm (Colles' fracture). The fracture was set by his father, a first by him (Azar, 2002).

He studied medicine with his father and later in the University of Cordoba. Upon completing his medical studies, he started his practice under his father, Abu Al-Ala' Zuhr (Al-Samerra'i, 1990; Freely, 2011; Tarabay, 2011).

Like his father, he was the court physician of the Moravid Amir Ali Ibn Yusef Ibn Tashfin (r. 1106–1143), who took him with him in 1130 AD to Morocco. However, having fallen out of favor with the Al-Moravid ruler Ali Ibn Yusef Ibn Tashfin, he was apprehended and jailed in Morocco. When the Al-Moravids were overthown by the Al-Mohad dynasty, who conquered Seville in 1143 AD, Ibn Zuhr returned to Seville in 1147 and was restored to favor by the new ruler, Abd Al-Mu'min (r. 1145-1163), who appointed him as his court physician and personal counsellor with the rank of vezier. Ibn Zuhr dedicated two medical works to Abd Al-Mu'min , one on antidotes to poisons and the other on dietetics (Al-Samerra'i, 1990; Athar, 1993; Azar, 2002; Freely, 2011; http://en.wikipedia.org/wiki/Ibn_Zuhr).

According to Ibn Abi Usaibiah, he held unorthodox views in medicine. For instance, he forbade hot baths because they had a poisonous action and they interfered with the composition of the humors (Al-Rubiay, 2005).

He was a tactful, experienced physician who practiced medicine in an autocratic manner, much more as a consultant than a practicing physician. He used the art of medicine to a very high degree of refinement (Haddad, 1993).

SCHOLARSHIP

Ibn Zuhr is considered the father of experimental surgery. He introduced human dissection and autopsy. He was the first physician to reject the theory of the four humors that dominated thinking for ages. Along with Al-Zahrawi, he developed (in Islamic Spain) modern anesthesia. The sponge used to be dipped and left in a mixture of cannabis, opium, hyocyamus, and a plant called zoan. It differed from the drinks forced by Indians, Romans, and Greeks into their patients for relief of pain. The claim of credit for the use of sponge to an Italian or Alexandrian has not been confirmed. He developed a special interest in simple drugs and wrote an early pharmacopeia, which later became the first Arabic book to be printed with movable type in 1491 (Al-Samerra'i, 1990; Tarabay, 2011; http://en.wikipedia.org/wiki/Ibn_Zuhr).

Kitab al-Tayseer fil Mudawah wal-Tadbeer (Early Guide to Therapy and Dietetics)

This is the main book written by Ibn Zuhr. It was written at the request of his friend Ibn Rushd to complement Ibn Rushd's book "Al-Kuliyyat fil Tibb" and is dedicated to Ibn Rushd (Al-Samerra'i, 1990; Freely, 2011). It is a book of clinical medicine and pathology, including a section "Al-Jami' ", a collection of prescriptions (Haddad, 1975; Al-Samerra'i, 1990; Ullman, 1997). It includes clinic-pathological correlations , diagnosis, and treatment of diseases starting from the head and neck, chest, upper abdomen, lower abdomen, then bones, then general affections, fevers and epidemics, followed by "Al-Jami'", a health education book for patients and their relatives (Abdel-Halim, 2005). It includes a clinical description of mediastinal abscess from which the author suffered personally and left a very careful record of his own symptoms (Haddad, 1975). In the book, Ibn Zuhr was the first to distinguish between a moist and a dry type of pericarditis (Bloomfield, 1983). The book was translated into Hebrew and from Hebrew into Latin (Myers, 1964; Ullmann, 1997; Abdel-Halim, 2005; Freely, 2011). The Latin edition was printed eight times between 1490 and 1554 (Haddad, 1993; Ullmann, 1997, Abdel-Halim, 2005) and was still in use until the European renaissance (Freely, 2011).

The book is in three volumes.

The first volume contains sixteen chapters. It covers disorders of the head, neck, heart, lungs, liver, spleen, and stomach (Al-Samerra'i, 1990).

The second volume contains seven chapters dealing with disorders of the intestine, kidneys, reproductive organs in males and females, skeleton, and joints (Al-Samerra'i, 1990).

The third volume contains three chapters dealing with infectious diseases (Al-Samerra'i, 1990).

Kitab al-Iqtisad fi Islah al-nufus wal-Ajsad (Book of Moderation Regarding the Restoration of Health of Souls and Bodies)

The book contains names of scholars who contributed knowledge to the subject of the book, including those of his contemporaries who wrote on the subject. The book was dedicated to Ibrahim Ibn Yusef Ibn Tashfin. An original copy of the book is in the National Library in Paris (Al-Samerra'i, 1990; Pormann, 2007).

Kitab al-Agthiyah (Book of Nutrition)

It was written for Abdel Mu'min Al-Muwahiddi. An original copy of the manuscript is kept in the National Library in Paris (Al-Samerra'i, 1990). The book was translated from Arabic into Hebrew by Nathan Hameati (Myers, 1964; Al-Samerra'i, 1990).

Kitab al-Zeina (Al-Samerra'i, 1990)

Misbah al-Shifa (Lamp of Healing)

This book was found in its Hebrew translation by Samuel Ibn Talmuk and Ya'coub Ibn Tibbon. The title of "Lamb of Healing" was chosen by Sarton (Al-Samerra'i, 1990).

Tathkara fil Dawa' al-Mushil (Notes on Laxative Drugs)

This book lists laxative drugs and methods of administering them, written to his son, Al-Hafid (Al-Samerra'i, 1990).

Maqala fi Ilal al Kila (Essay on Kidney Diseases)

This book covers disorders of the kidney, including description of kidney stones and methods of treatment (Al-Samerra'i, 1990).

Risala fil Baras (Letter on Leprosy) (Al-Samerra'i, 1990)

Tathkarah fi Ilag al Amrad (Note on Treatment of Diseases)

This book was written for his son Al-Hafid (Al-Samerra'i, 1990).

AL-Qanoun al Muqtadab (Abbreviated Canon of Medicine) (Al-Samerra'i, 1990).

SCABIES MITE

Ibn Zuhr is credited with the discovery of the itch mite of scabies (Ather, 1993; Haddad, 1993).

IBN ZUHR's CONTRIBUTIONS TO THE PROGRESS OF SURGERY

Ibn Zuhr made many contributions to the progress of the specialty of surgery. The most important contribution was his application for the first time of experimental methodology in evaluating new or contro-versial surgical procedures. Ibn Zuhr's application of an experimental animal model to a clinical problem was the forerunner of the method by which many current surgical procedures were developed. An example of such experiments is the indications and safety of tracheotomy, which he proved to be safe and which allowed physicians who came after him, such as Al-Baghdadi and Ibn al-Quff, to recommend tracheotomy without reservation (Abdel-Halim, 2005).

The second important contribution of Ibn Zuhr to the progress of sur-gery was his emphasis on the great importance of a practical knowledge of anatomy for the surgical trainee. Mastering anatomy, according to Ibn Zuhr, was essential training for a surgeon (Abdel-Halim, 2005).

The third contribution of Ibn Zuhr to the progress of surgery was his insistence on an adequately supervised and structured training program for the trainee in surgery before allowing him to operate independently (Abdel-Halim, 2005).

The fourth contribution of Ibn Zuhr was that he drew, in an emphatic way, the red lines at which a physician should stop during his general management of a surgical condition. An example of this, quoted from his book "Al-Tayseer," is: "If the wound caused by a sharp iron has taken into the bones and not extended to the interior, then the treatment I just mentioned is enough for you, so stick to it. However, if it did penetrate the bone then in such a case, the surgeon should come and see" (Abdel-Halim, 2005).

According to his grandson, al-Hafid, Ibn Zuhr was considered the founder of a famous medical school in Andalus (Al-Rubiay, 2005).

Ibn Zuhr died with an empyema and was buried near his father near the Victory Gate in Seville (Haddad, 1993).

IBN ZUHR, AL-HAFID (ABU BAKR MOHAMMAD IBN ABU MARWAN ABD AL-MALIK) (1110/11–1198/9)

Al-Hafid Ibn Zuhr was the son of Abi Al-Ala' Zuhr Ibn Abdel Malik. He was a physician and poet. He was born in Seville. He learned the Quran by heart and studied traditions and Arabic language and literature (Al-Rubiay, 2005). He matriculated in medicine with his father, abu Marwan , and became a distinguished physician. As a poet, he was famous for his muwashahat. He joined the court of Caliph Yacoub Ibn Yusef Al-Mansur, ruler of Morocco, and was favored by him, which raised the envy of other members of the court. The Vezier Abu Zayd 'Abd Al-Rahman Ibn yudian, a jealous and spiteful man had him and his niece poisoned (Al-Samerra'i, 1990; Al-Rubiay, 2005). Some of his poems, for which he was as famous as his medical skills, were preserved (Al-Rubiay, 2005).

SCHOLARSHIP

Al-Hafid wrote a valuable "Risala Fi Tubb Al-Oyoun" (Letter on Eye Diseases) (Al-Samerra'i, 1990; Al-Rubiay, 2005).

Adwiyah Al-Murakkabah (Compound Medicines) (Al-Rubiay, 2005)

Among Al-Hafid's poems "Ayyuha Al-Saki" (To the Provider of Drinks), on drinking, is still popular today (Al-Samerra'i, 1990).

IBN ZUHR, ABDULLAH IBN AL-HAFID (ABU MUHAM-MAD) (b.1181/2–1205/6 AD)

Abdullah Ibn Zuhr was born in Seville in 1181/2. He matriculated in medicine with his father, Al-Hafid Ibn Zuhr, and served in the court of Al-Nasir Ibn Al-Mansour Al- Muwahaddi in Morocco. He died in Morocco in 1205/6 AD at the age of twenty-five under mysterious conditions, possibly poisoned, as was his father. His body was later taken to Seville and buried beside his ancestors at the Gate of Victory. He left two sons who lived in Seville ; the younger, Abul-Al'a Muhammad, was the last physician of the Ibn Zuhr family of physicians who practiced the profession for over one and a half centuries (Al-Samerra'i, 1990; Al-Rubiay, 2005).

IBN ZUHR, ABU AL-ALA' MUHAMMAD

Abu Al-Ala' Muhammad, the younger, studied the works of Galen and became a famous physician. There are no books credited to him (Al-Rubiay, 2005).

BANI ZUHR FEMALE PHYSICIANS

The Banu Zuhr family of physicians included two female physicians, a sister of Abu Bakr Muhammad (Al-Hafid) and her daughter, who died poisoned in the way of Al-Hafid. Both women had good knowledge in women's diseases and labor (al-Rubiay, 2005).

IBN MAYMOUN (MAIMONIDES), ABU IMRAN MUSA (1135/36/38–1204)

Maimonides, a student of Ibn Rushd (Averros), was born in Cordoba (Spain, Al-Andalus) in 1135 AD. His father was an accomplished rabbinical scholar and judge, as had been five generations of his forefathers (Wakim, 1944; Al-Samerra'i, 1990; Freely, 2011).

Around 1159/1160, in the wake of the transition (in 1148) in Andalus from the liberal Al-Moravid rule to the restrictive Al-Mohad rule, his family moved first to the southern area of Spain (Almeria), a Muslim territory, instead of moving north to the Christian territory of Spain, where most Jews of the Andalus went. This move of the family to a Muslim territory suggested to some that the Maymoun family may have converted to Islam (Al-Samerra'i, 1990; Menocal, 2002).

From Almeria in the south of Spain, the Maymoun family moved to another Muslim country, Al-Maghrib (current Morocco) and settled in the town of Fez. It was in Fez where Maimonides received most of his education. He studied philosophy, astronomy, mathematics, and medicine, while he continued the study of rabbinical literature (Keys, 1953; Menocal, 2002; Freely, 2011).

After a stay of five or six years in Fez, the family moved in 1165 to Jerusalem, which at that time was under Crusaders rule. He stayed in Jerusalem for a short time of six months before settling in Egypt, first in Alexandria and later in Fustat, the name of old Cairo , where the family stayed until 1200 (Al-Samerra'i, 1990; Athar, 1993; Menocal, 2002; Al-Khalili, 2011; Freely, 2011; Tarabay, 2011).

In Egypt, Maimonides started his career as a gold merchant before becoming a rabbinical judge and the unofficial leader of the Jewish community. He later engaged in the practice of medicine, became an eminent physician, and served Saladin and his eldest son, Al-Malik Al-Afdal (Keys, 1953; Al-Samerra'i, 1990; Athar, 1993; Freely, 2011; Tarabay, 2011).

Because of his leadership in the Jewish community, he went on to be a revered figure in Jewish history, referred to as the "second Moses" (Menocal, 2002; Taylor, 2008).

During the crusades, Maimonides was sent by Saladin to treat the ailing King Richard the Lion Heart, leader of the Crusaders, who suffered from a poisoned arrow. After his recovery, Richard the Lion Heart asked Maimonides to join his court, but Maimonides declined the offer and stayed in the service of Saladin (Athar, 1993; Tarabay, 2011).

In Al-Fustat, Maimonides had a very busy schedule. In a letter to Ibn Tibbon, Maimonides described his day as beginning with a visit to the Sultan early every morning, and if he or his children and harem were sick, he spent most of the morning in the palace, returning to Fustat in the afternoon to see the yard of his house full of patients, theologians, judges, et cetera. He ate his only meal in the day and attended to visitors and patients until after midnight (Freely, 2011).

SCHOLARSHIP

During the time of Maimonides, Jews had a golden era in Spain, which contributed to the scholarly pursuits of Maimonides. Under Muslim rule in Spain, Jewish physicians came into close contact with learned Arabic medical culture and had access to written heritage of Arabic medicine in the original language. Thus, Maimonides's medical writings were written in Arabic and show extensive knowledge of Arabic versions of works of Hippocrates and Galen (Siraisi, 1990). A renowned scholar and an eminent rabbi wrote, "It was Maimonides Spain, the only land the Jews knew in nearly a thousand years of their dispersion, which made the genius of Moses Maimonides possible" (Tarabay, 2011).

Maimonides was an admirer of Andalusian Muslim philosophers, such as Ibn Bajja and Ibn Rushd, and was well versed in earlier philosophers from the East, such as Al-Farabi and Ibn Sina (Al-Khalili, 2011). What Maimonides took from Islamic philosophers and applied to Jewish theology was no different from what Thomas Acquinas did for Christian theology (Al-Khalili, 2011). Maimonides's writings include treatises on rabbinic theology, philosophy, and medicine (Goodman, 2003). He was to establish a model for the relationship between philosophy that meant not only speculative thought but rational and scientific thought, on the one hand, and theology, or faith-bound thought, which accepted the teachings of scripture and its official interpreters, on the other (Al-Samerra'i, 1990; Menocal, 2002). A fundamental part of Maimonides's makeup was his courageous stand against the concept of Jewish martyrdom, which was encouraged at the time by many religious leaders (Menocal, 2002). Maimonides developed an apophatic spirituality that denied any positive attributes to God. He argued that we could not say that God was good or existed. In his book "Guide to the Perplexed," he said a person who relied on this kind of affirmation would make God incredible and unconsciously lose belief in God (Armstrong, 2009).

Commentary on the Mishneh

This was the earliest of Maimonides's rabbinic writings. The writing of the book began at age twenty-three and was completed in seven years (Freely, 2011).

Book on the Commandments

This was the next major rabbinic work, which was completed in 1170. It was an attempt to codify the 613 commandments presented to Moses according to the Babylonian Talmud (Freely, 2011).

Mishneh Torah

This was Maimonides's major rabbinic scholarship. It was written in Hebrew in fourteen volumes, encompassing Talmudic and biblical law, and completed in 1178 (Taylor, 2008; Freely, 2011).

Treatise on Logic

This is considered Maimonides's earliest philosophical work, although questions have been raised about Maimonides's authorship of the book (Freely, 2011).

The Guide for the Perplexed

This is the major philosophical work by Maimonides, which laid the foundation for much of subsequent Jewish philosophical thought (Al-Khalili, 2011). It is an attempt to explain the fundamental theology of Judaism. It took him five years (1185–1190) to complete the work. The guide was translated into Latin in the thirteenth century (Freely, 2011).

Maimonides was the most prolific author of theMiddle Ages and the shining Jewish physician of the time. He wrote ten medical books (Keys, 1953; Taylor, 2008; Freely, 2011):

Kitab al Mukhtasar (Compendium of Galen's Books)

This book is a summary of medical books by Galen. He was assisted, in its writing, by his student Yousef Ibn Aqnin (Al-Samerra'i, 1990).

Maqala fi Bayan-al A'rad (Treatise on the Cause of Symptoms)

This book was written for Al -Sultan Al -Afdal Al- Ayyoubi following his illness and the different treatments offered by his physicians. The book was translated into Hebrew and Latin (Al-Samerra'i, 1990).

Maqala fi Sharh Fusul Apocrat (Commentary on the Aphorisms of Hippocrates)

This is a collection of more than four hundred brief statements on medicine attributed to Hippocrates. The book is based on a similar book by Hunayn Ibn Ishaq (Al-Samerra'i, 1990). The first aphorism and the best is "Life is short, the art is long, time is limited, experience is dangerous, and the judgment is difficult." This was a statement that spoke to the medical profession's long years of training and enormous number of complex subjects that had to be mastered (Freely, 2011). The book was translated into Hebrew by Samuel Ibn Tibbon (Al-Samerra'i, 1990).

Kitab al-Fusul fil Tibb, Fusul Musa (Medical Aphorisms of Maimonides)

These aphorisms were designed by Maimonides as a reference for physicians. The book includes about fifteen hundred topics dealing with almost every aspect of medical practice and medical theory, including general rules of health. He believed that man must control his passion and live moderately in order to have good health (Wakim, 1944).

One of the general rules of health included in the book concern sexual intercourse: "The indulgence in sexual intercourse is one of the requirements for the maintenance of health, provided that there should be adequate intervals of abstinence between periods of indulgence, so that no noticeable enfeeblement or weakness ensues; rather one's body should feel lighter than before the act. During the time one performs coitus, a person should not be filled with food, nor completely empty thereof, nor very cold, nor very warm" (Freely, 2011).

Another aphorism relates to nerve supply of sex organs: "The penis, genitalia, and neck of the uterus are reached by a surplus of nerves because of the extra sensation which they need during sexual intercourse" (Taylor, 2008).

"In treating the sick, the first thing to consider is the provision of fresh air, clean water, and a healthy diet" (Taylor, 2008).

On what we now call "nail clubbing," he wrote, "With an illness affecting the lung…namely phthisis, there develops rounding of the nails as a rainbow" (Taylor, 2008).

The chapter devoted to specific remedies contains many bizarre prescriptions such as "the brain of the camel, if dried, prepared in vinegar, and imbibed is of value against epilepsy", and "mouse excrement breaks bladder stones…"; "a cattle hoof, if burned and drunk with oxymel, shrinks an enlarged spleen and stimulates the drive to coitus…"; and "staring at the eyes of a wild donkey generates healthy vision, and helps against tearing of the eyes" (Freely, 2011).

The book includes material from Hippocrates and Galen, as well as contributions from six Arab medical writers, along with about forty-two critical remarks by Maimonides (Al-Samerra'i, 1990; Athar, 1993; Freely, 2011).

The aphorisms were translated from the original Arabic into Hebrew and Latin in 1279. It became a popular medical text and continued to be used until the sixteenth century (Al-Samerra'i, 1990; Freely, 2011). An original Arabic copy is kept in the library of Leyden (Al-Samerra'i, 1990).

Treatise on Hemorrhoids

This book was written for a Muslim nobleman who suffered hemorrhoids. In the book, Maimonides advised against surgery and recommended warm baths and bloodletting (Freely, 2011). The book was translated into German and published in Hebrew letters in 1911 (Al-Samerra'i, 1990). A copy of the book is kept in the Egyptian National Library (Al-Samerra'i, 1990).

Treatise on Asthma

In this book, Maimonides recommended treatment of asthma with proper diet, exercise, sleep, bathing, massage, and avoidance of sexual intercourse (Freely, 2011). The book was written for a nobility friend in Alexandria who suffered from asthma. Maimonides advised him to move to Cairo, where the air was dry (Al-Samerra'i, 1990). The book was translated into Hebrew three years after the death of Ibn Maynoun. It was also translated into Latin (Al-Samerra'i, 1990).

Maqala fi Tadbeer al-Sihha, Al-Maqala al-Afdaliyyah (Regimen Sanitarium, Regimen of Health)

This book was written in the form of letters to Saladin's eldest son Al-Afdal (hence the title Al-Afdaliyyah), who suffered from indigestion, constipation, and attacks of depression attributed to overindulgence of alcoholic drinks and life pleasures. In it he stressed personal hygiene and moderation in the pleasures of life. The treatments recommended by Maimonides were those for asthma (see above), in addition (for the treatment of depression) to listen to music and engage in pleasant conversation in the evening to relax prior to sleep. The book was translated from Arabic into Hebrew in 1244 and Latin in 1294 and became popular among Jews, Christians, and Muslims (Myers, 1964; Al-Samerra'i,

1990; Athar, 1993; Freely, 2011). Copies of the original Arabic manuscript are kept the Bodleian library in Oxford and the the Egyptian National Library (Al-Samerra'i, 1990).

Maqala fi al-Jima' (Short Untitled Treatise on Improving Sexual Intercourse)

This book was written for Sultan of Hamat (in Syria) Al-Malik Al-Muzaffar Abi Saad Omar Ibn Nur Al-Din (1179–1192). In the book, Maimonides recommended proper diet, positive mental attitude, massage, ointments, and proper choice of a partner (not in this order!). He also prescribed aphrodisiacal medications for deficient erection, weak semen, and weak desire. Such aphrodisiacal medications included fox testicles as one of its ingredients (Freely, 2011). The contents of the book included references to Avicenna's Book Al-Qanoun (The Canon) and Ibn Zuhr book Al-Tayseer (Al-Samerra'i, 1990). The book was translated into Hebrew (Al-Samerra'i, 1990).

Maqala Sharh Asma' al-A'qar (Treatise on Explanation of Names of Drugs)

This book contains a listing of about four hundred pharmaceutical items with names in Arabic, Greek, Syriac, Persian, and Castilian (Freely, 2011). At the beginning of the book, the author mentions his sources, which include material from Ibn Juljul Al-Andalusi, Al-Lakhmi, and Ibn Samjoun, all of whom are known for their contributions and knowledge of drugs (Al-Samerra'i 1990). A copy of this manuscript is kept in Istanbul (Al-Samerra'i, 1990).

Kitab al-Sumum Wal-Taharruz min al-Adwiyah al-Qatilah; Al-Risala al-Afdaliyyah (Book on Poisons and Their Antidotes)

This book was commissioned by Al Qadi Al-Fadil Abdul Rahim Al-Bisani, Saladin's Vezier (Al-Samerra'i, 1990; Freely, 2011). In the book, Maimonides recommended, for the treatment of snake bites, the use of a tourniquet above the wound, incision made, and venom sucked out, a practice still current today. For ingested poisons, he recommended induction of vomiting. The section on antidotes includes the "electuary of Mithridates," which king Mithridates VI (ruled 120–63 BC) took throughout all his life to immunize himself against poisons (Freely, 2011).

The Inner Secret: Memorandum for Noblemen, and Tried and True Devices for the Highborn

Doubt has been raised about the authenticity of authorship of this treatise by Maimonides (Freely, 2011).

It is a treatise dedicated to Al-Muzaffar Ibn Ayyoub, King of Hamat in Syria and cousin of Saladin. The book deals with sexual issues. He stated, "One select class of human males benefit from sexual intercourse, men who have a hot, moist, irascible disposition, have hairy bodies, eat and drink heartily, live idle lives, and lack intellectual interests" (Freely, 2011).

Kitab al-Tibb al-Qadeem (Book of Ancient Medicine)

A manuscript with this title was found in one of the old Coptic monasteries in Egypt. It includes quotes copied from those other than Maimonides (Al-Samerra'i, 1990).

On Epilepsy

Supported by examples from the Talmud, Maimonides stated, "As long as he has seizures, an epileptic is not admissible as a witness, irrespective of whether seizures occur only at certain times or constantly, but without a specific type. On the other hand, he is qualified to testify when he is healthy, provided that his mind at that time (i.e. between seizures) is completely clear; for there are epileptics whose intellect is disturbed even when they are healthy. One must scrupulously examine the testimony of epileptic individuals" (Rosner, 1975).

It is noteworthy that all of Maimonides's writings were in Arabic except for his "Mishneh Torah," which was written in Hebrew (Menocal, 2002).

FAMOUS QUOTES:

"Man should not cast his sound reason behind him, for the eyes are in front and not in the back" (Burge, 2008).

"The world's redemption would come with the annulment of oppression and of occupation" (Burge, 2008).

"Medical practice in not knitting and weaving and the labor of the hands, but it must be inspired with soul and be filled with understanding and equipped with the gift of keen observation: these together with accurate scientific knowledge are the indispensable requisites for proficient medical practice" (Taylor, 2008; Taylor, 2015). In this quote, Maimonides was echoing Avicenna (three centuries earlier), who said, "An ignorant doctor is the aide-de-camp of death."

MAIMONIDES'S PHYSICIAN'S PRAYER (PETITIONARY PRAYER)

The Physician's Prayer first appeared in print in a German periodical in 1783 under the title "Daily prayer of a physician before he visits his patients: from a Hebrew manuscript of a renowned Jewish physician in Egypt from the twelfth century." Scholars assumed that the "renowned Jewish physician in Egypt from the twelfth century" referred to Maimonides (Rosner, 1967).

Since the 1783 German edition, numerous versions, abbreviations, or excerpts thereof have been presented in English, German, Hebrew, French, Dutch, and Spanish (Rosner, 1967).

Much heated debate exists among the various writers concerning the true authorship of the prayer. Many scholars suggest that the author was not Maimonides but rather Dr. Markus Herz (1747–1802). The history of the prayer is extensively reviewed by Rosner (1967). Points in favor of each, Maimonides and Herz, are listed in Rosner's review. Rosner (1967) concluded from all the discussions presented in the review that "the evidence overwhelmingly favors the concept that the physician's prayer attributed to Maimonides is a spurious work, not written by Maimonides but composed by an eighteenth century writer, probably Marcus Herz.

Absolute proof that this is so is, however, lacking and may never be discovered" (Rosner, 1967).

Excerpts from the prayer include:

"Inspire me with love for my art and Thy creatures. Do not allow thirst for profit, ambition for renown and admiration, to interfere with my profession ....Preserve the strength of my body and of my soul that they are ever ready to cheerfully help and support rich and poor, good and bad, enemy as well as friend. May no strange thoughts divert my attention at the bedside of the sick...Should those who are wiser than I wish to improve and instruct me, let my soul gratefully follow their guidance... Never allow the thoughts to arise in me that I have attained sufficient knowledge, but vouchsafe to me the strength, the leisure and the ambition ever to extend my knowledge" (Rosner, 1967; Al-Samerra'i, 1990).

MAIMONIDES'S LAST DAYS

Maimonides suffered from poor health. In the last years of his life, he spent most of it in bed.

Maimonides passed away in Fustat (old Cairo) in December 1208 at the age of sixty-six to sixty-eight. Jews, Christians, and Muslims mourned him (Al-Samerra'i, 1990; Taylor, 2008; Freely, 2011). He was buried in Tiberias, Palestine, in accordance with his will (Al-Samerra'i, 1990). According to legend, his body was placed on a donkey, which was set free to wander in Galilee. Eventually, the donkey stopped in Tiberias (Taylor, 2008).

Maimonides's tomb in Tiberias can still be seen with the inscription "From Moses (the Prophet) to Moses (Maimonides) there has arisen no one like him" (Freely, 2011). His tomb has become a sanctuary for people to visit (Taylor, 2008).

Maimonides had one son, Abu Al-Muna Ibrahim Ibn Musa, a physician but not of the stature of his father (Al-Samerra'i, 1990).

IBN RUSHD (AVERROS, AVERROES, AVERRHOES), ABU AL-WALID MUHAMMAD IBN AHMAD IBN MOHAMMAD (1126–1198)

Ibn Rushd, a student of Ibn Zuhr (Avenzoar), is also known as Ibn Rushd the grandson to distinguish him from Ibn Rushd the grandfather, who was a distiguished judge in Al-Andalus and the imam of the Great Mosque (Al-Samerra'i, 1990; Freely, 2011).

Ibn Rushd was born and lived in Cordoba, Spain. He was the son and grandson of Muslim jurists in Cordoba (Landau, 1959; Al-Samerra'i, 1990; Lyons, 2009). He studied theology, philosophy, law, and medicine and dabbled with astronomy but did not believe in astrology (Wakim, 1944; Freely, 2011). He was the personal physician to Abu Ya'qub Yusuf after the death of his friend and mentor, Ibn Tufayl, and was appointed judge in Seville from 1169 to 1172 before assuming the role of chief judge of Cordoba and going back to Seville (Athar, 1993; Lyons, 2009; Freely, 2011). He retained his posts under Ya'qub Yusuf's son and successor Abu Yusuf Ya'qub Al-Mansur (r. 1184–1199). Though a physician, he is better known as a philosopher and jurist. He was greatly influenced by Aristotle, on whom he wrote several commentaries (Landau, 1959; Athar, 1993; Freely, 2011). He is considered the most important interpreter of Aristotle in the Islamic world in the Middle Ages (Keys, 1953; Landau, 1959; Ullmann, 1997; Haddad 2003; Lyons, 2009).

His life and work, like that of Maimonides, were shaped by the advent of Al-Mohads and the repression that they brought to the Andalusian society. With Maimonides, he shared a basic vision of the defense of human freedom (Menocal, 2002).

In the twelfth century, politics tipped the balance against Ibn Rushd in favor of theologians (Lyons, 2009). Among his most incendiary philosophical teachings was his belief in the doctrine of the eternity of the world, in contrast to Muslim, Christians, and Jewish beliefs that God made the universe at a time of his choosing and controlled each and every event in it (Lyons, 2009).

In 1195, Caliph al-Mansur confined him for two years in the predominantly Jewish town of Lucena outside of Cordoba because orthodox Islamic scholars had condemned his philosophical doctrines. His philosophical work was buried and the study of his teachings was banned (Lyons, 2009; Freely, 2011). Early in 1198, the caliph lifted the ban and took Ibn Rushd back to his court in Marakesh, where Ibn Rushd died in December of that year (Wakim, 1944; Al-Samerra'i, 1990; Athar, 1993; Freely, 2011).

Ibn Rushd's philosophical views about the soul made him declared, by both Muslims and Christians, a heretic. His students abandoned him. He believed that only weak intellects believed in religion (Wakim, 1944).

His death occurred under suspicious circumstances, and his body was returned to Cordoba for burial (Al-Samerra'i, 1990; Menocal, 2002; Stone, 2003; Freely, 2011).

Ibn Rushd complained about discrimination against women, which he considered one of the serious problems in Muslim society. He wrote, "Our society allows no scope for the development of Women's talents. They seem to be destined exclusively to childbirth and the care of children, and this state of servility has destroyed their capacity for larger matters. They live their lives like vegetables, devoting themselves to their husbands. From this stems the misery that pervades our cities, for women outnumber men by more than double and cannot procure the necessities of life by their own labor" (Freely, 2011).

SCHOLARSHIP

Ibn Rushd's scholarship can be divided into two categories: his "commentaries" on Aristotle and his own treatises on medicine and philosophy (Freely, 2011).

Ibn Rushd wrote at least sixty-seven original works, which included twenty-eight on philosophy, twenty on medicine, eight on law, five on theology, and four on grammar. In addition, he wrote thirty-eight commentaries on most of Aristotle's works and a commentary on Plato's "The Republic" (Freely, 2011; http://en.wikipedia.org/wiki/Averroes).

IN MEDICINE:

Al Kulliyyat fil Tibb (Colliget; Generalities)

This was an encyclopedic summary of medical science of the time based largely on the writings of Ibn Sina, with occasional references to Hippocrates. It is in seven parts (anatomy of organs, health, disease, symptoms, food and medicines, preservation of health, and treatment of illness). It is considered the best of what he wrote in medicine. It was translated from Arabic into Latin in Padua by a Jewish scholar named Bonacosa in 1255 and entitled "Colliget," with the first printed edition made in Venice in 1482 and in Strasburg in 1531 (Keys, 1953; Myers, 1964; Al-Samerra'i, 1990; Athar, 1993, Stone, 2003; Freely, 2011). Two Hebrew translations of the book were made; one was by Solomon Ben Abraham Ben David (Freely, 2011).

The book was a great success. Versions of the book were still appearing on medical school reading lists in Europe as recently as one hundred years ago (Stone, 2003). Upon completion of the book, he asked his colleague and friend Abu Marwan Abdul Malik Ibn Zuhr to write a book in medicine to complement Al-Kulliyat, upon which Ibn Zuhr wrote "Kitab Al-Tayseer Fi Mudawat wal-Tadbir" (Al-Samerra'i, 1990; Freely, 2011).

Al Tayseer (Practical Medicine)

This was a collection of useful excerpts and a clinical description of disease (Athar, 1993).

Damima li Mas'alat al-Ilm al-Qadeem (Supplement to Questions in Ancient Medicine)

This book addresses issues of ancient science, including the work of Ptolemy (Stone, 2003).

Sharh Urjusa of Ibn Sina (Explanation of Mnemonics Attributed to Avicenna)

This book was translated into Hebrew prose by Moses Ben Tibbon in 1260 and into Hebrew verse by Solomon Ben Ayyoub Ben Joseph in 1261. A Latin translation was done in 1280, and a printed edition was published in Venice in 1484. A revised Latin translation was done by Andrea Alpago (Al-Samerra'i, 1990; Freely, 2011).

Sharh Kitab al-Hayawan li Aristo (Explanation of Aristotle's Book on Animals) (Al-Samerra'i, 1990)

Most of the above explanations were translated into Latin by Michael Scott and into Hebrew by Moses Ibn Tibbon (Al-Samerra'i, 1990).

Treatise on Theriac (Antidotes to Poisons)

This book was translated into Latin by Andrea Alpago (Freely, 2011).

Ibn Rushd also made a compilation of the works of Galen (Al-Samerra'i, 1990; http:en.wikipedia.org/wiki.Averroes).

IN UROLOGY, Ibn Rushd identified the tissues of sexual dysfunction and erectile dysfunction and was among the first to prescribe medications for the treatment of these problems.

IN NEUROLOGY, he suggested the existence of Parkinson's disease.

In OPHTHALMOLOGY and OPTICS, he was the first to attribute photoreceptor properties to the retina (http://en.wikipedia.org/wiki/Averroes).

IN PHILOSOPHY:

Ibn Rushd is considered one of the most important philosophers of all times, and is considered by many as the father of secular thought in

Europe (Al-Khalili, 2011). He is famous for extending the work of the previous Islamic philosophers such as Al-Kindi, Al-Farabi, Al-Razi, and Ibn Sina in integrating Aristotle's philosophy with Islamic theology (Al-Khalili, 2011). He applied rational reasoning to theology, which stirred his colleagues against him. He considered Aristotle as "the best representative of philosophy and the most complete of human minds," calling him "the divine philosopher." Ibn Rushd considered that there was no difference between religion and philosophy. Religion, according to him, was aimed at humans to know absolute truth (God) through revelation, while philosophy was aimed at leading humans towards God through reason (Tarabay, 2011).

In Raphael's painting in the Vatican, *The School of Athens* (1510), depicting the world's greatest philosophers, the only Muslim in it is Ibn Rushd (Al-Khalili, 2011).

Of all Muslim physicians, it was Ibn Rushd who grasped what Aristotle meant by his analysis of "being." He saw the Aristotelian "being" to be the essence of a thing. He saw that he must sever the dependence of Islamic philosophy on Avicenna's synthesis, if he was to save the philosophy of Aristotle. In his writings on the subject, he attempted to isolate Avicenna as no true peripatetic (Goodman, 2003).

Ibn Rushd's philosophical work had direct influence on the writings of Albertus Magnus and Thomas Aquinas and in the development of Aristotelianism in the nascent universities of Europe (Landau, 1959; Ivry, 2002; Freely, 2011). Thomas Aquinas believed Ibn Rushd to be so important that he referred to him as "the Commentator," in contrast to Aristotle, who was known simply as "the Philosopher" (Al-Khalili, 2011).

THE COMMENTARIES

Ibn Rushd composed some thirty-eight book-length commentaries on Aristotle's (The First Teacher) corpus. All these commentaries, save two, refer to Aristotle's philosophical corpus. The "De anima" (On the Soul) received particular attention, being one of only five works that he treated fully in three separate formats: The "Jami' " (short commentary); "Talkhis" (middle commentary); and "Tafsir" (long commentary" (Ivry, 2002).

The "short commentaries" are generally considered to be early works and comprise summaries of Aristotle's ideas, based on the Greek commentators. The "middle commentaries" are simplified paraphrasings of Aristotle's writings and are thought to have been written in response to the request of Ibn Ya'qub Yusuf. The "long commentaries," the mature works of Ibn Rushd, deal with the entire Aristotelian corpus, beginning with the "Posterior Analytics," followed by "De anima", the "physics," "De Caelo," and the "Metaphysics."

In one of Ibn Rushd's Aristotelian commentaries, "The Epitome of the "Parva Naturalis", he supported Aristotle's intromission theory of light: "We maintain that the air by means of light receives the forms of objects first and then conveys them to the external coat of the eye, and the external coat conveys them to the remaining coats" (Freely, 2011).

The commentaries were translated into Latin in the thirteenth century and influenced intellectual figures in Europe (Freely, 2011).

Commentary on Plato's "Republic"

In his commentary on Plato's "Republic," Ibn Rushd argued that the ideal state described by Plato in the "Republic" was the same as that of the Arab caliphate (Myers, 1964; http://en.wikipedia.org/wiki/Averroes). He also stated that the government in Cordoba was a tyranny from 1145 onwards, for which he was exiled (Stone, 2003).

His commentary on Plato's "Republic" is believed to have inspired thinkers of the Renaissance such as Thomaso Campanella and Sir Thomas Moore to produce their theories of utopia or the ideal state (Stone, 2003).

Because of his commentaries, Ibn Rushd is referred to as "The Commentator" (Lyons, 2009).

DISSERTATIONS

Ibn Rushd also wrote three dissertations. The first two dealt with Avicenna's theory of the three modes of "being," the third with pre-science (Myers, 1964).

Tahafut al-Tahafut (Incoherence of the Incoherence).

This is the philosophical work that Ibn Rushd is best known for in Islam. It is a refutation of Al-Ghazali's "Incoherence of Philosophy"and in defence of Aristotelian rationalism and the two Muslim interpreters of Aristotle, Al-Farabi and Ibn Sina. It is an attempt by Ibn Rushd to resolve the dispute between Muslim theologians and philosophers (Landau, 1959; Myers, 1964; Al-Samerra'i, 1990; Freely, 2011; Tarabay, 2011).

Ibn Rushd was criticized by Muslim scholars for this book, which nevertheless had a profound influence on European thought.

Fasl al-Maqal

In this treatise, Ibn Rushd seemed to favor human dissection:"Knowledge of the ways of creation leads to an intimate knowledge of the Creator. The better you know these ways, the more intimate your knowledge of the Creator will be. The canonical law of Islam has urged people to ponder everything in existence." He is also quoted to have said, "Practice of dissection strengthens the faith" (Al-Samerra'i, 1990; http:// www.is-lamset.com/isc/nafis/otaga.html). In the "Fasl Al-Maqal," he argued against the proofs of Islam advanced by the Ash'arite school of jurisprudence. In spite of encouraging dissection and supporting the practice by his contemporaries like Ibn Zuhr, there is no evidence that he practiced human dissection (http://en.wikipedia.org/wiki/Averroes).

Kitab al-Jawami' al- Saghir fil Falsafah (Compendium of Philosophy)

This book was written during Ibn Rushd's exile in Morroco before

1158. It includes sections on physics, heaven and earth, generation and corruption, meteorology and metaphysics (Stone, 2003).

Kitab al-Akhlaq (Book of Character)

This is a paraphrase of the "Nicomachaem." It has not survived intact (Stone, 2003).

LAW AND JURISPRUDENCE

In law and jurisprudence, Ibn Rushd wrote:

Bidayat al-Mujtahid Wa Nihayat al-Muqtasid

This was a legal treatise dealing with Shari'a (law) and jurisprudence (fiqh). It is considered the best treatise ever written on the subject (http:// en.wikipedia.org/wiki/Averroes). This was his first book on fiqh (jurisprudence) and took him twenty years to complete. It detailed the principles of Islamic law, their use in each school of jurisprudence, and their practical application in the daily lives of Muslims (Stone, 2003).

ASTRONOMY

At age twenty-five, Ibn Rushd conducted astronomical observations near Marakesh (today's Morocco) during which he discovered a previously unobserved star (http://en.wikipedia.org/wiki/Averroes).

Several of Ibn Rushd's works were translated from Arabic into Hebrew in the 1200s by Jacob Anatoli. Many of these were later translated from Hebrew into Latin by Jacob Mantino and Abraham de Balmas. Other works were translated directly from Arabic into Latin by Michael Scott (http://en.wikipedia.org/wiki/Averroes).

Only a few of Ibn Rushd numerous writings in Arabic, the language in which they were written, survived. Most are preserved only in Latin and Hebrew translations. Among the works that have survived in Arabic is the commentary on the major medical poem (Urjusa) of Avicenna (http://www.nml.nih.gov/hmd/arabic/biol.html).

A manuscript at the Bibliotheque Nationale, dated 1243, contains almost all the works of Ibn Rushd known to the medieval West (Lyons, 2009).

In the Muslim world, Ibn Rushd is remembered as a medical pioneer. The West esteemed his philosophy for being a bridge between faiths (Stone, 2003).

Ibn Rushd is named by Dante in "The Divine Comedy"; he is briefly mentioned in the novel "Ulysses" by James Joyce, alongside Maimonides, and in Alamgir Hashimi's poem "In Cordoba." In addition, he is the main character in "Destiny," a film by Youssef Chahine. The Muslim pop musician Kareem Salama composed and performed a song in 2007 titled "Aristotle and Averros." Averroes is also the title of a play, "The Gladius and the Rose" by Tunisian writer Mohammad Ghozzi, which won first prize in the theater festival in Sharjah (United Arab Emirates) in 1955. Ibn Rushd also has an asteroid (8318 Averroes) named in his honor. (http://en.wikipedia.org/wiki/Averroes).

IBN AL-BAYTAR, ABU AHMAD DIYA' UD-DIN ABD ALLAH IBN AHMAD Al-MALQI (1190–1248)

Ibn Al-Baytar was born in the Spanish Muslim city of Malaqa or its neighborhood (hence the name Malqi), Kingdom of Granada in Spain, at the end of the twelfth century, between 1190 and 1197. He came from a family with a great scientific tradition, which settled in Malaqa. He lived his first years in Malaqa, and between eighteen and twenty years, he moved to Seville (Gorini, 2004). In Seville, he studied with the best botanic teachers of the period, Abd Allah Ibn Salih , Abul -Hadjdjadi, and particularly Abu Al -Abbas Al-Nabati Al- Andalusi (nicknamed Ibn Al-Rumiyya), with whom he started collecting plants and learned to distinguish and identify numerous species, often concentrating on the medicinal uses of the samples. In 1220, he left Spain and began to travel east across North Africa (Morocco, Algeria, Tunisia, Libya) to Egypt, Syria, Constantinople,

Iraq, and Persia, covering the same route as his teacher Abu Al-Abbas Al-Nabati Al-Andalusi. He finally settled in Cairo, Egypt, and shortly before his death, he left Cairo (where he saw people, especially Sufis, using hashish) to go to Damascus, where he met another luminary, Ibn Abi Usaibiah (some say that Ibn Abi Usaibiah accompanied him in his travels). He died in 1248 (Al-Samerra'i, 1990; Ulmann, 1997; Gorini, 2004; Freely, 2011; http://www.nlm.nih.gov/hmd/arabic/biol.html; http://www.al-hakawati. net/Arabic/arabpers.phil2.asp).

His travels were motivated by his interest in herbs and their medicinal use. He became known as the reference on herbal medicine (Wakim, 1944; Al-Samerra'i, 1990; Taraby, 2011). He contributed much that made pharmacy a special science separate from that of medicine (Wakim, 1944).

In Cairo, he served as chief herbalist under the Ayyoubid Sultan Al-Malik Al-Kamil (ruled 1218-1238/1240), nephew of Saladin, and his son and successor Al-Malik Al-Salih (ruled 1240–1249), to whom he dedicated most of his work (Gorini, 2004; Tarabay, 2011). After the death of Sultan Al-Kamil, he spent time in Palestine before returning to Egypt to serve Sultan Al-Malik al-Salih (Gorini, 2004).

SCHOLARSHIP

Ibn Al-Baytar was considered the most influential writer on botany and pharmaceuticals and, by some, the greatest compiler of pharmacological books in the Arab World (Gorini, 2004; Freely, 2011; Tarabay, 2011; http://www.nlm.nih.gov/hmd/arabic.biol.html).

His best pharmacology books are the following two (Freely, 2011; Tarabay, 2011):

Kitab al-Mughni fil Adwiyah al-mufradah (The Ultimate in Materia Medica)

The book is also known in the West as "Mufradat Ibn Al-Baytar". It was dedicated to the Ayyubid ruler of Egypt, Al-Malik Al-Afdal. It describes simple medicines used for various illnesses (Freely, 2011). In the book,

Ibn Al-Baytar addressed each organ of the body separately, with the appropriate medications for that organ (Wakim, 1944; Al-Samerra'i, 1990; Tarabay, 2011; http://al-hakawati.net/Personalities/PersonalityDetails/4/). In the book is the first attempt in history to treat cancer, and Ibn Al-Baytar discovered that Hindba (dandelion) had antibodies to the disease (Tarabay, 2011).

Kitab al-Jami' li Mufradat al-Adwiyah Wal-Aghthiyah (Corpus of Simple Remedies and Nutritionals)

This is considered his most important book. It is an enormous dictionary of simple medicaments and food stuff in tabulated form dedicated to Al Malik Al-Salih. It is an alphabetical guide of 1,400 medicaments (over three hundred discovered by the author and not found in Greek or Indian books) in 2,324 separate entries taken from his own observations as well as over 260 quoted from Greek, Persian, and Arabic predecessors. The book was originally known as "Mufradat Ibn Al-Baytar," but Ibn Abi Usaibiah changed the name to "Al-Jami' Li Mufradat Al Adwiyah and Al Aghthiyah" (Wakim, 1944; Al-Samerra'i, 1990; Freely, 2011; Tarabay, 2011;

http://www. Nml.nih.gov/hmd/arabic/biol, html; http:al-hakawati.net/ Personalities/PersonalityDetails/4/).

The author gave the names of simple medicines in all the languages known to him, as well as the Arabic names of almost all the simple medicines listed in the first-century AD work of Dioscorides (Dallal, 2010). The coexistence of foreign languages with Arabic represents an unprecedent occurrence among Arab Muslim scientific works (Gorini, 2004).

Among quotations in the book from Greek, Persian, and Arab predecessors are a number from the book of his mentor Ahmad Ibn Muhammad Ibn Mufrij "The Eastern Trip," about his travels to the East in search of new plants (http://al-hakawati.net/Personalities/PersonalityDetails/4/).

Kitab al-Jami' had considerable influence in the East among Muslims and Christians. It was translated from Arabic into German, French, and

Turkish. A copy of the book is kept in the Library of Mosul (Iraq) (Al-Samerra'i, 1990; Freely, 2011).

"Al-Jami' " is considered the most important and complete treatise of applied botany produced in the Middle Ages (Dallal, 2010).

Kitab Al Af'al Al Ghariba Wal-Khawas Al 'Ajiba (Book of Strange Actions and Peculiar Qualities) (Al-Samerra'i, 1990; http://al-Hakawati.net/Personalities/PersonalityDetails/4/).

Mizan al-Tibb (Balance of Medicine) (Al-Samerra'i, 1990)

Al-Durra al-Bahiyyah fi Manafi' al-Abdan al-Insaniyyah (The Shining Pearl in the Benefits to Human Bodies) (Al-Samerra'i, 1990)

AL-GHAFIQI, MUHAMMAD IBN QASSIM IBN ASLAM

Al-Ghafiqi was an Andalusian physician with very little known about his life.

SCHOLARSHIP

Guide to Ophthalmology

This book on eye diseases is enriched by illustrations of instruments used in ophthalmology (http://www.nlm.nih.gov/exhibition/islamic_medical/islamic_09 html).

SIX

Female Practitioners
in Medieval Islamic World

In pre-Islamic times, it was often women who acted as healers. The tradition continued in one way or another in the medieval Islamic world. Female physicians are rarely mentioned in the available literature on this period in Islamic history. Sporadic information is available about such female luminaries as the legendery Zaynab of Bani Awd, who is reported to have been a famous oculist. Many of female practitioners were similarly oculists. In North Africa, women are reported to have treated trachoma by scraping the eyelids with fig tree twigs and sugar. Few women practitioners were competent physicians and surgeons (Pormann, 2007). The sister of Abi Bakr Ibn Zuhr and her daughter were luminaries in medicine,and in particular, in obstetrics and gynecology.They were the consultants for the family of Al-Mansour Abi Yousef Ya'qoub Ibn Yousef and are reported to have delivered all their children. Um Al-Hasan, the daughter of Judge Ahmad Ibn Abdullah Ibn Abd Al-Mun'im Abi Ja'far Al-tanjali, was an Andalusian physician and poet *Ahmad Isa Bek, 1981).

Some women practitioners even assumed the post of chief physician, as in the case of the daughter of Shihab Al-Din Ibn Al-Sayigh, who replaced her father as chief physician of Baghdad's al-Mansouri Hospital after his death (Ahmad Isa Bek, 1981).

Women in Islam were also instrumental in establishing hospitals and shelters. Rufaida Bint Sa'ad al-Aslamiyyah (of the Bani Aslam tribe in Medina),daughter of a physician, was the first Muslim nurse. She was born in Yathrib (Medina) before the migration of the Prophet to it. She was among the first people in Medina to accept Islam. Rufaida's father was a physician. She learned medical care by working with him as his assistant. She did not limit her practice to a clinic but went out to the community to solve problems related to disease. As such, she was a public health nurse and social worker. When the Islamic state was established in Medina, Rufaida devoted herself to nursing the Muslim sick. She set up a tent outside the Prophet's mosque (first hospital in Islam) where she attended to the sick and trained nurses. Among those trained by her were Umm Ammara, Amineh, Umm Ayman, Safiyat, Umm Sulaim, and Hind. She also joined the Prophet in some battles to attend to the wounded and to divert casualties to her "hospital tent" in Medina. In some battles, she set up her "hospital tent" on the battlefield. Other Muslim women who were famous as nurses were: Ku'ayiba, Aminah Bint Abi Qays Al-Ghifariya, Umm 'Atiyyah Al-Ansariyya, and Nusaybah Bint A-Maziniyya (http:// en,wikipedia.org/wiki/Rufaida_Al-Aslamia).

The mother of Caliph Al-Mutawakkil (Shuj'a) increased endowment to a hospital in Baghdad to ensure its growth, and the mother of Caliph Al-Muqtadir (Shaghab) founded a hospital named after her in Baghdad (Pormann, 2007).

SEVEN

Luminaries' Firsts

AL-RAZI

He is credited with the oldest and most original work on smallpox and measles. The claim of earlier description, in the pre-Islamic period, by a priest physician who lived in Alexandria has not been documented (Ibn Abi Usaibiah, 1245/1246; Keys, 1953; Brown, 1962; Ullmann, 1997; Ligon, 2001; Lee, 2001; Souayah, 2005; Kaadan, 2005; Freely, 2011).

He was the first to describe "Rose Cold," "allergic rhinitis" (Ullmann, 1997; Ligon, 2001; Syed, 2002).

He was the first to use alcohol for medicinal purposes (as an antiseptic) (Ligon, 2001; Khan, 2006).

He was the first to introduce mercurial ointment in medical practice (Athar, 1993; Ligon, 2001; Syed, 2002). He was the first to refer to the use of mercury ointment for pediculosis (Laws, 1998; Syed, 2002).

He was the first to introduce opium for anesthesia (Ligon, 2001; Ramen, 2006).

The first book devoted to pediatrics "Practica Puerorum" was written by him (Ligon, 2001).

He is credited with the first detailed description of scrotal gangrene, one thousand years before Foumier (Ligon, 2001).

He was the first to describe the laryngeal branch of the recurrent laryngeal nerve and to note that it may be double on the right side (Khairallah, 1942; Ligon, 2001).

He is credited with the first description of bladder paralysis in spinal cord tumors (Ligon, 2001).

He was the first to use animal catgut in surgery (Al-Mahi, 1959; Laws, 1998; Syed, 2002; Souayah, 2005).

He was the first to describe the guinea worm disease and method (still used today) of extracting the worm (Al-Mahi, 1959; Souayah, 2005).

He is considered to have been the first to describe what is now called "Baker's Cyst," after the English surgeon William Baker, who described it in 1877 (Kaadan, 2005).

He was the first to recognize the reaction of the pupil to light (Syed, 2002).

IBN SINA

He was the first to describe the different parts of the eye (conjunctiva, sclera, choroid, iris, retina, lens, aqueous humor, optic nerve, and chiasma) in minute details (Al-Mahi, 1959; Al-Kurdi, 2004).

He was the first to describe the exact number of extrinsic muscles of the eyeball, namely six (Syed, 2002).

He was the first to differentiate obstructive from nonobstructive jaundice (Al-Mahi, 1959; Al-Kurdi, 2004).

He was the first to describe the symptoms of meningitis with such clarity and brevity that little has been added to it since (Athar, 1993), including differentiation between meningitis and meningismus (Laws, 1998).

He differentiated primary (cerebral) from secondary (extracerebral) paralysis (Al-Mahi, 1959; Al-Kurdi, 2004).

He was the first to recognize that tuberculosis was contagious, proved to be correct centuries later (Khan, 2006).

He was the first to correctly propose that ankylostomatitis (hookworm) was caused by intestinal worm (Khan, 2006).

He was the first to call attention to psychological factors in disease states by diagnosing "love sickness" in a person whose pulse increased when the girl's name he loved was mentioned (Keys, 1953; Khan, 2006).

He was the first to suggest that germs can be transmitted through air, water, or soil (Khan, 2006).

He was the first to draw attention to the necessity of not splinting the fracture immediately, advising postponing it beyond the fifth day. Today this is called the "theory of delayed splinting," considered to be pioneered by George Perkins (Kaadan, 2005).

He was the first to describe what is now called "Bennett's fracture" after the Dublin surgeon Edward H. Bennett, who described it in 1882 (Kaadan, 2005).

He originated the idea of the use of oral anesthetics and recognized opium as the most effective anesthetic (Mukhadir) (Syed, 2002).

His description of the surgical treatment of cancer still holds true today (Syed, 2002).

He was the first to mention caressing a woman's breast as erotic foreplay (Miles, 2008).

IBN ZUHR (AVENZOAR)

He was the first to distinguish between the moist and dry types of pericarditis (Bloomfield, 1983).

He introduced artificial feeding either by gastric tube or by nutrient enemas (Syed, 2002).

He discoverd the itch mite in scabies (Syed, 2002).

IBN MASAWEH, YUHANNA

He wrote the first book on epilepsy (Al-Kurdi, 2004; Al-Mahi, 1959)

He was the first Arab to write a book about anatomical dissection (Haddad, 1993).

He introduced into medicine the use of alum, aloes, and antimony (Haddad, 1993).

He was the first to write comprehensively about leprosy and its contagion (Haddad, 1993).

He was of the first to describe pruritis due to food allergy (Haddad, 1993).

IBN AL-RAHWI, ISHAQ

He wrote the first description of peer review process (Spier, 2003).

AL-KAHHAL

Ali Ibn Isa Al-Kahhal was the first to describe temporal arteritis and a detailed description of a surgical method for its treatment (Al-Samerra'i, 1990). The condition was not known to the Greeks and was not mentioned in the literature until the nineteenth century (Al-Samerra'i, 1990). Al-Kahhal wrote about it in the fourteenth century (Al-Samerra'i, 1990).

Al-Kahhal was also the first to suggest use of anesthesia in surgery (Freely, 2011).

AL-ZAHRAWI

He was the first to identify hemophilia as a hereditary disorder (Haddad, 1993; Syed, 2002; Ramen, 2006).

He was the first to develop the innovative use of catgut to stitch wounds (Haddad, 1993; Majeed, 2005; Ramen, 2006).

He was the first to describe surgery to treat breast cancer (Haddad, 1993; Ramen, 2006).

He was the first to introduce the lithotomy position (Athar, 1993; Haddad, 1993; Syed, 2002; Ramen, 2006).

He was the first to use mirrors to reflect light on a patient during an operation, such as during examination of cervices of women (Khairallah, 1942; Ramen, 2006).

He described the technique of patellectomy (Syed, 2002; Ramen, 2006).

He was the first to write on orthodontia (Khairallah, 1942; Keys, 1953).

He was the first to describe and treat mouth and palate malformations (Haddad, 1993).

Performance of transverse tracheotomy (Haddad, 1993).

He was the first to describe tennis ball (Ping-Pong ball) skull fractures in children (Al-Kurdi, 2004).

He was the first to describe "Kocher's technique" in the reduction of hip dislocation (Haddad, 1993).

He was the first surgeon to use cotton as surgical dressing in the control of bleeding, as padding in splinting of fractures, and as vaginal padding in the tearing of the pubes during delivery (Athar, 1993; Syed, 2002).

He was the first to use saline solution in irrigating wounds (Haddad, 2003).

He was the first to introduce a bevel-ended cannula, instead of the earlier straight one for draining off liquid, when treating dropsy (http://www.nlm.nih.gov/exhibition/islamic_medical/islamic_09.html).

He introduced a technique using a fine drill inserted through the urinary passages for treating impacted calculi in the urethra (Haddad, 1993; http://www.nml.nih.gov/exhibition/islamic_medical/islamic_09.html).

He designed a concealed knife for opening abscesses in a manner that would not alarm the nervous patient (http:// www.nlm.nih.gov/exhibition/islamic_medical/islamic_09.html).

He pioneered the preparation of medicines by sublimation and distillation (http://en.wikipedia.org/wiki/Al-Zahrawi).

He was the first to extract fetal bones from the abdomen (Haddad, 1993).

He was the first to describe extra uterine pregnancy (Haddad, 1993).

He was the first to describe placenta accrete and its extraction (Haddad, 1993).

He was the first to use of hooks to extract a dead fetus (Haddad, 1993).

AL-BAGHDADI

He was the first to suggest that the lower jaw is made up of one, not two, bones (Ullmann, 1997).

IBN AL-NAFIS

He was the first to describe the pulmonary circulation (Laws, 1998; Majeed, 2005; Freely, 2011; Raju, 2012; http://en.wikipedia.org.wiki/Ibn al Nafis).

IBN AL-QUFF

He is credited with description of the capillary vascular system (Huff, 2003; Freely, 2011).

IBN AL-HAYTHAM

He was the first to describe the law of refraction and the intromission theory of vision (Syed, 2002; Freely, 2011).

AL-HALABI

He was the first to use a magnet to remove foreign objects from the eye.

IBN AL-ASH'ATH

He was the first to demonstrate gastric physiology preceding Beaumont by about one thousand years (Syed, 2002).

EIGHT

Islamic Medical Encyclopedias

Several medieval medical authors who wrote encyclopedic works in Arabic had subsequently major influence in Western Europe. The following is a list of such leading encyclopedias (Siraisi, 1990):

FIRDAWS AI-HIKMA (PARADISE OF WISDOM)

This is the first encyclopedia of medicine in Arabic (860 AD), written by Ali Ibn Sahl Rabbani Al-Tabari.

AL HAWI FIL TIBB (COMPREHENSIVE BOOK OF MEDICINE)

Written by Al Razi in the ninth century, it was a very influential book in Europe.

KITAB AL-KAMIL AS-SINA'A AL-TIBBIYA (COMPLETE BOOK OF MEDICAL ART)

This book is better known as "Kitab Al-Malaki" in Arabic and "Liber Regalis" in Latin. It was written by Ali Ibn Abbas Al-Majusi in 980 AD.

KITAB AL-TASRIF (BOOK ON CONCESSIONS)

This is a thirty-volume encyclopedia written by Abu Al Qasim Al-Zahrawi (Abulcasis), c. 1000.

KITAB AL- QANOUN FIL TIBB (THE CANON OF MEDICINE)

This encyclopedic work was written by Abu Ali Ibn Sina (Avicenna), in 1020 AD.

KITAB AL-SHIFA (THE BOOK OF HEALING)

This is another encyclopedic work by Ibn Sina.

NINE

Completing the Circle

REVERSE TRANSLATION

Although some important translations appeared before the end of the eleventh century, they were few. In the twelfth century, Latin Christian communities had become aware of the technological and philosophical riches in the Muslim libraries and the exchange of cultural activities among Christians, Jews, and Muslims was never more intense (Myers, 1964; Menocal, 2002).

The groundwork had earlier been laid by Archbishop Raymond of Toledo (Raymond of Sauvetat), the powerful primate of all of Christian Spain, during his episcopate from 1125 to 1151. He was responsible for the patronage and organization of a loose body of scholars who made up the "Toledo School of Translation," which corresponded very closely to the Bayt al-Hikma (House of Wisdom) of Abbasisd Baghdad (Afnan, 1958). Thus, via Toledo, the rest of Europe had access to the vast body of philosophical and scientific materials translated from Greek to Arabic in the Abbasid capital of Baghdad (Menocal, 2002; http:www//absoluteastronomy.com/topics/Toledo_translation_Sc).

The main intellectual task of the thirteenth century was one of translations from Arabic to Latin but also from Arabic to Hebrew, Greek to Latin, Hebrew to Latin, Latin to French, and Celtic to Latin (Myers, 1964).

TRANSLATORS

Eleventh Century

Constantine the African

Constantine the African was born in Tunisia to a Muslim family and might have converted to Christianity. His original Muslim name is   reported to have been Abdallah (Abdilla in Latin) and his name became Constantine when he converted to Christianity (Al-Samerra'i, 1989). He went to Italy at the age of forty as a merchant. While in Italy, he saw the pitiful state of medicine and returned to Tunisia to study medicine. Upon completing his studies, he returned to Italy, became a monk, joined a Benedictine monastery, and spent the rest of his life there translating books from Arabic into Latin under his name without giving credit to the original authors (Ullmann, 1997). He is considered as one of the three scholars who introduced three languages to the school of Palermo namely Latin, Greek and Arabic (Al-Samerra'i, 1989). Among the most impportant of the books he translated was "Al-Malaki," ten volumes of theoretical and ten volumes of practical medicine by Ali Ibn Al-Abbas and a treatise in ophthalmology by Hunayn Ibn Ishaq. In the late eleventh century, he arrived in Salerno, where he organized the famous Salerno medical school along the pattern of Islamic medical schools. In addition to the books authored by Constantine the African, other teachers at Salerno Medical School authored books that resemble those of Arab authors (Hijazi, A. R.; http;//www.islamset.com/hip/Hijazi.html).

Twelfth Century

John of Seville

John of Seville was a Spanish Jewish translator. Most important of his translations are Al-Khawarismi's "Arithmatic", Al-Farghan's "Astronomy", and the "secrets of Secrets", as well as Qusta Ibn Luqa's "Kitab al Fasl Bayn al-Ruh Wal Nafs" (The Difference between Life and Soul) and Ibn Sina's "Kitab al-Shifa" (A philosophical Encyclopedia) (Myers, 1964; http://en.wikipedia.org/wiki/John_of_Seville).

Robert of Chester (of Ketton)

Robert of Chrester was an English Christian mathematician, astronomer, and alchemist who lived in Spain. He was the first translator of the Holy Quran from Arabic into Latin at the request of Peter the Vulnerable (Abbot of Cluny), who gave him a large amount of money for the purpose of refuting it (Myers, 1964). He was the first to translate Khawarizmi's book "Al Jabr" into Latin a few years before Gerard of Cremona's version. Robert was thus the first to introduce the word "algebra" into Europe. He also translated the first Latin text of the Arab art of Alchemy (Lyon, 2009; Al-Khalili, 2011).

Stephen of Antioch (of Pisa)

Stephen of Antioch was an Italian Christian born in Pisa and lived in Antioch, hence references in his name to Antioch and Pisa. He was also known by the name Stephen the Philosopher. At his time, Antioch was emerging as an important center for translations of Arabic texts into Latin, particularly in medicine. He translated Al-Majusi's (Haly Abbas) "Kitab al-Malaki" (The Royal Book). His translation of the book turned out to be better than that of Constantinus Africanus. He added to the text of the book a glossary of Arabic and Greek medical terms with their Latin equivalents.

He also translated part of Aristotle's "Organon" (Myers, 1964; Ullmann, 1997; Lyon, 2009).

Marc of Toledo

Mark of Toledo was a Spanish Christian physician and a canon of Toledo. He translated one of the earliest translations of the Holy Quran into Latin, as well as several treatises of Hunayn Ibn Ishaq, including "Liber Isagoganum," and works of Hippocrates and Galen from Arabic versions (Afnan, 1958; Myers, 1964; https://en.wikipedia.org/wiki/Mark_of_Toledo).

Gerard of Cremona

Gerard of Cremona was an Italian Christian from Lombardi in Northern Italy. He is considered the greatest of all translators, occupying in the West the same position that Hunayn Ibn Ishaq occupied in the East (Baghdad). In Europe, he was called "Father of Arabism" (Afnan, 1958; Ramen, 2006; Al-Khalili, 2011). He went to Toledo in about 1144, attracted by Ptolemy's "Almagest," which was not available in Latin. He was impressed by its libraries and remained there for the rest of his life. He learned Arabic and translated eighty to eighty-seven works of Archimedes from Arabic into Latin (Freely, 2011; Campbell, 2011; http://www..brittanica.com/biography/Gerard-of-Cremona). Some of the translated books credited to Gerard of Cremona are probably works of Gerard of Sabloneta (Sabbionetta), who lived in the thirteenth century.

Gerard's translations included Arabic versions of works by Aristotle, Euclid, Archimedes, Ptolemy, and Galen, as well as works by Al-Kindi, Ibn Sina (Avicenna), Ibn Al-Haytham, Thabit Ibn Qurra, Al-Farghani, Al-Razi, Al-Farabi and Qusta Ibn Luqa (Freely, 2011). The most important books were the Latin version of Ptolemy's "Al-Magest" (Kitab al-Medjisti), Avicenna's "Canon of Medicine," and Albucasis's "Al-Tasrif."

Most of Gerard's translations occurred between 1170 and his death in 1187.

Gerard of Cremona may have headed a school for translation (Afnan, 1958; Myers, 1964; Haddad, 2003; Ramen, 2006; Lyon, 2009; Al-khalili, 2011).

In total, Gerard translated eighty to eighty-seven books from Arabic, including Ptolemy's "Almagest," Al-Kindi's "On Optics," Al-Razi's "Liber ad Al-Mansoris", Al-Farabi's" On the Classification of the Sciences", medical and chemical works of Al-Razi, and the works of Thabet Ibn Qurra, Hunayn Ibn Ishaq, and Al-Zahrawi (Campbell, 2011; http://www. summagallicana.it/lessico/g/gherardo; https://en.wikipedia.org/wiki/ Latin_translation_of_the_12th-century).

A lunar crater located along the north-northwestern limb of the moon is named after Gerard of Cremona. It is a relatively old, worn crater (http:// en.wikipedia.orgwiki/cremona (crater)).

Gerard of Cremona died in Toledo in 1187 at the age of seventy-three and was buried in the church of St. Lucy at Cremona, to which he had bequeathed his valuable library (Ramen, 2006; Campbell, 2011; http:// summagallicana.it/lessico/g/gherardo).

Thirteenth Century

The age of translation from Arabic to Hebrew began in the thirteenth century. Three of the leading translators were Michael Scott, Samuel Ibn Tibbon, and Jacob Anatoli (Myers, 1964).

Michael Scott

Michael Scott was a Scottish Christian who translated from Arabic into Latin. He was drawn to the court of Emperor Frederick II of Sicily (1212–1250) who, in his struggle with the papacy, drew to his court scholars who were discouraged by the priesthood. Michael Scott's translations included: Avicenna's "Abridgment on Animals" dedicated to his emperor; Maimonides's "Guide for the Perplexed" and "Book on the Divine Precepts"; and Averros's (Ibn Rushd) commentaries on the scientific works of Aristotle.

Scott was the first translator of Averros (Ibn Rushd) and one of the founders of Latin Averroism, the school of thought of Averros (Myers, 1964; Campbell, 2011; https://en.wikipedia.org/wiki/ Latin_translation_of_the_12th_century).

Samuel of Tibbon

Samuel of Tibbon was a Spanish Jew who translated from Arabic into Hebrew.

He worked mainly in Alexandria and Marseilles. He translated several treatises for Maimonides, including "Guide for the Perplexed," "Treatise on Resurrection," and "Mishneh Ethics." The diffusion of Maimonides's philosophy in the West was largely due to Ibn Tibbon's effort (Myers, 1964).

Jacob Anatoli (Jacob Ben Abba Mari Ben Simson Anatoli)

Jacob Anatoli was a French Jew. He translated from Arabic into Latin and Hebrew. He went to Naples at the invitation of Frederick II, the most enlightened monarch at the time, to devote himself to the rendition of scientific Arabic literature into Hebrew language. Anatoli was the first to translate Averros's "Commentaries on Isagoge." He was one of the first to popularize Maimonides's philosophy. Anatoli's esteem of Maimonides knew no bounds (Myers, 1964; http://en.wikipedia.org/wiki/Jacob_Anatoli; http:/www.brittanica.com/biography/Jacob-Anatoli).

Fourteenth Century

During the fourteenth century, there was a gradual decline in translations from Arabic into Latin, replaced by Arabic to Hebrew translations (Myers, 1964).

Qalonymos Ben Qalonymos (Kalonymus Ben Kalonymus Ben Mreir

Ben Qalonymos was a French Jewish philosopher and translator. Among his translations are Thabit Ibn Qurra's "Kitab fi Shakl al Qatta" (On Anatomy); Hunayn Ibn Ishaq's "Kitab al Madkhal fil Tibb" (Introduction to Medicine); and Ali Ibn Radwan's "Kitab al-Umud fi Usul al-Tibb" (Principles of Medicine) (Myers, 1964; https://en.wikipedia.org/wiki/Kalonumus_ben_Kalonymus).

Samuel Ben Solomon Hameati

Samuel Ben Solomon Hameati was an Italian Jew who translated Hunayn Ibn Ishaq's "Tafsir li Kitab Tadbir al Amrad al-Hadda" (Book on Care of Acute Diseases) and Ibn Zuhr's medical work "Lamps of Healing" (Myers, 1964).

ROUTES TO EUROPE

The main channel by which the new learning reached Western Europe was the Al-Andalus (Spain).

Other routes included Africa, England, and the island of Sicily, where the Arabs ruled from 902 to 1091 AD (Myers, 1964; Lyons, 2009).

IMPACT

At the end of the twelfth century, anarchy dominated the practice of medicine in Europe. Anybody could open a school of medicine and treat patients. In 1220, Cardinal Conrad, the Legate of Pope Honorius the Third, brought this to an end by creating the medical school of Montpellier, organized along the pattern of the Arab Medical Schools. Islamic medicine continued to be the main subject in the teaching program at Montpellier medical school during all of the thirteenth and fourteenth centuries and even during the fifteenth century (Hijazi, A. R., http://www.islamset.com.hip/hijazi.html).

The program of the medical school of Paris was identical to the one in Montpellier. In 1935, the most remarkable jewel of the University of Paris library was the "Totum Continens" of Razes. It was loaned to Louis the XI for a deposit of twelve silver plate sets and one hundred gold crowns (Hijazi, A. R., http://www.islamset.com/hip/Hijazi.html).

Thus, Islamic medicine was an essential element of the European Renaissance. The translations of the eleventh and twelfth centuries laid the foundations of "Arabism" in the medicine of the West (Ullmann, 1997).

By the early thirteenth century, reverse translations from Arabic to Latin were used in Italy, France, and England, where the West's earliest universities were created in Bologne, Paris, and Oxford. Nowhere was this effect more profound than at the University of Paris (Lyons, 2009).

By the end of the fourteenth century, there was little of real importance in the Arabic literature that was not made accessible to Western Europe (Myers, 1964).

The absorption of Arab-Hellenic learning that started in Spain in the eleventh century continued down to the sixteenth and seventeenth centuries in various parts of Europe. Andrea Alpago (d. 1520) in Italy was deeply occupied with new translations of Avicenna, Averros, and other Islamic authors as late as the beginning of the sixteenth century (Afnan, 1858).

Latin versions of Arabic books became the subjects of study in several European medical schools such as in Bologna, Montpellier, Paris, and Oxford (Afnan, 1958).

SPONSORS OF TRANSLATIONS

Translations were ordered by rulers, churches, and government officials. Churchmen took a most active part in the translation of knowledge. One such churchmen is Gerbert Aurillac (Pope Sylvester Second), also known as "The Scientific Pope." To further his education, he went to Islamic Spain where the library of the Caliph of Cordoba contained forty thousand books (some said four hundred thousand), compared to his French monastery, which contained only four hundred books. Gerbert spread the science of Islamic Spain throughout Europe. Gerbert was the first Christian known to teach mathematics using the nine Arabic numerals and zero (Brown, 2010).

CENTERS OF TRANSLATION

Cordoba

The first Muslim leader of Al-Andalus Abdul Rahman established his royal court in Cordoba and set out to import books and attract scholars from the East in a bid to compete with his adversaries, the Abbasids Baghdad (Lyons, 2009).

Toledo

Toledo had been in Muslim hands from 712 to 1085, and a large number of its population (Jews, Christians, and Muslims) spoke Arabic as their own language. In addition, Toledo had a famous school for translation organized by Archbishop Raymond the First (Myers, 1964; Lyons, 2009).

The Toledo School of Translation

The Toledo School of Translation refers to a group of scholars in Toledo during the twelfth and thirteenth centuries who worked together to translate works from Arabic, Greek and Hebrew into Latin.

During its heyday, the school attracted scholars from all over Europe who came to Toledo to study knowledge from Arab, Greek, and Hebrew texts. Those translators subsequently helped spread texts to European universities, and Islamic experimental methods would prove crucial for the later development of the European Renaissance (Campbell, 2011; https://en.wikipedia.org/wiki/Toledo-School -of-Translators; https://en.wikipedia.org/wiki/Latin_translation_of_the_12th_century).

Sicily

The Sicilian School of Translation

In addition to the Toledo School of Translation, Latin Europe absorbed the knowledge of Arabian medicine through Sicily. Sicily was under Muslim rule from 878 to 1060. The Center of Translation in Sicily was considerably less active than that of Toledo. Sicilian translators generally translated directly from Greek. When Greek texts were not available, they would resort to translation from Arabic sources.

With the death of the Sicilian physician and translator Faraj Ibn Salem (Farragut) in 1285, the great period of translation may be said to come to a close (Campbell, 2011; https://en.wikipedia.org/wiki/Latin-translations_of_the_12th_century).

TEN

Medical Education

PATHS TO BECOME A PHYSICIAN:

There were three paths to become a physician (Huff, 2003; Pormann, 2007).

The first was to have the good fortune of being born into a medical family whose male heads were eager to pass on their knowledge.

The second was self-teaching through the study of medical books. This was the path taken by the Egyptian physician Ibn Radwan, who was too poor to afford to study medicine with a teacher and wrote a tract defending the method of self-teaching. The claim of Avicenna, in his autobiography, to have been an autodidact has been questioned in recent scholarship.

The third path was to learn from a local physician who held classes (majlis or sessions) at home, in the local hospital, in a mosque or other public place, or in the palace court. Notable among local physicians who conducted these classes were Yuhanna Ibn Masaweh in Baghdad and Al-Dakhwar in Damascus.

The different paths to learning were not mutually exclusive. Students of Al-Razi accompanied him on his rounds in the hospital as well as at home.

MEDICAL SCHOOLS (MADRASSAS):

Medical schools did not constitute venues for medical education before the thirteenth century. The first school devoted exclusively to teaching medicine was established in Damascus (Syria) by the famous physician and teacher of medicine Al-Dakhwar (Pormann, 2007).

To establish the medical school, Al-Dakhwar bequested his house as a charitable trust (waqf) and provided endowment for its maintenance, teachers' salaries, and students stipends. The school was opened on January 12, 1231, and was still in existence in 1417 (Pormann, 2007).

Besides Damascus, major medical schools were established in Baghdad, Cordoba, and Cairo (Lyons, 2009).

Islamic medical schools were built according to the pattern of that in Ghondi-Shapour (Persia) with beautiful surrounding gardens (Athar, 1993).

BASIC SCIENCES STAGE

Candidates for medical schools received their basic science preparation from private tutors through private lectures and self-study. Special schools for teaching required basic science courses were available only in Baghdad (Iraq) and Ghondi-Shapour (Persia) (Syed, 2002).

Alchemy was required for admission to medical schools. Other subjects included medicinal herbs and pharmacognosy.In Baghdad,anatomy was learned by dissecting apes, skeletal studies, and didactic lectures. Other medical schools taught anatomy through illustrations and lectures (Athar, 1993; Syed, 2002).

PRECLINICAL STAGE

Upon completion of their basic science (premedical) courses, students were admitted to the preclinical program. This phase of their medical education consisted of familiarization with library procedures and use, in addition to lectures on toxicology, pharmacology, and the use of antidotes (Athar, 1993; Syed, 2002).

CLINICAL STAGE

During the clinical years, students were assigned in small groups to famous physicians and experienced instructors who gave them lectures, discussion sessions, and reviews and took them along on hospital rounds.

Early in the clinical phase, lectures were mainly on therapeutics and pathology. Later in this phase, students were exposed to diagnosis and judgment, clinical observations and physical examination. Students were asked to examine a patient and make a diagnosis (Athar, 1993; Syed, 2002).

Following a period of time in the hospital wards, students were assigned to the outpatient clinics. After examining a patient, they presented their findings to the instructor. Treatment was decided and prescribed. Maintenance of records on every patient was the responsibility of students (Athar, 1993; Syed, 2002).

The mainstay of the clinical curriculum was internal medicine. Surgery was also part of the curriculum. Orthopedic surgery was widely taught, especially on the use of casts and fractures reduction. Ophthalmology was not a regular component of the curriculum, and obstetrics/gynecology was the domain of midwives (Athar, 1993; Syed, 2002).

Graduates were required to pass a licensing exam before starting a practice (Athar, 1993; Syed, 2002).

Following completion of the course of medical studies, some students went into further specialization under the mentorship of a famous specialist (Athar, 1993; Syed, 2002).

METHODS OF LEARNING

Memorization was the main method of learning. Students believed that knowing a text by heart must precede its understanding. The physician Al-Baghdadi advised his students, "When you read a book, make every effort to learn it by heart and master its meaning. Can you imagine the book to have disappeared and that you can dispense with it, unaffected by its loss."

Teachers also dictated their works to students, and the notes were frequently made into handbooks for students (Huff, 2003).

TEACHING HOSPITALS

By the first half of the tenth century, hospitals became important centers of medical education. Many of the best physicians practiced and trained their students there. Some physicians regarded the hospitals as the best place to receive medical instruction (Pormann, 2007).

In his book "Complete Book of the Medical Art," Al-Majusi stated that one of the requirements for the student of the art was "that he should be in attendance in a hospital (Bimaristan), that he consults with the most skilled teachers among the physicians about the patient's situation and circumstances, and that he frequently examines the condition of the patients and their symptoms, calling to mind what he had read about these conditions and what they indicate of good and ill. If he does this, he will reach a high degree of perfection in this art" (Athar, 1993; Pormann, 2007).

Al-Razi advised medical students that while they examine the patient, they should bear in mind the classic symptoms of disease as given in textbooks and compare them with what they find (Brown, 1962).

QUALIFYING EXAMINATIONS

In the early days of the Islamic empire, it was enough for a person to practice medicine that he or she learned the profession from books or by being mentored by one of the successful practitioners (Ahmad Isa Bek, 1981).

Qualifying examinations for physicians probably existed as early as 850 AD. They were certainly instituted in 931 AD by the Abbasid Caliph Al-Muqtadir. Following a case of malpractice that came to his attention, he issued an order legislating that no one should practice medicine in Baghdad unless he satisfied the chief physician, Sinan Ibn Thabet, of his competence and proficiency. In the first year of the decree, more than 860 practitioners were examined in Baghdad alone. Exempted from the examination were few physicians of recognizable reputation and physicians of the Royal court (Brown, 1962; Ahmad Isa Bek, 1981; Athar, 1993).

Among those who presented themselves before Ibn Thabet was a dignified and well-dressed old man of imposing appearance. When asked an examination question, he told the examiner, "I cannot read or write well, but I have a family whom I maintain by my professional labor, which I beg you not to interrupt." Ibn Thabet laughed and said, "On condition that you do not treat any patient with what you know nothing about." "This," said the old man, "has been my practice" (Brown, 1962).

The following day, among those who presented themselves before Ibn Thabet was a well-dressed young man of pleasing and intelligent appearance:

"With whom do you study?" asked Ibn Thabet. "With my father," answered the young man. "And who is your father?" asked Ibn Thabet. "The old man who was with you yesterday," replied the young man, "a fine old gentleman!" exclaimed Ibn Thabet. "And do you follow his method?" "Yes." "Then see to it that you do not go beyond it" (Brown, 1962).

Licensing boards were set up under a government official called

"Muhtasib" or "Inspector General," who, upon the recommendation of the chief physician, would administer the Hippocratic Oath and issue a license to those who passed the qualifying exam. A thousand years later, the West started to implement licensing of physicians (Athar, 1993; Syed, 2002; http://www.islamset.com/hijazi.html).

ELEVEN

Islamic Hospitals

The hospital was one of the greatest institutional achievements of medieval Islamic society (Dallal, 2010).

The first Islamic hospital was a tent set up next to the Prophet's mosque in Yathrib (today's Medina in Saudi Arabia) to treat the sick. It was run by a nurse named Rafeeda Al-Aslamiyyah and was known as Rafeeda's Tent (Al-Samerra'i, 1990).

Health care in Islam was provided in different forms, such as (Al-Samerra'i, 1990; Haddad, 2003):

1. Clinics, the first of which was established by Ahmad Ibn Tolon (868 AD), attached to the mosque that carried his name; it had a cabinet full of medicine and a physician to attend to the praying public

2. Shelters for patients with chronic intractable diseases, such as lepers (built in 706 by Walid Abdel Malik in Damascus), and the mentally ill, the blind, and the aging populations

3. Hospitals for prisoners and the military, both stationary and mobile

4. General public hospitals

Hospitals were called bimaristan, a Persian word (bimar, sick; stan , place) for "place for the sick." In the thirteenth century, the bimaristans were used by the Crusaders to house their sick soldiers in Jerusalem. Because of the name, Hospitaliers, of the Crusaders, those places became known as hospitals. During the Ottoman Empire, those places became known as Khista Khana (Al-Samerra'i, 1990; Haddad, 2003).

Before the Islamic era, medical care was largely provided by "physician" priests in convents, sanatoriums, and annexes to temples (Al-Samerra'i, 1990; Azeem, 2005).

Islamic hospitals were paid for and maintained by endowments from caliphs, other rulers, philanthropies, and religious foundations (Al-Samerra'i, 1990; Turner, 1995; Dallal, 2010).

In addition to medical facilities, hospitals contained or were attached to a mosque, school (Madrassa), and sometimes mausoleum honoring the founder. Separate wards were provided for males and female patients. Special wards were maintained for internal diseases, ophthalmic and orthopedic disorders, as well as for surgical patients, the mentally ill, and patients with contagious diseases (Athar, 1993; Turner, 1995; Syed, 2002; Azeem, 2005; Lyons, 2009; Dallal, 2010). Male and female wards were staffed with nurses and ancillary staff of the same sex (Athar, 1993). Libraries and conference rooms were included within hospitals. The Toulon hospital library in Cairo contained one hundred thousand volumes (Athar, 1993, Syed, 2002). Libraries were the place where the chief physician met after daily rounds with other physicians, students, and staff to discuss patients' disorders, followed by didactic sessions for medical students (Al-Samerra'i, 1990; Haddad, 2003).

Some hospitals had bathhouses nearby and accommodations (Takiyyehs) for the relatives of patients to stay in them (Haddad, 2003). Many hospitals had readers with good voices to sing religious songs one hour every evening (Haddad, 2003).

On admission, patients were bathed and given special apparel. Their clothes, money, and valuables were stored away and returned to them upon discharge from the hospital. Upon discharge, patients received enough money to tie them over until they could support themselves (Al-Samerra'i, 1990; Athar, 1993; Syed, 2002; Haddad, 2003).

Convalescent centers and housing for students and house staff were attached to the hospitals (Athar, 1993; Syed, 2002).

The bed/population ratio in tenth-century Baghdad city was equivalent to what the whole country of Pakistan had in 1998. The bed/population ratio in Damascus in the thirteenth century surpassed that of Pakistan in 1998 (Turner, 1995).

Islamic hospitals served all citizens for free, without regard to color, religion, gender, age, or social status (Al-Samerra'i, 1990; Athar, 1993; Syed, 2002). Taxation and philanthropy produced free health care in Baghdad in the tenth century as they did in London in the twentieth century (Souweif, 2004).

Each hospital had an administrator/accountant and chief physician, whose main responsibility included examining each of the physicians to ensure his qualifications and specialty (Al-Samerra'i, 1989; Haddad, 2003; Dallal, 2010).

At the beginning, Islamic hospitals were built in large cities such as Mecca, Medina, Baghdad, and Cairo (Haddad, 2003).

The number of hospitals increased dramatically during the Abbasid dynasty.

The first hospital was built in the eighth century in Baghdad during the rule of Caliph Al-Rashid. It was soon followed by similar hospitals throughout the Islamic empire (Turner, 1995).

There were twenty-one hospitals in Iraq (seventeen in Baghdad, one in each of Mosul, Harran, Al-Raqqa, and Nasibin); ten in Egypt (nine in

Cairo and one in Alexandria); eight in Syria (six in Damascus and two in Aleppo); four in Palestine (one each in Jerusalem, Safad, Ramleh, and Akka); four in Tunisia (one each in Al-Qayrawan, Susa, Safaqes, and the city of Tunis); three in Morroco (one each in Marakesh, Salla, and Fas); two in Saudi Arabia (one each in Mecca and Medina); one in Lebanon (Beka Valley), one in Jordan (Karak); and one in Granada, Spain (Hamarni, 1962; Jadon, 1970; Ahmad Isa Bek, 1981, 1989; Al-Samerra'i, 1989, 1990; Athar, 1993; Syed, 2002; Haddad, 2003; Dallal, 2010).

The most prominent hospital in Syria was the Greater Al-Nuri Hospital. It was sort of a university hospital attached to a medical school (Jadon, 1970; Athar, 1993).

Similar to the Greater Al-Nuri Hospital in Damascus were the Al-Muqtadiri Hospital in Baghdad, described by the Arab traveler Ibn Jubayr as a royal palace, and the Al-Mansuri Hospital in Cairo, considered the greatest example of Muslim architecture (Al-Khalili, 2011).

TWELVE

Medical Ethics

HISTORICAL PERSPECTIVE

Babylonian

The Babylonians treated physicians as they did other professionals. A surgeon who caused a patient to lose his vision was punished by cutting his hand. Punishment was part of Hammurabi's Law. Hammurabi's Law recognized only surgeons, since medical conditions were treated by priests. If surgery on a slave resulted in his death, the surgeon was required to provide a replacement slave to the master (Kaadan, A. N.; http://www.ishim.net/articles.htm).

Persian

The Persians were more lenient with surgeons. They did not practice the Babylonian rule of bodily harm on physician (Kaadan, A.; http://www.ishim.net/articles.htm).

Chinese

The Chinese practiced the punishment rule in dealing with physicians' errors, including the penalty of death of a physician. If the dead person was from the nobility, the responsible physician was buried with him (Kaadan and Mahrouseh; http://www.ishim.net/articles.htm).

Jewish

In Jewish medical ethics, the physician was fined an amount of money comparable to the harm done to the patient (Kaadan, A. N. & Mahrouseh, M. N.; http://www.ishim.net/articles.htm).

Indian

Physicians were given special treatments in Indian medical ethics. The Indians believed that life and death were decided by the gods. Priests thus practiced medicine without fear of punishment. Indian practitioners were expected to cut their hair short, to keep their nails short and clean, and to dress neatly and use perfumes to smell good. The Indian code of medical ethics contained many of those later written in the Hippocratic Oath. (Kaadan, A. N.; http://www.ishim.net/articles.htm).

Egyptian

Physicians in Pharaonic Egypt were highly respected. Emhotep the physician was made the God of Medicine. In later Egyptian dynasties, codes of medical ethics were written and physicians were required to abide by them or risk death (Kaadan; http://www.ishim.net/articles.htm).

Greek

Like the Egyptians, the Greeks made Aesculapius their God of Medicine, and his daughters, gods of health and healing. Medical practice remained in the hands of priests belonging to the family of Aesculapius until the advent of Hippocrates, who, although a member of Aesculapius family, started teaching medicine to commoners. According to Ibn Abi Usaibiah, the motives for the action of Hippocrates was that he was afraid that the medical profession could dwindle in time if it remained limited to the children of one family, the Aesculapius family (Kaadan; http://www.ishim. net/articles.htm).

Roman

The Romans were late in instituting codes of medical ethics. When they did, in the last century BC, they regulated the relationships between the public and professions, including the medical profession. They stipulated that children should practice their father's profession and introduced a system of examinations for physicians prior to their licensure to practice. They also instituted procedures to deal with professional negligence or ignorance. These codes of ethics remained in use in the Byzantine kingdom as well (Kaadan; http://www.ishim.net/articles.htm).

MEDICAL ETHICS IN ISLAM

Medical ethics issues were handled in a sophisticated manner in Islam. One of the first medical books and the oldest known surviving work in Arabic treats the subject of medical ethics, "Adab Al-Tabib" (The Physician's Code of Ethics) by Ishaq Ibn Ali Al-Rahawi (Rahwi) (854–931). It is a twenty-chapter book written in the ninth century and based to a great extent on Hippocrates and Galen. It had much information for interns, in particular. Rahawi was a Christian who converted to Islam (Athar, 1993; Turner, 1995; Al-Kawi, 1997; Prioreschi, 2004; Al-Ghazal, 2004).

The titles of the twenty chapters reflect the contents of the book:

1. The loyalty and faith of the physician, and ethics he must follow to improve his soul and morals.

2. Care of the physician's body.

3. What the physician must avoid and be ware of.

4. Directions of the physician to the patient and servant.

5. Manners of the visitors.

6. Care of remedies by the physician.

7. What the physician asks the patient and the nurse.

8. What the patient may conceal from the physician.

9. How the healthy and ill must take orders of the physician.

10. Training of servants by the patient before the illness.

11. Patient and visitors.

12. Dignity of the medical profession.

13. Respect for the physician.

14. Physicians and peculiar incidents to aid treatment.

15. Medical art for moral people.

16. Examination of physicians.

17. Removal of corruption of physicians.

18. Warning against quacks.

19. Harmful habits.

20. Care of the physician himself.

Rahawi's book reflects the author's religious traditions and his Islamic scholarship. The word "Allah" is used hundreds of times, along with the attributes of Allah (exalted, beneficent, compassionate, life-giver, healer, creator, etc). In the introductory part of the first chapter of the book, the author outlines the primary qualities of the physician (Aksoy, 2003):

1. The first thing in which the physician must believe is that all in this world has only one able creator, who performs all deeds willfully.

2. The second article of faith in which a physician must believe is that he has credence in the great Allah with a firm affection and is devoted to Him with all his reason, soul, and free will.

3. The third faith that a physician must possess is that Allah sent His messenger to mankind to teach them what is good since the mind alone is not sufficient. The book described the process of licensing physicians, keeping patients records and their use in education, quality control, and litigation (Al-Kawi, 1997). The physician was told to be "Hasib," that is, honest, generous, noble of character, and righteous, and seek God's favor and mercy. He should be "Alim," that is, proficient, learned, savant, capable, and skillful. He ought to be "War'i," a pious and God-fearing devotee or a deeply religious person. He should not be "Ajoul"; that is, he should take his time and not be in a rush but rather be congenial. The physician must in addition possess three traits: "Aql," to have a sane mind, reason, common sense, and intelligence; "Razanah," that is, having self-control and being sober, calm, composed, sedate, and serious; and finally "Iffah," to possess abstinence, chastity with purity and decency with integrity and   modesty. He should protect himself against the following vices, evils, malpractices, and wickedness (Prioreschi, 2004):

1. "Al-fujur," which means debauchery, licentiousness, or fornication

2. "Al-khubth," which means malevolence and malice

3. "Al-danawah," lowliness, meaness

4. "Al-ghadab," wrath, anger

5. "Al-jaz'a," anxiety, apprehension and uneasiness

6. "Al-shahwah," craving, carnal appetite, lust for sexuality

Al-Rahawi listed the following virtues the physician should possess (Prioreschi, 2004):

1. "Miqdam," which means bold, daring

2. "Afif," chaste, decent, and pure in heart

3. "Sabur," patient and tolerant

4. "Mutawassiq bil-haq," unprejudiced and candid

5. "Waqur," dignified and venerable

The physician should be virtuous, kind, and merciful and avoid money-grubbing, slander, and addiction to wines and drugs (Turner, 1995). The physician was advised to avoid losing his temper and to answer patiently when asked many questions by the patient and family (Turner, 1995). The physician was urged to render his best professional services to rich and poor alike. Moreover, he was urged to give consent courteously if a patient requested a second opinion (Turner, 1995). The book includes the first description of the peer review process. It stated that it was the duty of a physician to make duplicate notes of the condition of the patient on each visit with the patient. The record was to include the name of the patient, the place of encounter and the date, the diagnosis, the basis upon which the diagnosis was made, the pulse and positive signs, the prescribed treatment, and the diet prescribed (Al-Kawi, 1997). A copy of the record was to be left with the patient's family. On subsequent visits, the physician should enter in the record any changes in the patient's condition or in management (Al-Kawi, 1997). When the patient is discharged, cured or dead, from the hospital the notes of the physician were examined by a local council of physicians (peers) who would adjudicate as to whether the physician had performed according to the standards that then prevailed. On the basis of their rulings, the practicing physician could be sued for damage by the maltreated patient. The Islamic medical records were adapted and modified from Greek medical heritage. This is probably the first documented reference to peer review (Ajlouni, 1997; Al-Kawi, 1997; Spier, 2002).

In 931 AD, it was reported to Caliph Al-Muqtader that a certain man died as a result of a physician's error. The caliph ordered the prevention of any physician from practicing the profession except those who were examined, beforehand, by the chief physician Sinan Ibn Thabet, and that a license be issued in their names with the chief physician's signature affixed to it (Hamarneh, 1983; Al-Kawi, 1997).

Muslim physicians recognized the validity of the Hippocratic Oath and were required to take the Hippocratic Oath prior to practicing their profession and to adhere to certain ethical standards and customs (Ajlouni, 2003; Prioreschi, 2004; Pormann, 2007). The oath was translated and adapted to the Islamic religion, in the same way as it was modified in the West to reconcile with Christianity (Prioreschi, 2004). The reference to Aesculapius in the Islamic version of the oath at first is surprising but must be understood in light of the fact that in the Islamic world Aesculapius was not a god but simply a legendary originator and discoverer of medicine (Prioreschi, 2004).

Students of medicine were expected to learn medical ethics. In Ibn Hindu's book "The Book of Taking Care of One's Health," he stated "that the medical student should learn, not only logic to enable him to discern truth from falsehood, but also some ethics so that he may cleanse his own soul from impurities and prepare it for admission and acceptance of excellence" (Farhadi, 1989).

Quality control (Hisbah) was highly developed in the Arab/Islamic world during the eighth and ninth centuries AD. A handbook for the Muhtasib (quality controller with the power of a judge) was written in the eleventh century (Ajlouni & Al-Khalidi, 1997). The purpose of the Hisbah system was the supervision of the application of the standards of practice of medicine which were already established (Al-Kawi, 1997).

Contrary to general belief, dating informed medical consent to the nineteenth century, informed medical consent was actually recorded as early as 1677 AD. A document signed on November 1677 stated "that the patient asked people to duly and legally bear witness that if he (the patient) died as a result of fate, and God's divine decree because of his being treated by the surgeon, the latter shall not be held as guarantor for him. The patient has also relieved the surgeon from any responsibility for his death and blood money, and that the patient or his heir after him shall not be entitled to any related claims made against the surgeon" (Al-Kawi, 1997).

As for medical fees, it is known that physicians were, in general, relatively affluent. There was the possibility for famous physicians to accumulate considerable fortunes, which led to an ethical dilemma. The general view on medical fees was that the physician should earn enough so that he did not need to do anything else than practice his profession. In spite of that, accusations of greed on the part of physicians were common in medieval Islamic literature (Prioreschi, 2004).

Another source for the Islamic code of ethics is found in Abu Al-Hasan Al-Tabari's book "Firdous Al-Hikma" (Paradise of Wisdom), in which the Islamic Code of Ethics was described as (Al-Ghazali, 2004):

1. Personal Character of the Physician:

The physician ought to be modest, virtuous, merciful, and un-addicted to liquor. He should wear clean clothes, be dignified, and have well-groomed hair and beard. He should not join the ungodly, nor sit at their table. He should be careful of what he says and should not hesitate from asking forgiveness if he made an error. He should be forgiving and never seek revenge. He should be friendly and a peace-maker. He should not make jokes or laugh at the improper time or place.

2. Obligations towards Patients:

The physician should avoid predicting whether the patient will live or die. Only God knows. He should not lose his temper when patient keeps asking questions, but should answer gently and compassionately. He should treat alike the rich and the poor, the master and the servant, the powerful and the powerless, the elite and the illiterate. He should be punctual and reliable. He should not wrangle about his fees. He should be decent towards women, and should not divulge secrets of his patients.

3. Obligations towards His Community:

The physician should not be critical of any one's religious belief, and should speak no evil of reputable men of the community.

4. Obligations towards His Colleagues:

The physician should speak well of his acquaintances and colleagues. He should not honor himself by shaming others.

5. Obligations towards Assistants:

If his assistant does wrong, he should not rebuke him in front of others, but privately and cordially.

THIRTEEN

Rise and Fall of Islamic Civilization

RISE

Several factors contributed to the rise and success of Islamic Civilization in science and medicine as described in the pages above. These include:

Islam, the religion and system of values

Arabic language

Tolerance

Translation

Education and paper industry

Islam, the religion and system of values

Muslims and Arabs were inspired by the calls of Prophet Muhammad to seek knowledge:

"Seek knowledge from the cradle to the grave."

"Search for knowledge, even if you must go to China to find it."

"The ink of the scholar is more sacred than the blood of a martyr" (Craig, 1977).

"Seeking knowledge is an obligation upon every Muslim" (Lunde, 1982; Deuraseh, 2004).

"Verily the men of knowledge are the inheritors of the prophets" (Eknoyan, 1994).

He who leaves his home in search of knowledge walks the path of God to paradise" (Eknoyan, 1994).

"Seek knowledge, for seeking it is worship, reference to it is extolment (of God), searching for it is jihad, and teaching it is charity" (Geha, 2012).

"Knowledge is of two kinds. The science of bodies and the science of religion" (Farhadi, 1989).

The Quran states:

"He who restored life to a man shall be accounted as if he had restored life to humanity," Sura 5:35 (Athar, 1993).

"Are those who know equal to those who know not," Sura 39:9 (Athar, 1993).

In the Quran, there is repeated reference to the "Rasikhuna fil Ilm" ,those who are well grounded in Knowledge (Athar, 1993).

The Prophet is reported to have set free prisoners captured in battle if they taught ten Muslims to read and write (Lunde, 1982; Tarabay, 2011).

Muslim scholars are reported to have loved to repeat a quote by Aristotle "Let no one enter who does not have knowledge of mathematics" (Lunde, 1982).

Arabic language

An Arab proverb says, "Wisdom has aligned upon the three things, the brain of the Franks, the hands of the Chinese, and the tongue of the Arabs" (Landau, 1959).

The Arabic language was key to seeking knowledge from the seventh century AD, being the language of the Quran. Being flexible to development, Arabic was able to evolve to become the language of science. Scholars from different ethnic origins and languages found it easier to write in Arabic than in their own languages. One prominent bishop complained that young Christian men were devoting themselves to the study of Arabic, rather than to Latin, a reflection of the fact that Arabic had become the international language of science (Lunde, 1982).

Tolerance

One of the values of Muslim culture was tolerance and encouragement of secular and religious learning, creating the climate for the exchange of ideas. Under Islam, Muslims, Christians, and Jews of different ethnicities worked together in the development of science and the arts (Lunde, 1982; Tarabay, 2011). Isolated acts of intolerance committed by some Islamic rulers were the exception, not the rule (Tarabay, 2011).

Translation

Translation of knowledge of cultures and civilizations that preceded Muslim civilization was essential for the development of Muslim contributions in science and art.

Most translations were made by non-Muslims and non-Arabs, including Christians, Jews, Nestorians, and Persians who were welcomed and integrated into Islamic civilization.

Extensive translations into Arabic peaked in Baghdad during the rule of Caliph Al-Mamoun in the first half of the ninth century (Tarabay, 2011).

Besides the encouragement and generous support of translation by Islamic rulers, the success of translations was principally due to its development in a culture and various social classes eager to acquire new knowledge (Dallal, 2010).

Education and paper industry

The introduction of paper mills by Muslims in mid-eighth century facilitated the spread of knowledge and education. Muslims learned the process of papermaking from captured Chinese soldiers in the war of 751. Soon afterwards, paper mills spread throughout the Arab Islamic world (Landau, 1959; Al-Khalili, 2011; Tarabay, 2011; Houston, 2016).

The first paper mill in the Abbasid Empire was built in Samarkand, in modern-day Uzbekistan. The first paper mill opened in Baghdad during the golden days (786-795) of Caliph Haroun Al-Rashid (Al-Khalili, 2011).

As papermaking spread across the caliphate, it was refined. By the time papermaking had traversed the caliphate in the East, and reached Morocco and Spain, the Arabs had transformed it from a cottage industry into a manufacturing enterprise (Houston, 2016).

Though Muslims did not adopt printing until centuries after Europe, they get the credit for introducing the paper book shortly after learning from the Chinese in the eighth century how to manufacture paper. Europe, on the other hand, did not replace parchment with paper until the fourteenth century (Landau, 1959).

THE FALL

For more than a thousand years, the Islamic empire remained the most advanced and civilized in the world. Islam stressed the importance of learning and respect of the learned, forbade destruction, and nurtured respect of other religions (Syed, 2002).

Eventually, the Islamic empire became weak, and its civilization went into decline.

In the East, new powers arose. The Mongols in 1258 devastated Baghdad, the greatest Arab city of the time. Most of the books in the House of Wisdom in Baghdad were destroyed by Hulago's army.

Later, from the fourteenth century onward, large parts of the Arab world were brought under Ottoman Turks Empire (Syed, 2002; Majeed, 2005; Al-Khalili, 2011).

In the West, the demise of the Andalus finally came in 1031. Many petty states mushroomed, and the Franks attacked from the North.

To rescue Muslims in Spain from the Franks, al-Moravids, a confederation of Sufi Berber tribes who had established their rule in Morocco, came to Spain and, for nearly a century (1090–1147), ruled Spain.

In 1150, al-Moravids were succeeded by another Sufi Berber tribe, the al-Mohads, who ruled North Africa and Spain until the middle of the thirteenth century. They were in turn defeated by the Franks in a battle northeast of Cordoba, in 1212 AD (Landau, 1959; Tarabay, 2011).

Besides the demise of science centers in Baghdad and Cordoba, some historians attribute the decline of Muslim science and scholarship to political factors such as Western colonization, which dominated the Muslim world from the eighteenth century onward. It is argued that Western colonialists felt it necessary to belittle the achievements of the great centers of learning such as those of the Abbasid Baghdad and Umayyad Cordoba in order to rationalize their superiority over the colonized people (Al-khalili, 2011).

Another factor claimed to have contributed to the decline was the reluctance of Muslim world to employ the printing press quickly enough. The early typesetters were faced with great problems in setting the cursive Arabic letters, as compared to Latin letters, and the different shapes the letters take depending on their position in the word (Al-Khalili, 2011).

Muslims also resisted printing because it would not match with the flowing and artistic calligraphy style of writing that defined their identity (Al-Khalili, 2011).

The first book to be printed in Arabic was the Quran, in 1537, by the Paganinis of Venice. The sole surviving copy of the book was discovered in the 1980s in the library of the Franciscan Friars of San Michele in Isola, Venice. The copy was reviewed by Dr. Jim Al-Khalili, who found several typographical errors. Although seemingly trivial, misspelling words in the Muslim holy book would have been regarded sacrilegious and would explain why the Ottomans refused to accept the many copies sent to them by the Venice printer (Al-Khalili, 2011). When Arabic printing was introduced in Turkey in 1727, it was limited to books of geography, history, and languages. Printing of religious books was not authorized (Al-Khalili, 2011).

References

Abdel-Halim, R.E. Contributions of Ibn Zuhr (Avenzoar) to the Progress of Surgery: A Study and Translation from His Book Al-Taisir. Saudi Medical Journal 26 (9): 1333–1339, 2005.

Abokrysha, N. Ibn Sina (Avicenna) on pathogenesis of Migraine compared with the Recent Theories. Headache 49:923-927, 2009.

Abu al-Qasim al-Zahrawi http://en.wikipedia.org/wiki/Al-Zahrawi, accessed April 22, 2017.

Abu-Asab, M., Amri, H., Micozzi, M.S. Avicenna's Medicine, A New Translation of the 11th Century Canon with Practical Applications for Integrative Health Care. Healing Art Press, 2013.

Abuelaish, Izzeldine. I will Not Hate, Walker and Co., 2010.

Afnan, S.M. Avicenna. His Life and Works. Ruskin House. London. First Ed., 1958.

Ahmad Isa Bek. Tarikh al-Bimaristans in Islam (History of Hospitals in Islam), 2nd Edition. 1981, Dar al-Ra'ed al-'Arabi, Beirut, Lebanon.

Ajlouni, K. M. History of Informed Medical Consent. The Lancet 346: 980, 1995.

Ajlouni, K. M. Al-Khalidi, U. Medical Rounds, Patient Outcome, and Peer Review in Eleventh Century Arab Medicine. Annals of Saudi Medicine 17: 326–327, 1997.

Ajlouni, K. M., Values, Qualifications, Ethics and Legal Standards in Arabic (Islamic) Medicine. Saudi Medical Journal 24: 820–826, 2003.

Aksoy, S. The Religious Tradition of Ishaq ibn Ali al-Ruhawi: The Author of the First Medical Ethics Book in Islamic Medicine. Journal of the International Society of the History of Islamic Medicine, 3: 9–11, 2003.

Al-Ghazal, S. K. The Discovery of the Pulmonary Circulation-Who Should Get the Credit: Ibn Al-Nafis or William Harvey. Journal of the International Society of the History of Islamic Medicine (JISHIM) 1(2):46–48, 2002.

Al-Ghazal, S. K. Medical Ethics in Islamic History at a Glance. Journal of the International Society of the History of Islamic Mediciine 3:12–13, 2004.

Al-Kawi, M. Z. History of Medical Records and Peer Review. Annals of Saudi Medicine 17:277–278, 1997.

Al-Khalili, J . The House of Wisdom. How Arabic Science Saved Ancient Knowledge and Gave Us the Renaissance. The Penguin Press, NY, 2011.

Al-Kurdi, A., Khoury, S., Role of Arabs and Muslims in Neuroscience (500–1516 AD). Neuroscience 9 (1): 1–33, 2004.

Al-Mahi, T. History of Arabic Medicine, Egypt Press, Khartoum, 1959.

Al-Rhodan, N.; Fox, J. L. Al-Zahrawi and Arabian Neurosurgery, Surgical Neurology 26:92–96, 1986.

Al-Rubiay, K.K. Banu Zuhr Family in Andalus: Six Physicians and two Women Doctors: Their Scholarship Status. Journal of the International Society of the History of Islamic Medicine (JISHIM)4(8): 1-7, 2005.

Al-Samerra'i, K. Mukhtasar Tarikh Al-Tib Al-Arabi (Summary of History of Arab Medicine) Vol. I, 1989, Dar Al- Nidal, Publisher, Beirut, Lebanon.

Al-Samerra'i.K. Mukhtasar Tarikh Al-Tib Al-Arabi (Summary of Hitory of Arab Medicine) Vol. II, 1990, Dar Al-Nidal, Publisher, Beirut, Lebanon.

Ardekani, M.R.S., Moatar, F.A. Research Conducted on the Life and Works of Hakim Sayyid Esmail Jurjani. Journal of the International Society of the History of Islamic Medicine (JISHIM)4(7):1-12, 2005.

Armstrong, K. The Case for God, Anchor Publ, 2009.

Aschoff, A., Kremer, P., Hashemi, B., Kunz, S. The Scientific History of Hydrocephalus and its Treatment. Neurosurgery Review 22: 67–93, 1999.

Athar, s. Islamic Perspectives in Medicine. A Survey of Islamic Medicine: Achievements and Contemporary Issues. American Trust Publication, 1993.

Averroes. http: //en.wikipedia.org/wiki/Averroes, accessed April 22, 2017.

Avicenna Crater http://en.wikipedia.org/wiki/Avicenna_Crater, accessed April 22, 2017.

Azar, H.A. When I Was Young. Excerpts from Ibn Zuhr's (Avenzoar) Kitab al-Taysir. Journal of the International Society of the History of Islamic Medicine (JISHIM) 1(2):21-26, 2002.

Bayon, H. P. Arabic Philosophers-Physicians and Christian Doctors of Medicine. Proceedings of the Royal Society of Medicine, March 5, 310–314, 1952.

Bloomfield, R. L., Chandler, E. T. Pocket Mnemonics for Practitioners. Harbinger Medical Press, 1983.

Bosmia, A., Watanabe, K., Shoja, M.M., Loukas, M., Tubbs, R.S. Michael

Servetus (1511–1553): Physician and Heretic Who Described the Pulmonary Circulation. International Journal of Cardiology 167: 318–321, 2013.

Brown, N. M. The Abacus and the Cross. The Story of the Pope Who Brought the Light of Science to the Dark Ages, Basic Books, 2010.

Browne, E. G. Arabian Medicine, Cambridge University Press, 1962.

Burg, A . The Holocaust Is Over. We Must Rise from Its Ashes. Palgrave Macmillan, 2008.

Burr, D.B. AAA News Letter, June, 2, 2008.

Bushrui, S. Wisdom of the Arabs (Oneworld of Wisdom). Oneworld Publications, 2002.

Campbell, D. Arabian Medicine and Its Influence on the Middle Ages, Volume I. Routledge, London, 2011.

Cortas, W.M. A World I Loved. Nations Books, 2009.

Craig, H. A. L. Bilal. T. J. International Ltd, 1977.

Cumston, C.G. A Brief Historical Summary of the Treatment of Trachoma with Special Reference to the Arabian School and the Writings of Ali Ibn Issa (Jesu Hali). Annals of Medical History 3: 244–251, 1921.

Dallal, A. Islam, Science, and the Challenge of History. Yale University Press, 2010.

Deuraseh, N. Ahadith of the Prophet on Healing in three Things (al-Shifa fi Thalatha): An Interpretational. Journal of the International Society for the History of Islamic Medicine 3 (6): 10–16, 2004.

Deuraseh, N .The Contribution of the Arabs to Medical Science during the Abbasid Period, 132-655 A.H. (750–1258 C.E.), http://www.e-imj. com/vol 2-no 1/vol 12-no 1-13, accessed December 23, 2011.

Dunn, P. M. Avicenna (AD 980–1037) and Arabic Perinatal Medicine. Archives of Diseases of Childhood 77: F75–F76, 1997.

Ead, H.A. http://www.levity.com/alchemy/islam 14.html, accessed April 22, 2017.

Eknoyan, G. Arabic Medicine and Nephrology. American Journal of Nephrology 14:270–278, 1994.

Erolin, C., Shoja, M. M., Loukas, M. Shokouhi, G., Rashidi, M. R., Khalili, M., Tubbs, R. S. What Did Avicenna (Ibn Sina, 980–1037 AD) Look Like. International Journal of Cardiology167:1660–1663, 2013.

Farhadi, M. A Survey of the Views of Ibn Hindu Based on Research about the Programs of Medical Instruction. Medical Journal of the Islamic Republic of Iran, Vol 3 No. 1 & 2, 47–50, 1989.

Feiler, B. Generation Freedom. Harper Collins, 2011.

Freely, J. Light from the East. How the Science of Medieval Islam Helped to Shape the Western World, L. B. Tauris, 2011.

Geha, S. Al-Tadween al-Musiqi al Mu'Arrab (The Arabized Musical Notations) American University of Beirut Press, 2011.

Geha, S. Al-Wajh Al Adabi of Shafiq Geha, Geha Family Publishing, 2012.

Goodman, L. E. Islamic Humanism. Oxford University Press, 2003.

Gorini, R. Al-Haytham the Man of Experience. First Steps in the Science of Vision. Journal of the International Society of the History of Islamic Medicine (JISHIM) 2 (4): 53–55, 2003.

Gorini, R. An Andalusian Muslim Scientist: Ibn al-Baytar. Journal of the International Society of History of Islamic Medicine 3 (6):69–71, 2004.

Gorini, R. Medical Poetry in the Arabic Tradition: A Glimpse. Journal of the International Society of the History of Islamic Medicine (JISHIM) 4 (8):1–4, 2005.

http://al-hakawati.net/Personalities/PersonalityDetails/4/, accessed on April 24, 2017.

http//en.wikipedia.org.wiki/cremona_(crater), accessed April 22, 2017.

http://en.wikipedia.org/wiki/Bukhtishu, accessed April 22, 2017.

http://en.wikipedia.org/wiki/User:Onciaoncia, accessed May 27, 2013.

http://syriacstudies.com?AFSS/Syriac_Scholars_and_writers, accessed May 27, 2013.

http:www//summagallicana.it/lessico/g/Gerardo, accessed April 22, 2017.

http://www.nlm.nih.gov/hmd/arabic/med_islam.html, accessed April 22, 2017.

http://www.nlm.nih.gov/exhibition/islamic_medical/islamic_09.html, accessed April 22, 2017.

http://www.nlm.nih.gov/hmd/arabic/biol.html, accessed April 22, 2017.

http://nih.gov/hmd/arabic/biol.html, accessed April 22, 2017.

http://www.nlm.nih.gov/hmd/arabic/prophetic_med 1.html, accessed April 22, 2017.

http://www.nlm.nih.gov/hmd/arabic/prophetic_med 3.html, accessed April 22, 2017.

http://www.nlm.nih.gov/hmd/arabic/mon 3.html, accessed April 22, 2017.

http://www.nlm.nih.gov/hmd/arabic/mon 4.html, accessed April 22, 2017.

http://en.wikipedia.org/wiki/Al-Dakhwar, accessed April 22, 2017.

http://en.wikipedia.org/wiki/Rufaida-Al-Aslamia, accessed April 22, 2017.

http://en.wikipedia.org/wiki/Rashidun_al-Suri, accessed April 22, 2017.

http://www.angelfire.com/md/takrouti/ibn_alnafis.htm, accessed April 22, 2017.

http:www//absoluteastronomy.com/topics/Toledo_translation__Sc, accessed April 22, 2017.

http://wzzz.tripod.com/RAZI.html, accessed April 22, 2017.

http://encyclopedia.the free dictionary.com/Islamic+medicine, accessed April 22, 2017.

http://www.en.wikipedia.org/wiki/yahya_ibn_sarafyun, accessed April 22, 2017.

http:en.wikipedia.org/wiki/Ibn_juljul, accessed April 22, 2017.

http://en.wikipedia.org/wiki/masarjawaih, accessed April 22, 2017.

http://en.wikipedia.org/wiki/Zayn_al_Din_Gorgani, accessed April 22, 2017.

http://www.daralhadith.org.uk/?=164, accessed April 22, 2017.

http://theislampath.com/smf/index.php?topic=6955.0, accessed April 22, 2017.

http://en.wikipedia.org/wiki/Galen, accessed April 22, 2017.

Haddad, S.I. History of Arab Medicine, Publications of the Orient Hospital, Beirut, Lebanon, 1975.

Haddad, F. Pioneers of Arabian Medicine. Bulletin De La Societe Libanaise D'Histoire De La Medicine (Lebanese Society for the History of Medicine)3: 74–83, 1993.

Haddad, F.S., Haddad, S.I. Arabic Medicine and Islamic Hospitals (Al-Tibb Al-Arabi Wa Al-Mashafi Al-Islamiyeh). Masa'd Odeh Press, Tempe, Arizona, 2003.

Hamarneh, S. Development of Hospitals in Islam. Journal of the History of Medicine and Allied Sciences 17:366–384, 1962.

Hamarneh, S. The Physician and the Health Professions in Medieval Islam. Bulletin of the New York Academy of Med, 47 (9), 1971.

Hamarneh, S., Anees, M.A. Health Sciences in Early Islam. A Noor Health Foundation and Zahra Publication, Vol. I, 1983.

Hamarneh, S.; Anees, M.A. Health Sciences in Early Islam. A Noor Health Foundation and Zahra Publication, Vol. II, 1983.

Hijazi, A.R. The Islamic Medicine: its Role in the Western Renaisance. http://www.islamset.com/hip/hijazi.html, accessed April 22, 2017.

https://en.wikipedia.org/wiki/John_of_Seville, accessed April 22, 2017.

https://en.wikipedia.org/wiki/Jacob_Anatoli, accessed April 22, 2017.

https://en.wikipedia.org/wiki/Mark-of-Toledo, accessed April 22, 2017.

http://www.brittanica.com/biography/Gerard-of-Cremona, accessed April 22, 2017.

https://www.brittanica.com/biography/Jacob-Anatoli, accessed April 22, 2017.

https://en.wikipedia.org/wiki/Kalonymus_ben_Kalonymus, accessed April 22, 2017.

https://en.wikipedia.org/wiki/Toledo_School_of_translators, accessed April 22, 2017.

https://en.wikipedia.org/wiki/Latin_translations_of_the_12th_century, accessed April 22, 2017.

Hillenbrand, C. The Crusades, Islamic Perspective. Routledge, New York, 2000.

Hosseini, S. F. Alakbarli, F., Ghabili, K., Shoja, M. M. Hakim Esmail Jorjani (1042–1137 AD): Persian Physician and Jurist. Archives of Gynecology and Obstetrics 284: 647–650, 2011.

Houston, K. The Book, A Cover-to-Cover Exploration of the Most Powerful Object of Our Time, W. W. Norton & Co. New York, London, 2016.

Huff, T. E. The Rise of Early Modern Science. Islam, China, and the West, 2nd Ed. Cambridge University Press, 2003.

Hunayn ibn Ishaq. http://en.wikipedia.org/wiki/hunayn_bin_Ishaq, accessed April 22, 2017.

Ibn Abi Usaibia http://en.wikipedia.org/wiki/Ibn_Abi_Usaibia, accessed April 22, 2017.

Ibn Abi Usaibiah, Muwafak Al-Din, Uyoun al-Anba fi Tabaqat al-Atibba (Sources of Information on Classes of Physicians). Complete Biography of 400 Arab Physicians. Ist Edition, 1245/1246.

Ibn al-Jazzar (Algizar) http://en.wikipedia.org/wiki/Ibn_Al_Jazzar, accessed April 22, 2017.

Ibn Al-Thahabi http://en.wikipedia.org/wiki/ibn Al-Thahabi, accessed April 22, 2017.

Ibn Hubal http://en.wikipedia.org/wiki/ibn_Hubal, accessed April 22, 2017.

Ibn-Qayyim al Jouzieh, al-Tibb al-Nabawi (Prophetic Medicine), revised by al-Harastani, I.F., and Abdul-Manan, H.Dar Al-Jeel, Beirut, Lebanon, undated

Ibn Zuhr http://en.wikipedia.org/wiki/Ibn_Zuhr,accessed April 22, 2017.

Ivry, A. L. Averroes' Middle Commentary on Aristotle's De anima, Brigham Young University Press, 2002.

Jadon, S. the Physicians of Syria during the Reign of Salah Al-Din, 750-789 AH, 1174–1193 AD. Journal of the History of Medicine and Allied Sciences, 25 (3), 323–340, 1970.

Kaadan, A. N. Ibn Hindu and His book in Medicine (Miftah Ttib). Journal of the International Society of the History of Islamic medicine (ISHIM-NET), 2003.

Kaadan, A. N. Some of Arab and Muslim Physicians Achievements Attributed to Western Physicians. Journal of the International Sciety of the History of Islamic Medicine. 4 (8) 1–10, 2005.

Kaadan, A. N. & Mahrouseh, M. N. (http://www.ishim.net/articles.htm), accessed April 22, 2017.

Karenberg, A., Hort, I. Medieval Description and Doctrines of stroke: Preliminary analysis of select sources. Part II: Between Galenism and Aristotelism-Islamic Theories of Apoplexy (800–1200). Journal of the History of the Neurosciences 7 (3): 174–185, 1998.

Keys, T. E., Wakim, K.G. Contributions of the Arabs to Medicine, Proceedings of Staff Meeting of Mayo Clinic 28: 423–437, 1953.

Khairallah, A. A. Arabic Contributions to Anatomy and Surgery. Annals of Medical History 3: 409–415, 1942.

Khairallah, A. A. Outline of Arabic Contributions to Medicine and Allied Sciences. American Press, Beirut, Lebanon, 1946.

Khalidi, M. A. Medieval Islamic Philosophical Writings. Cambridge University Press, 2005.

Khalidi, T. Images of Muhammad. Narratives of the Prophet of Islam Across the Centuries. Doubleday, New York, 2009.

Khalidi, T. Abu Hatim al-Razi, The Proofs of Prophecy. Brigham Young University Press, 2011.

Khan, A. Avicenna (Ibn Sina) Muslim Physician and Philosopher of the Eleventh Century. Rosen Publishing Co., NY, 2006.

Koehler, P. J., Bruyn, G. W., Pearce, J. M. S. Neurological Eponyms. Oxford University Press, 2000.

Krueger, H.C. Avicenna's Poem on Medicine. Charles C. Thomas. Publishers, 1963.

Landau, R. Islam and the Arabs. The Macmillan Co. 1959.

Laws, E. R. Jr. Udvarhelyi, G. B. The Genesis of Neuroscience by A. Earl Walker. American Association of Neurologicall Surgeons, 1998.

Ligon, B.L. Biography: Rhazes: His Career and His Writings. Seminars in Pediatric Infectious Diseases, 12:266–272, 2001.

Loukas, M., Lam, R., Tubbs, R.S., Shoja, M., Apaydin, N. Ibn al-Nafis (1210–1288): The First Description of the Pulmonary Circulation. The American Surgeon 74 (5): 440–442, 2008.

Lunde, P. Science. The Islamic Legacy. Science in the Golden Age. Saudi Aramco World 33(3): 6-13, May/June, 1982.

Lunde, P. Science. The Islamic Legacy. Saudi Aramco World 33(3):2-5, May/June, 1982.

Lyons, J. The House of Wisdom. How the Arabs transformed Western Civilization. Bloomsbury, 2009.

Majeed, A. How Islam Changed Medicine. Arab Physicians and Scholars Laid the Basis for Medical Practice in Europe. British Medical Journal 331:1486–1487, 2005.

Masoud, M., Masoud, F. How Islam Changed Medicine. British Medical Journal 332:120, 2006.

Mayer, C. F. The Collection of Arabic Medical Literature in the Army Medical Library. Bulletin of Medical Library Association 30(2) January: 96–108, 1942.

McCrory, P. R., Berkovic, S.F. Concussion: The History of Clinical and Pathophysiological Concepts and Misconceptions. Neurology 57:2283–2289, 2001.

Meadows, I. Historical Markers. Saudi Aramco World, 44 (1) Jan/Feb, 10-11, 1993.

Menocal, M. R. The Ornament of the World, Back Bay Books, 2002.

Mernissi, F. The Forgotten Queens of Islam. University of Minnesota Press, 2006.

Meyerhof, M. The Ten Treatises On the Eye Ascribed to Hunayn Ibn Ishaq, Dar Al-Maa'rif, Soouse, Tunisia, 1989.

Miles, S. H. The Hippocratic Oath and the Ethics of Medicine, Oxford University Press, 2004.

Miles, M. R. A Complex Delight. The Secularization of the Breast 1350–1750. University of California Press, 2008.

Morgan, M. H. Lost History. The Enduring Legacy of Muslim Scientists, Thinkers, and Artists, National Geographic Society Publishers, 2007.

Morton, L . T., Moore, R . J . A Chronology of Medicine and Related Sciences, Ashgate Publishers, 1997.

Mujais, S. K. Nephrologic Beginnings: The Kidney in the Age of Ibn Sina (980-1037 AD). American Journal of Nephrology 7: 133–136, 1987.

Myers, E. A. Arabic Thought and the Western World in the Golden Age of Islam, . Frederick Ungar Publishing Company, Inc. 1964

Nagamia, H. F. Ibn al-Nafis. A biographical Sketch of the Discoverer of Pulmonary and Coronary Circulations. Journal of the International Society of the History of Islamic Medicine 1(3):22–28, 2003.

Nasser, M., Tibi, A. Ibn Hindu and the Science of Medicine. J. R. Soc. Med. 100:55–56, 2007.

Nusseibeh, H. Z. Jerusalemites: A Living Memory, Rimal Publications, 2009

Otaya, S. Ibnul-Nafees Has Dissected the Human Body. http://www.islam-set.com/isc/nafis/oataya.html, accessed April 22, 2017.

Otri, A. M., Singh, A.D., Dua, H.S. Abu Bakr Razi. British Journal of Ophthalmology 92:1324, 2008.

Pormann, P. E., Savage-Smith, E. Medieval Islamic Medicine, Georgetown University Press, 2007.

Prioreschi, P. Medical Ethics in Medieval Islam. Journal of the international Society of the History of Islamic Medicine, 3:44–48. 2004.

Radbill, S.X. The First Treatise on Pediatrics, American Journal of Diseases of Childhood 122:369–376, 1971.

Rafida Al-Aslamia. http://en.wikipedia.org/wiki,Rufaida_Al-Aslamia, accessed April 22, 2017.

Raju, T. K. The Importance of Having a Brain. Tales from the History of Medicine, Outskirts Press, 2012.

Ramen, F. Albucasis (Abu Al-Qasim Al-Zahrawi), Renowned Muslim Surgeon of the Tenth Century, Rosen Publishing Co., NY, 2006.

Rosenthal, F. Physicians in Medieval Muslim Society. Bulletin of the History of Medicine 52:475–491, 1978.

Rosner, F. The Physician's Prayers attributed to Moses Maimonides. Bulletin of the History of Medicine, 41: 440–454, 1967.

Rosner, F. Neurology in the Bible and Talmud. Israel Journal of Medical Science 11 (4): 385–397, 1975.

Sahih al-Bukhari http://www.usc.edu/dept/MSA/ , accessed April 22, 2017. fundamentals/hadithsunna/bukhari/ 071.S B 1.

Savage-Smith, E. Dissection in Medieval Islam. Journal of the History of Medicine and Allied Sciences 50: 67–110, 1995.

Scott, W.A. Cervical Cancer, Canadian Medical Journal 29 (3): 290–293, 1933.

Shadid, A. House of Stone. Mariner Books, 2012.

Shama'a, M., Al-Khalidi, U. The Victims of Ignorance: Who Are the Arabs? (Translated from Arabic by Fneish, R.), 2010.

Shoja, M., Tubbs, S. The Disorder of Love in the Canon of Avicenna (AD 980-1037). The American Journal of Psychiatry, 164: 228–229, 2007.

Shoja, M. M., Tubbs, R.S., Ardalan, M. R., Loukas, M., Eknoyan, G., Salter, E.G., Oakes, W.J. Anatomy pf the Cranial Nerves in Medieval Persian Literature: Esmail Jorjani (1042–1137) and the Treasure of the Khwarazm Shah. Neurosurgery 61 (6) 1325–1331, 2007.

Shoja, M., Tubbs, R. S., Loukas, M., Khalili, M., Alakbarii, F., Cohen-Gadol, A. Vasovagal Syncope in the Canon of Avicenna: The First Mention of Carotid Artery Hypersensitivity. International Journal of Cardiology, 134(3): 297–301, 2009.

Shoja, M. M., Tubbs, R. S., Loukas, M., Ghaffar, S., Ardalan, M. Facial Palsy and its Management in the Kitab al-Hawi of Rhazes. Neurosurgery 64 (6):1188–1191, 2009.

Shoja, M., Tubbs, R. S., Khalili, M., Khodadoost, K. , Loukas, M. , Cohen-Gadol, A. Esmail Jorjani (1042–1137) and His Description of Trigeminal Neuralgia, Hemifacial Spasm, and Bell's Palsy, Neurosurgery 67 (2): 431–434, 2010.

Shoja, M. M., Rashidi, M. R., Tubbs, R.S., Etemadi, J., Abbasnejad, F., Agutter, P.S. Legacy of Avicenna and Evidence-Based Medicine. International Journal of Cardiology 150: 243–246, 2011.

Sinan ibn Thabit http://en.wikipedia.org/wiki/Sinan_ibn_Thabit, accessed April 22, 2017.

Siraisi, N.G. Medieval and Early Renaissance Medicine. An Introduction to Knowledge and Practice. The University of Chicago Press, 1990.

Skinner, H.A. The Origin of Medical Terms. Williams & Wilkins, 1961.

Souayah, N., Greenstein, J.I. Insight into Neurologic Localization by Rhazes, A Medieval Islamic Physician. Neurology 65:125–128, 2005.

Souweif, A .Mezzatera, Fragments from the Common Ground, Penguin Random House. 2005.

Spier, R. The History of the Peer Review Process. Trends in Biotechnology 20 (8): 357–358, 2002.

Stone, C. Doctor, Philosopher, Renaissance Man. Saudi Aramco World 54 (3): 8–15, 2003.

Syed, I. B. Islamic Medicine: 1000 Years Ahead of the Times. Journal of the International Society of the History of Islamic Medicine (ISHIM) 2: 2–10, 2002.

Tarabay, A., Wakim, J. An Overview of Arab Islamic Civilization. Early 7th to Late 15th Century. Dar Nelson Publisher, 2011.

Taylor, R. B. White Coat Tales. Medicine's Heroes, Heritage, and Misadventures, Springer, 2008.

Tschanz, D. W. Hunayn Bin Ishaq: The Great Translator. Journal of the International Society of the History of Islamic Medicine (JISHIM):1 (3), 39–40, 2003.

Tschanz, D. W. Ibn-Sina: "The Prince of Physicians". Journal of the International Society of the History of Islamic Medicine (JISHIM):1 (3), 47–49, 2003.

Tubbs, R. S., Shoja, M. M. Abubakr Muhammad Ibn Zakaria Razi, Rhazes (865–925 AD). Childs Nervous System 23:1225-1226, 2007.

Tubbs, R. S., Loukas, M., Shoja, M., Ardalan, M., Oakes, W. J. Ibn Jazla and his 11th Century Accounts (Taqwim al-Abdan fi Tadbir al-Insan) of Disease of the Brain and Spinal Cord. Historical Vignettes. Journal of Neurosurgery Spine 9: 314–317, 2008.

Turner, H. R. Science in Medieval Islam. University of Texas Press, 1995.

Ullmann, M. Islamic Medicine. Edinburgh University Press, 1997.

Vernet, J. Ibn Juljul, Sulayman Ibn Hasan. Complete Dictionary of Scientific Biography, 2008.

Wakim, Kh. G. Arabic Medicine in Literature. Bull. Med. Libr. Assoc. 32: 96–104, 1944.

Whitaker, B. Centuries in the House of Wisdom. The Guardian, September 23, 2004.

Williams, H. Days that Changed the World. The 50 Defining Events of World History, Metro Books, N.Y. 2006

Index

Surnames starting with "al-" are alphabetized by the subsequent part of the name.

A

B

CPSIA information can be obtained
at www.ICGtesting.com
Printed in the USA
BVHW060319030222
627685BV00003B/62

9 781478 789277